C000302852

Abbie

For Elsevier

*Content Strategist:* Alison Taylor
*Content Development Specialist:* Veronika Watkins
*Project Manager:* Louisa Talbott
*Designer:* Amy Buxton

THIRTEENTH EDITION

# BAILLIÈRE'S MIDWIVES' DICTIONARY

**Denise Tiran** MSc, RM, PGCEA

Educational Director, Expectancy; Visiting Lecturer,
University of Greenwich, London, UK

ELSEVIER

# ELSEVIER

© 2017 Elsevier Ltd. All rights reserved.

First edition 1951
Sixth edition 1976
Seventh edition 1983
Eighth edition 1992
Ninth edition 1997
Tenth edition 2003
Eleventh edition 2008
Twelfth edition 2012

ISBN: **978-0-7020-6906-2**
International ISBN: 978-0-7020-7016-7
eISBN: 978-0-7020-6954-3

**Notices**

Knowledge and best practice in this field are constantly changing. As new research and experience broaden our understanding, changes in research methods, professional practices, or medical treatment may become necessary.

Practitioners and researchers must always rely on their own experience and knowledge in evaluating and using any information, methods, compounds, or experiments described herein. In using such information or methods they should be mindful of their own safety and the safety of others, including parties for whom they have a professional responsibility.

With respect to any drug or pharmaceutical products identified, readers are advised to check the most current information provided (i) on procedures featured or (ii) by the manufacturer of each product to be administered, to verify the recommended dose or formula, the method and duration of administration, and contraindications. It is the responsibility of practitioners, relying on their own experience and knowledge of their patients, to make diagnoses, to determine dosages and the best treatment for each individual patient, and to take all appropriate safety precautions.

To the fullest extent of the law, neither the Publisher nor the authors, contributors, or editors, assume any liability for any injury and/or damage to persons or property as a matter of products liability, negligence or otherwise, or from any use or operation of any methods, products, instructions, or ideas contained in the material herein.

your source for books,
journals and multimedia
in the health sciences
www.elsevierhealth.com

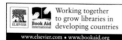

Working together
to grow libraries in
developing countries

www.elsevier.com • www.bookaid.org

The Publisher's
policy is to use
paper manufactured
from sustainable forests

Printed in China

Last digit is the print number: 9  8  7  6  5  4  3  2  1

# CONTENTS

# PREFACE

The profession of midwifery is continually evolving and changing. Since my last revision of *Bailliére's Midwives' Dictionary* the UK birth rate rose to an all-time high of almost 700,000 in 2013, but fell again by 2015 to around 650,000.

Midwives are faced with the challenges of a changing population which is now more multi-ethnic than ever before. Conditions such as morbid obesity and diabetes affect maternity services, whilst advances in technology have enabled improved diagnostics and management of compromised pregnancies. There are huge managerial challenges such as staff shortages, budgetary cuts and rationalization of services. An ageing workforce and less recruitment to training compound these issues. The role of the midwife is changing, and other professionals are increasingly becoming involved in maternity care.

In other countries, whilst the problems may be different, challenges persist. In some areas midwives are persecuted simply for doing their job. In others, particularly in the developing world, basic resources are minimal and war, famine and lack of basic facilities such as clean water add to the difficulties.

Despite this, midwives all over the world continue to provide individualized, compassionate, responsive and nurturing care for women at the most significant time in their lives. Although mortality and morbidity rates are unjustifiably high in some parts of the world, statistics would be worse without the skill and knowledge of midwives. The relationship that an expectant and birthing mother has with her midwife is unique and deserves to be protected.

It is vital that midwifery education encompasses the changes and challenges in order to grow and to be fit for purpose. The *Bailliére's Midwives' Dictionary* has long been the dictionary of choice for student and qualified midwives, and each edition has changed to reflect contemporary practice. Other professionals will also find it invaluable in their work, for example, doulas, antenatal teachers, maternity support workers and maternity nurses.

In this edition I have endeavoured, as always, to keep in mind that the *Dictionary* needs to be user friendly, portable for use in practice and suitable for those in all midwifery settings, from high-tech obstetric units to home births to remote isolated areas in developing countries. I hope it serves its purpose in preparing students and supporting practising midwives all around the world.

**Denise Tiran, MSc, RM, PGCEA**
**Educational Director, Expectancy**
*London, 2017*

# ACKNOWLEDGEMENTS

As always, my grateful thanks go to everyone at Elsevier, especially Veronika Watkins and Alison Taylor for the invitation to revise, for the fifth time, the world-famous *Baillière's Midwives' Dictionary*.

I would also like to thank the numerous student and qualified midwives I have met while teaching and lecturing around the country and via my LinkedIn contacts, who have provided feedback on the previous editions of the *Dictionary* and helped to focus my thoughts on what was required in this revision. Midwives on our Expectancy courses have been keen to help too, as have our lecturers, including Charlotte Kenyon and Dr Harry Chummun.

Finally, as with all my books, this edition of *Baillière's Midwives' Dictionary* is dedicated to my son, Adam, now 27, working in the African music industry in London. He makes it all worthwhile.

**Denise Tiran**
*London, 2017*
**www.expectancy.co.uk**

# ILLUSTRATION ACKNOWLEDGEMENTS

The illustrations on the pages below have been reproduced or adapted with permission from the following publications.

**Pages 30, 40, 57, 81, 187, 191**
Fraser D M & Cooper M A (eds), 2009, *Myles Textbook for Midwives* 15e, Churchill Livingstone, Elsevier.

**Pages 1, 32, 33**
MacDonald S & Magill-Cuerden J (eds), 2011, *Mayes' Midwifery* 14e, Baillière Tindall, Elsevier.

**Page 249**
Sandberg E C, 1985, The Zavanelli maneuver, *American Journal of Obstetrics and Gynaecology* 152: 479-487.

**Page 172**
Tiran D, 2004, *Nausea and Vomiting in Pregnancy*, Churchill Livingstone, Elsevier.

The illustrations on the pages below have been adapted from the following publications.

**Page 147**
Bryan, E M, 1984, *Twins in the Family: A Parent's Guide*, Constable.

**Page 76**
Yerby M (ed), 2000, *Pain in Childbearing*, Baillière Tindall, Elsevier.

**Page 253**
Figure 3.1 in Appendix 3 has been reproduced with the kind permission of Brendan Ellis, Medical Illustrator, Royal Group of Hospitals, Belfast.

**abdomen** cavity between diaphragm and pelvis, lined by peritoneum; contains stomach, intestines, liver, gallbladder, spleen, pancreas, kidneys, suprarenal glands, ureters. Bladder, uterus become abdominal organs in pregnancy. ***Pendulous a.*** anterior abdominal wall hangs down over pubis. ***Scaphoid a.*** sunken abdomen in low-birthweight babies due to shrinkage of liver and spleen in utero.

**Abdomen**

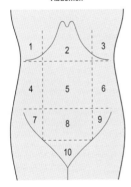

1, Right hypochondrium;
2, epigastrium; 3, left hypochondrium;
4, right lumbar region; 5, umbilical region; 6, left lumbar region; 7, right iliac fossa; 8, hypogastrium; 9, left iliac fossa; 10, suprapubis.

**abdominal** pertaining to the abdomen. ***A. aortic compression*** short-term measure to control severe third-stage haemorrhage; fist is placed above fundus, below renal artery level, pressure directed towards spine to compress aorta and reduce blood flow to uterus. ***A. enlargement*** abdomen becomes progressively larger as pregnant uterus increases in size; if excessive, may be due to multiple pregnancy, POLYHYDRAMNIOS, FIBROIDS, abnormal ovum development. ***A. examination*** systematic examination of abdomen: antenatally, visual inspection for shape, scars, STRIAE GRAVIDARUM, skin tension, symphysis–fundal height measurement; PALPATION; uterus palpable above symphysis pubis by 12 weeks' gestation, reaches diaphragm by 36 weeks' gestation, drops slightly with ENGAGEMENT. PRESENTATION palpated. Fetal heart auscultated for rate, rhythm, regularity. Postnatally, to monitor uterine INVOLUTION, identify deviations from normal, check return of uterus to non-pregnant size, position. ***A. pain*** minor discomfort due to growth, stretching, changing position; severe pain may be due to threatened miscarriage, ECTOPIC PREGNANCY, FIBROIDS, TORSION, PLACENTAL ABRUPTION. ***A. pregnancy*** rare; occurs when fertilized ovum embeds in fallopian tube; tubal rupture causes extrusion of ovum into peritoneal cavity; chorionic villi on surface of ovum attach to abdominal

http://dx.doi.org/10.1016/B978-0-7020-6906-2.00001-2

**Abdominal examination: fundal height assessed on palpation**

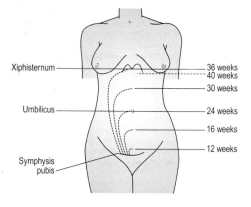

Xiphisternum — 36 weeks
40 weeks
30 weeks
Umbilicus — 24 weeks
16 weeks
12 weeks
Symphysis pubis

organs, fetus develops in abdominal cavity. **A. wall** structure covering abdominal organs: skin, fat, fascia, muscles, peritoneum. Neonatal defects, developing in utero, include EXOMPHALOS, GASTROSCHISIS.

**abduction** drawing away from centre, e.g. of legs for vaginal birth.

**aberrant** wandering or deviating from normal site or course.

**ABO blood groups** blood group classification according to whether they contain agglutinogens A, B, A and B (AB) or none (O). Serum may contain antibodies, anti-A or anti-B agglutinins or both; donor blood for transfusion must not contain same antibodies as recipient's blood group because fatal reaction occurs. Group AB people have no serum agglutinin or antibody so can receive blood from anyone, i.e. *universal recipients*;

group O people have no agglutinogens, i.e. *universal donors*. *See also* RHESUS FACTOR.

ABO *incompatibility* occurs in about 1 in 200 pregnancies when maternal blood group is O, serum contains anti-A and anti-B antibodies. If fetus is group A, B or AB, antibody differing immunologically from normal anti-A and anti-B may cross placenta, causing neonatal haemolysis with mild jaundice within 24 hours of birth; treated with phototherapy or exchange transfusion. Serum bilirubin level rises rapidly, anaemia less obvious. COOMBS' TEST usually negative. *See also* ABO BLOOD GROUPS, ISO-IMMUNIZATION, RHESUS FACTOR.

**abortifacient** chemical substance e.g. drugs, aromatherapy oils, or surgical means e.g. dilatation and curettage, causing inducing miscarriage.

**abortion** expulsion from uterus of products of conception before 24 weeks' gestation. *Therapeutic a.* induced termination of pregnancy before 24 weeks' gestation in line with Abortion Act. Methods: vacuum extraction, dilatation and curettage (first trimester); drugs, e.g. prostaglandins (second trimester). *See* MISCARRIAGE.

**abrachia** congenital absence of arms.

**abrasion** skin cut or scratch. *Neonatal a.* skin damage due to birth trauma from forceps blades, vacuum extraction cups, electrodes.

**abruption** tearing asunder. *Placental a.* partial or complete separation of placenta from uterine wall after 24 weeks of pregnancy, causing pain, haemorrhage.

**abscess** localized accumulation of pus in space or cavity. *Pelvic a.* in pouch of Douglas.

**abuse** deliberate inflicting of physical, emotional or sexual injury, trauma, pain on individual. *Child a.* physical or emotional maltreatment, neglect or sexual molestation of a minor *Domestic a.,* threatening behaviour, violence or abuse between intimate partners or family members.

**acardiac twin** *See* TWIN REVERSED ARTERIAL PERFUSION.

**acceleration** speeding up. *Fetal heart a.* may indicate fetal distress. *A. of labour. See* AUGMENTATION OF LABOUR.

**accessory** extra, supplementary. *A. nipple* extra nipple, commonly axillary.

**accountable** liable to be held responsible for a course of action.

**accreditation** process of evaluation for official recognition of standards set against agreed-on criteria, e.g. education.

**ACE inhibitors** *See* ANGIOTENSIN.

**acetabulum** cup-shaped socket in pelvic innominate bone into which head of femur fits.

**acetoacetic acid** abnormal fat metabolism product; occurs in diabetic and dehydrated mothers.

**acetone** by-product of acetoacetic acid, produced in abnormal amounts in uncontrolled diabetes mellitus, metabolic acidosis, resulting in characteristic ketotic odour on mother's breath or in urine.

**acetylcholine** chemical transmitter released by nerve endings at synapse between two neurons, or between cholinergic nerve ending and effector organ it supplies; rapidly destroyed by cholinesterase; antagonized by cortisol.

**achlorhydria** absence of hydrochloric acid in gastric juice; associated with pernicious anaemia, stomach cancer.

**achondroplasia** failure to form cartilage. Autosomal-dominant genetic condition; dwarfism, due to shortening of long bones, very short limbs, large head, normal trunk; normal mentality.

**acid** substance that forms salt when combined with alkali; turns blue litmus paper red; assists in body's chemical processes. *Hydrochloric a.* colourless hydrogen, chlorine compound; present in gastric juice; causes MENDELSON SYNDROME if inhaled.

**acid–base balance** equilibrium between acidity and alkalinity of body fluids; hydrogen ion (H+) balance. Positively charged H+ is active constituent of all acids. Most metabolic processes produce acids as end products, but alkaline body fluid is required as medium for vital cellular activities; continuous chemical exchange of H+

vital to maintain equilibrium and optimal pH (H+ concentration) between 7.35 and 7.45.

**acidaemia** acid accumulation in blood that alters pH (acidity), normally slightly alkaline. Occurs with dehydration, prolonged labour, diabetes mellitus. *Fetal or neonatal a.* may result from HYPOXIA, leading to coma, death if untreated.

**acidosis** pathological acid accumulation or depletion of alkaline reserve (bicarbonate) in blood and body tissues; increased hydrogen ion concentration (decreased pH below 7.30). *Adj* acidotic. *Metabolic a.* serum accumulation of ketoacids from fat metabolism at expense of bicarbonate; diminished ability to neutralize acids. Occurs in diabetic ketoacidosis, lactic acidosis, failure of renal tubules to reabsorb bicarbonate. *Respiratory a.* due to ventilatory impairment, serum carbon dioxide accumulation, uniting with water as carbonic acid; occurs in baby with severe birth asphyxia, other respiratory conditions; in mother with either acute airway obstruction or chronic respiratory condition.

**acini** alveoli; minute hollow structures, lined by secreting cells, with duct. Acini in breast secrete milk. *Sing* acinus.

**acquired immune deficiency syndrome (AIDS)** severe progressive disease due to HUMAN IMMUNODEFICIENCY VIRUS (HIV); fever, weight loss, diarrhoea, lymphadenopathy. Opportunistic infections, e.g. herpes simplex, *Pneumocystis carinii* or tumours, e.g. Kaposi's sarcoma eventually lead to death.

**acridine orange** stain used in fluorescence microscopy; causes bacteria to fluoresce green to red.

**acromegaly** chronic disease due to over-functioning pituitary gland, excess growth hormone; often due to pituitary tumour. Causes enlargement of bones and tissues of hands, feet, face.

**acromion** distal process of scapula, forming point of shoulder.

**acrosome** cap-like, membrane-bound structure over anterior part of spermatozoon's head; contains enzymes involved in penetration of ovum. *A. reaction* during fertilization, acrosomal layer becomes reactive, releases HYALURONIDASE, which disperses CORONA RADIATA, allowing access to ZONA PELLUCIDA of oocyte.

**active birth** style of birth preparation and care empowering mother to take active part in labour and decisions needed for her care.

**active management of first-stage labour** intervention to prevent prolonged labour and complications e.g. artificial membrane rupture, intravenous oxytocin. *A. m. of third-stage labour* oxytocin injection (e.g. SYNTOMETRINE) to facilitate placental separation plus manual delivery of placenta by CONTROLLED CORD TRACTION.

**active transport** ion or molecular movement across cell membranes and epithelial layers, usually against concentration gradient, due to expenditure of metabolic energy; process of maintaining normal differences in electrolyte composition between intracellular fluids.

**acupressure** Chinese medicine technique; thumb or finger pressure applied to specific points on body to balance internal energies.

**acupuncture** Chinese medicine technique based on internal energy lines linking one part of body to another. Needles applied to specific points to balance energy flow, assisting homeostasis. Useful for pregnancy discomforts, labour pain.

**acute** developing rapidly, running short course; reverse of chronic. *A. fatty liver of pregnancy (AFLP)* acute yellow atrophy; rare complication, unknown aetiology; rapidly progressive liver atrophy, massive fatty necrosis; over 80% mortality. Typically, obese woman in third trimester with vomiting, headache, malaise, drowsiness, tender but not enlarged liver, no jaundice; fulminating pre-eclampsia can mask diagnosis; liver enzymes slightly raised; hypoglycaemia and renal failure follow quickly; liver biopsy contraindicated due to coagulopathy risk. Management: correction of coagulopathy, immediate delivery. *A. inversion of uterus* See INVERSION OF UTERUS. *A. renal failure* sudden, severe, reversible, interrupted kidney function, often complication of haemorrhage or shock. OLIGURIA; fluid and electrolyte imbalance, anaemia, hypertension, uraemia; dialysis to monitor fluid and electrolyte imbalance until kidney function improves. *A. tubular necrosis* kidney tubule cell damage, blood transfusion reaction or severe hypotension; renal dialysis needed.

**acyclovir** oral or intravenous antiviral agent to treat herpes simplex.

**adactylia, adactyly** congenital absence of fingers or toes.

**addiction** physical or psychological dependence e.g. alcohol, drugs.

**adduct** to draw towards centre or median line; opposite of ABDUCT.

**adenine** purine derivative; one of four constituent bases of nucleic acids,

paired with thymine in double-stranded DNA.

**adherent placenta** placenta firmly attached to uterine wall; fails to separate during third-stage labour. *See* PLACENTA.

**adhesion** union between two normally separated surfaces, usually due to inflammation when fibrous tissue forms, e.g. after surgery.

**adipose tissue** *See* TISSUE.

**adnexa** appendages. *Uterine a.* ovaries and fallopian tubes.

**adnexal mass** enlarged area between uterus and ovaries; suggests ECTOPIC PREGNANCY in first trimester, especially if fluid in pouch of Douglas, no visible intrauterine pregnancy; may be due to physiological follicular or corpus luteal pregnancy, tumours.

**adolescence** developmental stage from puberty to cessation of physical growth.

**adoption** legal procedure, responsibility for child transferred from natural parents to adopting parents, regulated in UK by Adoption and Children Act and overseen by social services departments. *See also* FOSTERING.

**adrenal** pertaining to adrenal glands, two complex endocrine glands at upper pole of each kidney. *A. cortex* outer adrenal gland, produces steroids to regulate carbohydrate and fat metabolism and mineralocorticoids to regulate salt and water balance *Congenital a. hyperplasia* autosomal-recessive condition, 21-hydroxylase enzyme deficiency; adrenal glands overproduce androgens, needed for steroid production from cholesterol; causes rapid salt loss; ambiguous genitalia.

**adrenaline** neurotransmitter that increases heart rate, constricts blood vessels, dilates air passages, aids fight-or-flight response of sympathetic nervous system; produced naturally or synthetically for emergency use. *See also* PHAEOCHROMOCYTOMA.

**adrenocortical** pertaining to adrenal cortex. *Neonatal a. insufficiency* due to congenital hypoplasia, adrenal haemorrhage, enzyme defects or secondary to pituitary gland problems; presents with hypoglycaemia, poor feeding and weight gain, vomiting, prolonged jaundice; hyponatraemia, hypoglycaemia, hyperkalaemia, acidosis. Treatment: intravenous glucose, replacement of corticosteroid and mineralocorticoid hormones. *A. hyperfunction* congenital adrenal hyperplasia; inherited disorders due to enzyme deficiency, leads to excess androgenic hormones, glucocorticoid and mineralocorticoid deficiency; characterized by genital malformations, vomiting, diarrhoea, vascular collapse, hypoglycaemia, hyponatraemia, hyperkalaemia.

**adrenocorticotrophic hormone** anteriorpituitary gland hormone that stimulates adrenal cortex.

**adrenogenital syndrome** adrenocortical hyperplasia or malignant tumours causing abnormal adrenocortical hormone secretion; characterized by female masculinization, male feminization, precocious sexual development in children.

**adult respiratory distress syndrome** *See* RESPIRATORY DISTRESS SYNDROME.

**Advanced Life Support in Obstetrics** specialist training courses for midwives, doctors, other staff; cover advanced methods of dealing with emergency situations. *See* APPENDICES 1, 2 and 3.

**aerobe** organism requiring air or oxygen to sustain life. *Adj* aerobic.

**aetiology** science of causes, e.g. of disease.

**afebrile** without fever.

**affective** pertaining to emotional tone or feeling. *A. disorder* mental disorder with mood disturbance, manic or depressive symptoms or both e.g. bipolar disorder, depression, cyclothymic disorder.

**afferent** towards centre. *A. nerve* sensory nerve fibre carrying impulses from periphery to central nervous system.

**affiliation order** court order by which absent father is required to make regular payments towards his child's maintenance.

**afibrinogenaemia** absence of fibrinogen in blood.

**afterbirth** lay term for placenta and membranes expelled from uterus after birth of baby.

**aftercoming head** fetal head (coming after trunk) in breech birth. *See* BREECH.

**afterpains** early postnatal painful uterine contractions, common in multiparae, often felt when breastfeeding. If severe, persistent, may be blood clot, membrane or placental fragment retained in uterus.

**agenesis** absence of organ.

**agglutination** aggregation of separate particles into clumps or masses. 1. red blood corpuscles clumping in serum; occurs if incompatible cells transfused. Agglutination of sensitized red blood cells by urine reveals presence of human chorionic gonadotropin (hCG) in pregnancy test.

2. platelet clumping due to platelet agglutinins. 3. bacteria clumping when in contact with specific immune serum.

**agglutinin** substance reacting with AGGLUTINOGEN, causes agglutination.

**agglutinogen** substance that stimulates specific agglutinin to cause agglutination.

**agnathia** failure of jaw development.

**AIDS** *See* ACQUIRED IMMUNE DEFICIENCY SYNDROME.

**air** atmosphere surrounding earth, mainly two gases: OXYGEN (21%), NITROGEN (79%). *A. hunger* deep, sighing respiration occurs when oxygen supply depleted, as in haemorrhage, shock.

**airway** 1. passage by which air enters lungs. 2. mechanical device to secure unobstructed respiration during general anaesthesia or if woman not ventilating or exchanging gases efficiently.

**ala** wing, e.g. sacral ala. *Pl* alae.

**alanine aminotransferase** liver function test assessed in mothers with pre-eclampsia or HELLP SYNDROME.

**alba, albicans** white. *Linea a.* midabdominal white line in Caucasians.

**albumin** protein, soluble in water and salt solutions, coagulable by heat. *Serum a.* plasma protein formed in liver; maintains colloidal osmotic pressure of blood; regulates water exchange between plasma and interstitial compartments; reduced plasma albumin causes increased water flow from capillaries to interstitial compartment, increasing tissue fluid, oedema. Transports fatty acids, bilirubin, drugs, some hormones.

**albuminuria** presence of albumin in urine; occurs in renal or severe cardiac disease, some pregnancy complications.

**alcohol** in pregnancy women should discontinue alcohol consumption, especially in first trimester. Consuming large amounts may lead to low-birthweight babies, neonatal feeding, sleeping problems. *See* FETAL ALCOHOL SYNDROME.

**aldosterone** adrenal cortex hormone, regulates electrolyte and water balance by promoting sodium and water retention, potassium excretion; water retention increases plasma volume and blood pressure; secretion is stimulated by angiotensin II.

**alimentary** pertaining to nutrition. *A. tract* gastrointestinal passage.

**alkalaemia** increased blood alkalinity (pH) due to accumulation of alkaline substances or excessive acid loss, e.g. vomiting.

**alkali** substance capable of uniting with acid to form salt, turns red litmus paper blue; forms carbonates, combines with fatty acids to form soaps, maintains normal body chemistry. *See also* ACID–BASE BALANCE *and* BASE. *A. reserve* ability of blood's combined buffer systems to neutralize acid; blood pH normally slightly alkaline, 7.35–7.45; represented by plasma bicarbonate concentration; haemoglobin, phosphates, other bases also act as buffers. If low, indicates acidosis; if increased, alkalosis. Assessed as amount of carbon dioxide bound as bicarbonate by blood.

**alkaline** *Adj* pertaining to alkali. *Serum a. phosphatase* liver function measurement; by late pregnancy, levels are approximately double non-pregnant levels; upper limit of normal is three times greater than non-pregnant range.

**alkaloids** organic nitrogenous substances forming active principle of certain drugs, e.g. morphine, atropine.

**alkalosis** condition due to accumulation of base or loss of acid without comparable loss of base in body fluids; decreased hydrogen ion concentration (increased pH). Opposite of ACIDOSIS.

**allantois** membranous sac projecting from ventral surface of embryo; eventually helps to form placenta.

**all-fours position** labour position to relieve backache, e.g. with occipitoposterior position; increases pelvic outlet, facilitates normal birth.

**allele** one of two or more alternative forms of gene at same site in chromosome; determines alternative characters in inheritance.

**alloimmunization** immune response to donated blood, bone marrow or transplanted organ; rhesus-negative pregnant woman with rhesus-positive fetus can be alloimmunized after a sensitizing event, e.g. antepartum haemorrhage, miscarriage; antibodies target foreign material, cause newborn haemolytic disease.

**alongside midwifery unit** maternity unit sited adjacent to main obstetric unit (co-located), in which women at low risk of birth complications are cared for by midwives.

**alpha-adrenergic mechanism** autonomic nerve pathway mechanism through which excitatory responses occur due to release of adrenergic substances, e.g. adrenaline, noradrenaline

**alpha-fetoprotein (AFP)** plasma protein produced by fetal liver, gastrointestinal tract and in YOLK SAC; crosses placenta from fetal to maternal circulation; assessed in second trimester with HUMAN CHORIONIC GONADOTROPHIN (HCG), UNCONJUGATED OESTRIOL (UE₃). If raised, indicates open neural tube or abdominal wall defects; if low, may be chromosomal anomalies, e.g. EDWARD SYNDROME, DOWN SYNDROME; levels dependent on gestation, number of fetuses, maternal weight, diabetes mellitus.

**alpha thalassaemia** See THALASSAEMIA.

**alveoli** hollowed-out structures e.g. air sacs in lungs, acini in breasts. *Sing* alveolus.

**amelia** developmental anomaly with absence of limbs.

**amenorrhoea** absence of menstruation. *Primary a.* absence of menstruation in woman who has never menstruated after puberty. *Secondary a.* cessation of normal menstrual periods, usually due to pregnancy, or due to stress, environment, weight loss, disease.

**amino acid** organic substance from proteins, essential to nutrition.

**aminoglycosides** gram-negative antibiotics; molecules contain amino-modified glycoside (sugar) e.g. streptomycin, gentamicin.

**aminophylline** oral, intravenous or rectal alkaloid; relaxes bronchiole and coronary artery muscle spasm in asthma, heart failure.

**amitriptyline** See TRICYCLIC ANTIDEPRESSANTS.

**ammonia** alkaline gas from decomposition of proteins, amino acids, other nitrogen-containing substances; converted to urea in liver.

**amniocentesis** extraction of AMNIOTIC FLUID from intrauterine cavity by insertion of fine-gauge needle through abdomen under continuous ultrasound guidance. Desquamated skin, gastrointestinal, urinary tract fetal cells isolated from sample; used to assess fetal karyotype, detect inherited genetic disorders; determine fetal bilirubin levels when fetal HAEMOLYTIC disease from ALLOIMMUNIZATION suspected; as therapeutic procedure to drain polyhydramnios. One per cent miscarriage risk (operator dependent). Rhesus-negative mothers may need anti-D immunoglobulin.

**amniocytes** desquamated fetal cells obtained via amniocentesis are isolated, cultured or multiplied via FLUORESCENT IN SITU HYBRIDIZATION (FISH) or POLYMERASE CHAIN REACTION (PCR) to determine fetal KARYOTYPE and for genetic analysis.

**amnion** innermost membrane enveloping fetus, produces, encloses amniotic fluid. *A. nodosum* fetal amniotic surface condition, as in OLIGOHYDRAMNIOS; often due to fetal kidney atresia.

**amnionicity** presence/absence of AMNION for each fetus in MULTIPLE PREGNANCY; diamniotic twins each have amnion and amniotic cavity, but shared by monoamniotic twins so risk of entangled umbilical cords increases fetal morbidity and mortality.

**amniotic** pertaining to amnion *A. band syndrome* amnion wraps around developing fetal limb, causing necrosis, strangulation and/or amputation, possibly due to amnion rupture. *A. fluid* liquor amnii; clear, straw-coloured amniotic sac fluid; surrounds and swallowed by fetus; 99% water, 1% solids; allows fetus to grow and move freely, equalizes pressure and temperature, acts as shock absorber, provides some nutrition. Volume: approximately 1 L at 37–38 weeks' gestation, reduced by half at term. *See* also AMNIOCENTESIS, POLYHYDRAMNIOS, OLIGOHYDRAMNIOS. *A. fluid embolism* amniotic fluid escapes through uterine wall or placental site into maternal circulation, triggers life-threatening anaphylactic shock. *See also* ANAPHYLACTOID SYNDROME. *A. fluid index* measurement of amniotic fluid volume; if below 5 cm indicates OLIGOHYDRAMNIOS, if above 25 cm indicates POLYHYDRAMNIOS. *A. sac* fetal membrane bag, contains fetus and amniotic fluid.

**amniotomy** *See* ARTIFICIAL RUPTURE OF MEMBRANES.

**amoxicillin** oral penicillin analogue more efficiently absorbed from gastrointestinal tract than ampicillin, requires less frequent dosage, less likely to cause diarrhoea.

**amphotericin** anti-fungal drug.

**ampicillin** broad-spectrum synthetic oral, intramuscular or intravenous penicillin, active against many gram-negative pathogens and gram-positive ones affected by penicillin.

**ampulla** dilated end of canal, e.g. of fallopian tube.

**Amsel criteria** system to diagnose bacterial vaginosis; thin, white-yellow homogeneous discharge, pH 4.8 or higher, presence of clue cells, 'fishy' odour; three criteria present confirms diagnosis.

**anaemia** reduction in red blood cells, or amount of haemoglobin in them, due to haemorrhage, excessive red cell breakdown or failure to manufacture red blood cells. *Iron deficiency a.* common anaemia, may be due to poor nutrition; iron supplementation may be given if low serum ferritin; intramuscular or intravenous iron if severe; blood transfusion may prevent labour complications (e.g.

major haemorrhage). Anaemia not responding to iron therapy may be MEGALOBLASTIC ANAEMIA, i.e. folic acid deficiency. *Physiological a.* apparent anaemia in which red blood cell count reduces but remains within acceptable limits; due to normal HAEMODILUTION of pregnancy. *See also* SICKLE CELL ANAEMIA.

**anaerobe** micro-organism not requiring oxygen to exist e.g. *Clostridium welchii.*

**anaesthesia** state in which whole or part of body is insensible to pain or sensation, induced to permit surgical or other painful procedures.

**anaesthetic** agent that induces ANAESTHESIA. *General a.* renders person unconscious; *local a.* induces anaesthesia of local area.

**anal** pertaining to anus. *A. atresia* congenital absence or closure of anal opening *A. cleft line* pigmented mark in buttock cleft, progresses up anal cleft as labour progresses. *A. dilatation* in late first-stage labour, deep engagement of presenting part may cause anal gaping, suggests impending full cervical dilatation. *A. fissure* split or tear in anal canal skin; can occur postnatally due to straining to defaecate *A. sphincter* muscles encircling anus, attached posteriorly to coccyx.

**analgesia** insensibility to pain.

**analgesic** pain-relieving drug capable of inducing ANALGESIA.

**anaphylactoid syndrome** rare, potentially fatal entry of amniotic fluid into maternal circulation via placental sinuses triggers anaphylactoid response: pulmonary vasospasm causes hypoxia, hypotension, pulmonary oedema, cardiovascular collapse; followed by left ventricular failure, uncontrollable haemorrhage, coagulation disorders; high risk of maternal morbidity and mortality. Rare cause of intrapartum collapse or HYPOFIBRINOGENAEMIA.

**anaphylaxis** unusual, exaggerated acute allergic reaction to foreign substances, e.g. drugs; diagnostic agents; vaccines; foods; insect venom; pollens. Histamine release causes bronchospasm, peripheral vasodilatation, increased capillary permeability, bronchiole and bronchial constriction. Immediate adrenaline administration aims to produce bronchodilatation, reduce laryngeal spasm, raise blood pressure; later, steroid therapy aims to counteract histamine effects, decreasing capillary permeability; intravenous fluids and plasma restore intravascular fluid volume; dopamine, noradrenaline, isoprenaline increase and maintain blood pressure. *Adj* anaphylactic.

**anastomosis** communication between two vessels or other structures, either natural or established operatively. *Pl* anastomoses.

**anatomical conjugate** measurement of bony pelvis between sacral promontory and upper border of symphysis pubis, average 12 cm.

**anatomy** science of bodily structure of humans or animals.

**Anderson forceps** obstetric forceps for low- or mid-cavity delivery when sagittal suture of fetal skull is in anteroposterior diameter of outlet or cavity of maternal pelvis.

**andragogy** principles and practice of teaching adult learners.

**androgens** steroid hormones promoting male characteristics, i.e.

androsterone, testosterone, produced by testes under pituitary gland stimulation; aid growth and development of penis, scrotum, secondary sexual characteristics, muscle, bone. *Adj* androgenic.

**android** male-like, masculine. *A. pelvis see* PELVIS.

**anembryonic pregnancy** *See* BLIGHTED OVUM.

**anencephaly** gross congenital malformation, incompatible with life; cranial vault and cerebral hemispheres fail to develop; usually diagnosed by antenatal ultrasound scan; if undetected, may cause primary face presentation in labour.

**aneuploidy** incorrect number of chromosomes, e.g. monosomy (missing chromosome in pair) or trisomy (extra chromosome in pair, e.g. trisomy 21, DOWN SYNDROME).

**angina pectoris** severe chest pain and constriction, often radiating down left arm, caused by inadequate blood flow to heart.

**angiography** radiography of vessels of body after introduction of suitable contrast medium.

**angioma** tumour composed of blood vessels, e.g. naevus on skin.

**angiotensin** vasoconstrictor principle formed in blood when RENIN released from kidney; vasopressor action raises blood pressure, diminishes fluid loss in kidney by restricting blood flow. *A. converting enzyme inhibitors* drugs to control hypertension; contraindicated in pregnancy due to possible teratogenicity.

**angular pregnancy** fertilized ovum implantation at junction where fallopian tube enters uterus.

**anhydramnios** absence of amniotic fluid.

**ankyloglossia** tongue tie; congenital oral anomaly due to unusually short, thick frenulum; may reduce tongue-tip mobility.

**ankylosis** abnormal fixation or union of bones forming articulation, causes stiff joint. Sacrococcygeal joint ankylosis is rare cause of obstructed delivery.

**anococcygeal** pertaining to anus and coccyx. *A. body* muscular and fibrous tissue mass between anus and coccyx; part of insertion of levator ani muscles.

**anode** positive electrode to which negative ions are attracted.

**anodyne** pain-relieving agent.

**anomaly** marked deviation from normal. *A. scan* ultrasound scan, usually between 18 and 21 weeks' gestation, to detect fetal structural anomalies; examination of central nervous system (skull, brain, spine), thorax, heart, abdomen, urogenital tract, skeleton, extremities, face. *Adj* anomalous.

**anorexia** loss of appetite. *A. nervosa* complete lack of appetite with extreme weight loss, causing ANOVULATION, subfertility.

**anovulation** absence of ovulation.

**anoxia** OXYGEN deprivation. *See also* ASPHYXIA. *Adj* anoxic.

**antacid** substance that neutralizes acid. *A. drugs* reduce stomach acidity, as in indigestion, heartburn, acid reflux; most based on magnesium, calcium or aluminium salts; often combined with alginates which coat stomach and oesophageal lining. Avoid sodium bicarbonate: causes systemic alkalosis.

**ante-** prefix meaning 'before'.

**anteflexion** bending forwards, e.g. of body of uterus on cervix.

**antenatal** before birth. *A. care* bio-psycho-social midwifery and obstetric pregnancy care to assess fetomaternal well-being, enable early detection and treatment of deviations from normal. *A. education* midwifery advice and information for parents; preparation for birth sessions, usually in group settings, but may be one to one.

**antepartum** before PARTURITION *A. haemorrhage* genital tract bleeding after 24 weeks of pregnancy, caused by PLACENTA PRAEVIA, PLACENTAL ABRUPTION or incidental causes, e.g. cervical polyps, erosion, carcinoma. Midwife must call doctor, maintain observations, administer analgesia, take blood for cross-matching, provide emotional support. Never perform internal examination, may precipitate fatal haemorrhage.

**anterior** before, in front of. *A. obliquity of uterus* uterus tilts forwards due to lax abdominal muscles, often with pendulous abdomen *A. fontanelle* on fetal skull, junction of sagittal, coronal and frontal sutures; bregma 3–4 cm long, 1.5–2 cm wide; closes around 18 months of age.

**anteroposterior** from front to back.

**anteversion** turning forwards, e.g. of uterus in relation to vagina. *Adj* anteverted.

**anthropoid** man-like *A. pelvis see* PELVIS.

**anti-** prefix meaning 'against', 'opposite'.

**antibiotics** drugs derived from living micro-organisms, destroy or inhibit growth of pathogenic bacteria. Safe antibiotics in pregnancy include penicillins, cephalosporins, erythromycin, trimethoprim, clindamycin.

Others may cause adverse fetal effects e.g. tetracyclines, gentamicin, chloramphenicol, nitrofurantoin, quinolones, e.g. ciprofloxacin.

**antibody** specific substance formed in body, counteracts effects of antigens or bacterial toxins; can be transferred passively from one person to another, e.g. transfer of maternal antibodies across placenta to fetus. In neonate, antibody production completed some months after birth.

**anticardiolipin antibodies** antiphospholipid antibodies can cause hypercoagulation, venous and arterial thrombosis, thrombocytopenia, recurrent fetal loss; often occur with other autoimmune disorders, e.g. systemic lupus erythematosus; in pregnancy, may react against trophoblast, causing subplacental clots, placental thrombosis, causing growth restriction, fetal loss. *See also* ANTIPHOSPHOLIPID ANTIBODIES.

**anticoagulant** agent preventing or delaying blood clotting, e.g. heparin. May be required in pregnancy if history of previous thromboembolic disorders, thrombophilia, heart valve prosthesis; warfarin normally changed to heparin, as does not cross placenta. Women on anticoagulants must avoid all herbal remedies because they may potentiate anticoagulation.

**anticonvulsant** drug preventing fits, convulsions e.g. phenobarbital.

**antigalactogogue** substance inhibiting lactation. Drugs adversely affecting milk production include oestrogen, bromocriptine, cabergoline, thiazide diuretics, ergotamine.

**anti-D immunoglobulin** derived from human plasma, contains antibodies to rhesus factor D in blood. Nonsensitized women are given anti-D after 12 weeks' gestation, after any vaginal bleeding or potentially sensitizing incident, e.g. stillbirth, amniocentesis. Routinely administered intramuscularly to mother at 28 and 34 weeks' gestation and within 72 hours of birth if baby is rhesus positive.

**antidepressants** drugs to relieve depression symptoms, usually discontinued in pregnancy or dose reduced. Paroxetine, other SSRIs may cause fetal abnormality. Third-trimester administration may cause neonatal withdrawal, for example, respiratory distress, jitteriness, cyanosis, hyper-reflexia, irritability, sleeping problems. Tricyclic antidepressants generally considered safer in pregnancy.

**antidiuretic** 1. pertaining to or causing suppression of urinary secretion rate. 2. agent causing suppression of urine formation. *A. hormone* vasopressin; hormone suppressing urinary secretion; stimulates water reabsorption independently of solids, resulting in concentrated urine. Secreted by hypothalamus, stored and released by posterior PITUITARY GLAND, has vasopressor activity.

**antidote** agent counteracting effects of poison or drug.

**antiemetic** drug to prevent or treat vomiting. In severe pregnancy sickness, antihistamines, anticholinergics, antidopaminergics or 5HT3 receptor antagonists may be used. Metoclopramide or promethazine used in labour, often with intramuscular analgesia.

**antigen** substance conferring immunity by stimulating antibody production.

**antihaemophilic factor** factor VIII plasma protein essential for blood clotting. Deficiency causes haemophilia.

**antihistamine** substance that blocks tissue receptors for histamine, synthetic versions used to treat various allergic conditions, e.g. hyperemesis gravidarum.

**antihypertensive** agent that reduces high blood pressure. Some act on sympathetic nervous system, reducing peripheral vascular resistance, e.g. methyldopa; vasodilators act directly on arterioles; beta-blockers act on heart and kidneys, reducing cardiac output and renin secretion, e.g. propranolol. Some contraindicated in pregnancy: ACE inhibitors; diuretics (e.g. furosemide, bendroflumethiazide). Relatively safe: hydralazine, methyldopa; beta-blockers (propranolol, labetalol), calcium channel blockers (nifedipine).

**antiphospholipid antibodies** autoimmune anticardiolipin antibodies and lupus anticoagulant; cause antiphospholipid syndrome, abnormal coagulation and thrombosis; associated with fetal loss, poor placentation, thrombosis, autoimmune thrombocytopenia. Risks: preterm labour, hypertension, fetal or maternal mortality. Treatment: aspirin or heparin to improve pregnancy outcomes.

**antiretroviral therapy** drug therapy that attacks retrovirus, particularly HUMAN IMMUNODEFICIENCY VIRUS. *Highly active ART* three drugs combined to attack virus at different stages of replication. In pregnancy, reduces risk of vertical transmission to fetus.

**antiseptics** agents used to prevent sepsis, i.e. infection.

**antiserum** serum derived from blood of animal or human with a specific disease, having properties that are antagonistic to the bacteria that produce the disease. *Pl* antisera.

**antispasmodic** relieving spasm.

**antithrombin** naturally occurring or therapeutically administered substance; neutralizes thrombin, limits or restricts coagulation.

**antithromboplastin** substance preventing or interfering with interaction of blood-clotting factors that generate prothrombinase (thromboplastin).

**antitoxin** antibody produced to neutralize bacterial toxins. Serum from animals immunized with specific antitoxin is used to prevent and treat DIPHTHERIA and TETANUS.

**antral fluid** liquid surrounding the ovum in ovarian follicle, rich in hyaluronic acid.

**anuresis** lack of diuresis; retention of urine in bladder.

**anuria** failure of kidneys to secrete urine; may complicate severe concealed uterine haemorrhage, eclampsia, septic miscarriage, leading to CORTICAL NECROSIS OF KIDNEYS.

**anus** distal end of alimentary canal through which faeces are expelled. *Imperforate a.* congenital defect, non-patent anus.

**Anusol** rectal cream or suppositories to relieve haemorrhoid pain.

**aorta** large artery proceeding from left ventricle of heart.

**aortic** pertaining to aorta *A. stenosis* narrowing of aortic valve in heart; restricts blood flow through valve; heart needs to work harder to pump blood into aorta.

**aortocaval compression** abdominal aorta and inferior vena cava compression by gravid uterus when woman lies supine; causes hypotension and may cause fetal distress, especially in labour.

**aperient** drug that stimulates bowel action.

**Apert syndrome** congenital abnormality; fusion of all cranial sutures, syndactyly; increased risk with older fathers.

**Apgar score** scoring system devised by Dr Virginia Apgar to assess baby's condition in first few minutes of life; aids diagnosis of severe ASPHYXIA NEONATORUM. Mnemonic: Appearance (colour), Pulse, Grimace (response to stimulus), Active (tone), Respirations.

**aphthae** whitish spots caused by fungus *Candida albicans*; THRUSH. *Adj* aphthous.

**aphthous vulvitis** thrush (*Candida albicans*) infection of vulva.

**aplastic** relating to incomplete or defective structural development.

**apnoea** absence of breathing; intermittent periods occur in neonates with immature or depressed respiratory centre. *A. monitors* emit audible signal when periods of apnoea occur. *Adj* apnoeic.

**aponeurosis** flat sheet of fibrous connective tissue attaching muscle to bone or other tissues.

**apoplexy** sudden cerebral function failure due to cerebral vessel haemorrhage or thrombosis; leads to coma, stertorous breathing, paralysis.

**apoptosis** cell self-destruction process marked by fragmentation of nuclear DNA, activated by presence or removal of stimulus; eliminates DNA-damaged, superfluous or unwanted cells.

**Apgar score**

| SIGN | SCORE | | |
|---|---|---|---|
| | 0 | 1 | 2 |
| Colour | Blue to pale | Body pink, limbs blue | Pink |
| Respiratory | Absent | Irregular gasps | Strong cry effort |
| Heart rate | Absent | Less than 100/minute | Over 100/minute |
| Muscle tone | Limp | Some flexion of limbs | Strong active movements |
| Reflex | Nil | Grimace or sneeze | Cry irritability |

**appendicitis** appendix inflammation; in pregnancy appendix becomes abdominal organ so inflammation spreads rapidly.

**appendix vermiformis** worm-like tube with blind end, projecting from caecum in right iliac region of abdomen.

**Apresoline** *See* HYDRALAZINE.

**aqueduct** canal for passage of fluid. *A. of Sylvius* canal leading from third to fourth ventricle of brain; stenosis may cause hydrocephalus. Obstruction of absorption of cerebrospinal fluid occurs after meningitis or subarachnoid haemorrhage.

**arachidonic acid** long-chain polyunsaturated fatty acid in human breast milk; may aid neonatal retina and visual cortex development.

**arachnoid** web-like membranous middle brain covering between dura mater and pia mater. Cerebrospinal fluid circulates in subarachnoid space beneath it.

**arbor vitae** literally, tree of life. 1. branching appearance of white matter in cerebellum. 2. folds of columnar epithelium lining of uterine cervix.

**arcuate** arched, bow shaped. *A. ligament* strong ligament across subpubic arch of pelvis.

**arcus tendineus** thickening, 'white line', in pelvic fascia, giving rise to part of levator ani muscle.

**areola** pigmented area surrounding nipple, darkens in pregnancy.

**arnica** homeopathic remedy to treat bruising, shock, trauma; does not act pharmacologically, so will not interact with drugs; midwives must be adequately trained to advise on homeopathic remedies.

**Arnold Chiari malformation** condition in which brain tissue extends into spinal canal; occurs when skull is abnormally small or misshapen, causing downwards pressure on brain.

**aromatherapy** use of concentrated plant oils, administered via skin, respiratory tract or mucous membranes; chemicals in oils have positive (therapeutic) or negative (side) effects; many contraindicated in pregnancy, birth, may cause adverse maternal/fetal effects; never use on babies under 3 months. Midwives must be adequately trained to use/advise on aromatherapy.

**aromatic amino acid decarboxylase deficiency** rare metabolic neurotransmitter disease. AADC is essential enzyme involved in decarboxylation of aromatic amino acids; if enzyme is defective, dopamine and serotonin formation is impaired, passage and signalling within brain is disrupted.

**artefact** artificially produced lesion.

**arterial** pertaining to arteries.

**arteriography** radiography of artery or arterial system after injection of contrast medium into bloodstream.

**arteriole** small artery.

**arteriosclerosis** hardening and thickening of artery walls due to atheromatous plaques deposited on inner surface; causes ischaemia of organs or tissues, leads to hypertension, organ degeneration, mainly in old age.

**artery** vessel carrying blood from heart to other part of body.

**arthritis** inflammation affecting joints, as in disseminated gonorrhoea.

**artificial feeding** 1. feeding via orifices other than mouth, e.g. gastrostomy, jejunal, nasal, oesophageal, rectal feeding; sometimes used to feed preterm or sick babies. 2. infant feeding with fluids other than human milk.

**artificial insemination** mechanical conception; insertion of viable semen into uterus; semen may be produced by partner/husband who may adopt baby, or from known or unknown donor who has no legal rights over, or responsibility for, child.

**artificial respiration** artificial maintenance of respiration; mouth to mouth (mouth to mouth and nose in babies). OXYGEN administration mechanical maintenance of respiration may be necessary. *See also* APPENDICES 2 and 3.

**artificial rupture of membranes** surgical rupture of forewaters of amniotic sac for induction/acceleration of labour; instrument passed through cervix to pierce membranes. May aid observation of amniotic fluid, prevent cord prolapse if cord below fetal part.

**ascites** accumulation of free fluid in peritoneal cavity, rarely seen in pregnancy. In fetus or neonate, associated with HYDROPS FETALIS.

**aseptic** free from pathogenic bacteria. *A. technique* steps to avoid introducing infection; procedure under sterile conditions.

**asexual** without sexual organs.

**aspartate transaminase** serum glutamic oxaloacetic transaminase, enzyme normally in liver and heart cells; released into blood when liver or heart is damaged.

**asphyxia** suffocation. *A. neonatorum* failure of baby to breathe at birth; blood oxygen deficiency; increase in carbon dioxide in blood and tissues. *See also* APGAR SCORE *and* APPENDIX 3.

**aspiration** suction and withdrawal of fluid or air from cavity. *Meconium a.* fetal inhalation of meconium-stained liquor; causes chemical pneumonitis, airway obstruction, consolidation, under-aeration, hyper-inflation of lungs, contributing to meconium aspiration syndrome. Suction under direct vision and intubation at birth, preferably before baby breathes, may prevent it. *Chorionic villus a.* late first-trimester transvaginal or transabdominal aspiration of sample of chorionic villi under ultrasound guidance to aid DNA or chromosomal analysis, metabolism disorders diagnosis. *Vacuum a.* termination of pregnancy by removing uterine contents using vacuum via hollow curette or cannula introduced into uterus.

**aspirator**  apparatus for withdrawing air or fluid from cavity of body.

**aspirin**  salicylic acid, drug to relieve pain, fever, inflammation; contraindicated in pregnancy as increased risk of maternal, fetal, neonatal bleeding Antithrombotic action, thought to inhibit production of platelet-aggregating thromboxane $A^2$; low doses used preventatively if history of recurrent miscarriage, thromboembolism, pre-eclampsia, intrauterine growth restriction. May prolong bleeding time, discontinued at 36 weeks' gestation to prevent postpartum haemorrhage.

**assessment**  critical analysis and judgement of status or quality of particular condition, situation or subject.

**assimilation**  process whereby food is changed into body tissue.

**assimilation pelvis**  variation in normal sacral development *High a. p.* fifth lumbar vertebra fused into sacrum, pelvis is deep, causes difficulty in labour. *Low a. p.* first sacral vertebra assumes characteristics of lumbar vertebra, pelvis shallow, does not affect labour.

**assisted birth**  birth of baby assisted with FORCEPS, VACUUM EXTRACTOR, SYMPHYSIOTOMY for cephalic vaginal birth, manipulation for vaginal BREECH birth, operative birth by CAESAREAN SECTION.

**assisted reproduction, assisted conception**  artificial aid to conception in subfertility; regulated by Human Fertilisation and Embryology Authority *A. R. techniques* include ovulation-inducing drugs, intrauterine insemination, IN VITRO FERTILIZATION, embryo transfer, intracytoplasmic sperm INJECTION, GAMETE or ZYGOTE INTRA-FALLOPIAN TRANSFER.

**asthma**  allergic disease, recurrent paroxysmal dyspnoea, wheezing, cough, sense of suffocation; due to foreign proteins causing bronchiolar spasm. Stabilizes or worsens in pregnancy. Risk: preterm labour, reduced fetal oxygenation. Antenatal care shared between obstetrician, chest physician and general practitioner. In labour, materno-fetal condition closely monitored. Regional analgesia reduces hyperventilation and stress response to pain. Postnatally, breastfeeding encouraged to protect baby from developing allergic conditions. Asthma drugs considered safe in pregnancy, breastfeeding: bronchodilators, corticosteroids, theophyllines.

**asylum seeker**  person who has applied for refugee status in another country, awaiting decision. Pregnant asylum seekers may be at risk of physical, psycho-emotional and social problems.

**asymmetrical**  having parts that are not equal or symmetrical. *A. growth restriction* fetal growth restriction due to reduced placental nutrition, hypertension, genetic syndromes; head circumference normal (brain sparing), abdominal circumference reduced; vital organ growth maintained but subcutaneous fat deposition, glycogen storage in liver stops. More common (70%) than SYMMETRICAL GROWTH RESTRICTION. *A. pelvis* pelvis with one side distorted due to disease, injury; may be congenital e.g. Naegele's pelvis. *A. tonic neck reflex* neonatal reflex assessed in newborn examination; with baby in supine position, limbs should extend on side of body to which head is turned; those on opposite side flex.

**asymptomatic bacteriuria** presence of >105 bacteria/mL in midstream urine specimen without symptoms of infection; may cause pyelonephritis, preterm labour.

**asynchronous breathing** neonatal breathing in which diaphragm and abdominal muscles do not work in unison due to increased muscle fatigue and compliant chest wall; can occur with artificial ventilation.

**asynclitism** parietal presentation of fetal head; transversely placed sagittal suture lies close to symphysis pubis or sacrum; sideways rocking mechanism of fetal descent in labour in flat pelvis. *Anterior a.* anterior parietal bone moves behind symphysis pubis until parietal eminence enters brim. Movement then reversed, head rocks back until posterior parietal bone passes sacral promontory. *Posterior a.* posterior parietal bone negotiates sacral promontory before anterior parietal bone passes behind symphysis pubis.

**atelectasis** incomplete lung expansion due to respiratory obstruction or respiratory muscle weakness at birth, especially in preterm baby. *Primary a.* present from moment of birth; *Secondary a.* may be due to aspiration of meconium, infected liquor, vaginal discharge or maternal blood.

**atenolol** antihypertensive drug; long-term use in late pregnancy contraindicated, as may affect fetal growth.

**athetosis** condition involving involuntary limb movements; may occur after intracranial birth trauma, kernicterus.

**atlas** first cervical vertebra, articulating with occipital bone of skull.

**atonic** pertaining to atony. *A. uterus* uterus lacking efficient muscle tone, either in labour or early puerperium.

**atony** lack of muscle tone.

**atosiban** oxytocin antagonist to suppress preterm contractions.

**atresia** absence of opening of natural canal, e.g. oesophagus or vagina; usually congenital malformation.

**atrial** pertaining to atrium. *A. fibrillation* cardiac arrhythmia, with rapid, randomized contractions of atrial myocardium, leads to irregular, rapid ventricular rate. *A. septal defect* congenital heart defect; foramen ovale fails to close, persistent atrial septum patency.

**atrium** chamber of heart. *Pl* atria.

**atrophy** wasting of part of body due to cell degeneration from disuse, lack of nourishment or nerve supply.

**atropine** alkaloid that depresses salivation and respiratory secretions, relaxes muscular spasm, accelerates heart rate, dilates pupils; used before administration of general anaesthesia.

**attitude** relationship of fetal head, spine, limbs to each other; normally flexed; deflexed or extended when occiput not anterior.

**atypical** varying from normal pattern.

**audit** evaluation of care, management and organization to ensure quality and cost effectiveness. *Clinical a.* cyclical event to evaluate every aspect of healthcare.

**auditory** concerning hearing. *A. response cradle* device to screen infants for hearing impairment. Baby is played noises via headphones, and response movements are assessed by computer.

**augmentation of labour** acceleration when labour not progressing adequately; by AMNIOTOMY or intravenous oxytocin e.g. Syntocinon.

**aura** premonition prior to epileptic fit but not eclamptic fit. *See* ECLAMPSIA.

**aural** pertaining to ear.

**auricle** external portion of ear.

**auscultation** means of examining internal organs, listening to sounds given out. In pregnancy and labour FETAL HEART auscultated with Pinard stethoscope, cardiotocography.

**autistic** withdrawn; child with triad of impairment, i.e. difficulties with language and communication, social relationships, emotional understanding.

**autoclave** hermetically sealed apparatus using steam at high pressure to sterilize equipment.

**autogenous** generated within body, not acquired from external sources.

**autoimmune disease** disease caused by immunological action of individual's own cells or antibodies on components of body.

**autoimmune thyroiditis** *See* HASHIMOTO'S DISEASE.

**autoinfection** self-infection, transferred from one part of body to another by fingers, towels, etc.

**autolysis** self-digestion; tissue breakdown e.g. uterine INVOLUTION in puerperium. Surplus muscle broken down, absorbed into bloodstream, excreted in urine.

**automated auditory brainstem response test** part of Newborn Hearing Screening programme; records brain activity in response to clicking sounds via sensors placed on baby's head; babies failing to respond referred for full auditory assessment.

**autonomic** self-governing. *A. nervous system* sympathetic and parasympathetic systems, controlling involuntary muscle.

**autonomy** self-governing, independent. Midwives are personally responsible for their actions, legally permitted to oversee total care of childbearing women without complications. *Adj* autonomous.

**autopsy** post-mortem examination.

**autosomal inheritance** inheritance pattern of autosomal (non-sex) chromosomes; *A. dominant i.* dominant altered gene from one parent causes related disorder; 50% chance of inheriting altered genes and disorder; *A. recessive i.* two altered genes inherited, one from each healthy parent; carriers inherit one healthy and one altered gene set; 25% chance of inheritance if both parents carriers.

**autosome** chromosome other than X or Y sex chromosomes.

**avascular** not vascular; bloodless.

**avitaminosis** vitamin deficiency.

**axilla** armpit. *Pl* axillae. *Adj* axillary.

**axillary tail of Spence** mammary tissue extending into axilla.

**axis** 1. imaginary line passing through centre of body. 2. second cervical vertebra. *A. of birth canal/pelvis* imaginary line representing course taken by fetus in passage through pelvic canal, downwards and backwards through pelvic brim and major part of cavity; at level of ischial spines, turning through right angle to proceed downwards and forwards. *See also* PELVIS. *Pl* AXES.

**azithromycin** antibiotic for treatment of chlamydia infection.

**azoospermia** absence of spermatozoa in semen.

# b

**Babinski reflex (sign)** normal neonatal reflex, triggered by stroking sole of foot; large toe bends upwards instead of downwards; flexion develops later when infant learns to walk.

**Baby Friendly Hospital Initiative** World Health Organization and United Nations Children's Fund campaign to ensure all mothers are encouraged to breastfeed. UK standards incorporate Ten Steps to Successful Breastfeeding and Seven-Point Plan for Sustaining Breastfeeding in the Community, but also reflect the evidence base on delivering best outcomes for mothers and babies.

**baby-led feeding** infant feeding initiated in response to demand from baby. Also applies to weaning, when solid foods are introduced.

**baby massage** infant touch; enhances mother–baby relationship; relaxes, improves physical, cognitive development, enhances immune system, reduces stress in preterm babies.

**bacille Calmette–Guérin (BCG)** vaccine against tuberculosis, given in first week of life if mother has or is at risk of tuberculosis.

**bacilluria** presence of bacilli in urine.

**bacillus** rod-shaped organism, mostly gram-negative; *Koch's b.* and *Döderlein b.* are gram-positive (*see* GRAM STAIN). Pl. *bacilli*.

**backache** common pregnancy symptom, from exaggerated lumbar lordosis due to increased progesterone and relaxin; worsens as weight increases; often with SCIATICA and/or symphysis pubis dysfunction. Postural correction, wearing lumbar support and/or physiotherapy, osteopathy, chiropractic may help.

**bacteraemia** bacteria in blood.

**bacteraemic shock** rare condition associated with septicaemia caused by gram-negative organisms; endotoxins cause arteriolar dilatation in liver, lungs, elsewhere; reduced venous return causes profound shock; signs similar to hypovolaemic shock, rigours also occur. Requires urgent antibiotic administration.

**bacteria** microscopic unicellular gram-positive or gram-negative organisms, universally distributed. Beneficial when part of normal flora, e.g. DÖDERLEIN BACILLUS. Pathogenic bacteria produce toxins, cause inflammation, granulomas, hypersensitivities; aerobic bacteria require oxygen; anaerobes only grow in absence of oxygen; facultative anaerobes adapt to either environment. Some gram-positive bacteria produce endotoxins, causing hypotension, fever, disseminated intravascular coagulation, shock. Other toxins, haemolysins and leukocidins destroy red and white blood cells; kinases lyse blood clots; enzymes attack tissue. Sing. *bacterium*.

**bacterial** pertaining to bacteria. *B. vaginosis (BV)* vaginal flora overgrowth, e.g. *Gardnerella vaginalis*, causes vaginal discharge with fishy

http://dx.doi.org/10.1016/B978-0-7020-6906-2.00002-4

odour; not sexually transmitted but may relate to increased sexual activity, stress, other infections, feminine hygiene products; occurs in 15%–29% of pregnant women. Risks: pelvic inflammatory disease, preterm labour, recurrent urinary tract infections, uterine infection; treated with antibiotics.

**bacteriology** science of study of bacteria.

**bacteriophage** virus that infects bacteria.

**bacteriostatic** able to prevent multi-plication of bacteria.

**bacteriuria** bacteria in urine, 105 organisms/mL is significant. *Asymp-tomatic b.* occurs in 5% of pregnant women; if untreated, can progress to pyelonephritis.

**bag of membranes** amnion and chorion containing amniotic fluid and fetus; amniotic sac.

**Ballard score** technique to assess baby's gestational age from 26–44 weeks' gestation. Assessment: pos-ture, square window, arm recoil, popliteal angle, scarf sign, heel to ear; skin, ear/eye, lanugo hair, plantar sur-face, breast bud, genitals. *New B. S.* extension of scoring system to allow for preterm babies to be assessed.

**ballottement** literally, bouncing. Tap-ping structure in fluid causes it to rebound against examining fingers. *Internal b.* elicited by inserting two fingers per vaginam at 16–18 weeks' gestation to tap fetus, causing it to float away, quickly returning to exam-ining fingers. *External b.* elicited in examination per abdomen when head not engaged; fetal head tapped on one side, floats away, returns against examining fingers.

**Bandl's ring** extremely thickened RETRACTION RING in obstructed labour; transverse ridge felt across abdomen; imminent risk of uterine rupture.

**barbiturates** large group of hypnotic drugs, derivatives of barbituric acid; dependence and tolerance occur readily.

**Barlow test** neonatal diagnostic test for congenital hip dislocation; baby lies on back, feet pointing towards examiner, who abducts knees and hips, places middle fingers over greater trochanters and thumbs on inner thighs. Thighs abducted, middle fingers push greater trochanter forward; if hip dislocated, femoral head 'clicks' as enters acetabulum; femoral head can be displaced backwards out of aceta-bulum by exerting slight pressure when hips are flexed and adducted (Barlow sign). *See* ORTOLANI'S TEST.

**Barr bodies** small dark-staining bodies in normal female cell nuclei; obtained from buccal cavity smear, examined microscopically.

**barrier contraception** mechanical barrier to prevent sperm from enter-ing cervical canal, e.g. condom, diaphragm.

**barrier nursing** staff precautions to prevent infection from one patient spreading to others, or to staff. *Reverse b. n.* protects patient from external infection, e.g. after organ transplantation.

**bartholinitis** BARTHOLIN'S GLAND inflam-mation with abscess or cyst.

**Bartholin's glands** two labia majora glands; ducts open into vagina just external to hymen; secrete lubrication for vulva.

**Barts hydrops** most severe form of alpha-THALASSEMIA, usually fatal; fetal oedema; pleural, pericardial effusions; severe hypochromic anaemia.

**basal body temperature** temperature of body at rest.

**basal metabolic rate** minimum heat produced by resting person after 18-hour fast; measures amount of oxygen consumed, expressed as percentage above or below norm; increases 30% in pregnancy.

**base** 1. lowest part, foundation. *B. of fetal skull* two temporal, one ethmoid, one sphenoid bone, fused, part of OCCIPUT. 2. non-acid part of compound. 3. non-acid part of a salt; combines with acids to form salts, essential to maintain ACID–BASE BALANCE; in excess leads to ALKALOSIS and pH rises.

**baseline** measurement of clinical factors as basis for comparison *B. variability* on cardiotocograph, fluctuations in fetal heart rate of more than two cycles per minute, based on amplitude, i.e. peaks and troughs. If persistently minimal or absent, significant sign of fetal compromise.

**basic life support** measures taken in life-threatening events e.g. cardiac arrest; all midwives trained to provide basic life support to international standards or ADVANCED LIFE SUPPORT IN OBSTETRICS. A. airway; B. breathing; C. circulation. *See* APPENDIX 2.

**basophil** leucocyte with affinity for basic dyes.

**battledore placenta** placenta with umbilical cord attached to margin. *See also* PLACENTA.

**Bell's palsy** facial paralysis due to oedema of facial nerve; may occur in pregnancy; usually temporary.

**beneficence** ethico-legal term dictating that healthcare practitioner

should act in best interests of patient/client.

**Benefits Agency** UK governmental department; provides up-to-date information on financial and practical benefits for those in need, including pregnant women, children, new mothers. Online at https://www.gov.uk/browse/benefits.

**benzodiazepines** group of drugs including sedative-hypnotics, anti-anxiety drugs, anticonvulsants; prolonged use causes dependence.

**bereavement** loss through death, separation, adverse change in health, wealth, position (e.g. redundancy); produces psychological reaction with stages of anger, denial, disbelief, acceptance.

**beta-** β, second letter of Greek alphabet; denotes second position in classification system. *B.-adrenergic* receptors specific cell sites that respond to adrenaline. *B.-blockers* drugs blocking adrenaline at beta-adrenergic receptors, e.g. antihypertensives. Adverse effects: reduced fetal growth, neonatal hypoglycaemia, bradycardia; contraindicated in asthmatic women, may cause bronchoconstriction. Excreted in breast milk but safe. *B. haemolytic streptococcus See* STREPTOCOCCUS. *B. sympathomimetics* tocolytic drugs, e.g. ritodrine, salbutamol; high doses may cause maternal palpitations, tremor, nausea, vomiting, headaches, chest pain, breathlessness, tachycardia, pulmonary oedema, raised blood sugar; ketoacidosis possible in diabetic women. Monitor serum potassium, urea, electrolytes. *B. thalassaemia See* THALASSAEMIA.

**betamethasone** synthetic anti-inflammatory glucosteroid; given intramuscularly for preterm labour to reduce neonatal respiratory distress syndrome: increases lecithin levels in fetal alveoli.

**bi-** prefix meaning 'two'.

**bias** influences on a research study that may lead to invalid conclusions about a treatment or intervention.

**bicarbonate** carbonic acid salt ($H_2CO_3$); one hydrogen atom replaced by base, e.g. sodium bicarbonate, $NaHCO_3$, corrects ACIDAEMIA.

**bicornuate** having two horns. *B. uterus* congenital partial or complete vertical division of uterus; normal pregnancy, labour possible but associated with miscarriage, malpresentation, retained placenta.

**bifid** cleft into two parts or branches. In SPINA BIFIDA, spinous processes of one or more vertebrae fail to unite, remain divided.

**bifidus factor** present in human milk; promotes growth of gram-positive bacteria in gut flora, particularly *Lactobacillus bifidus*, preventing multiplication of pathogens.

**bifurcation** fork or separation into two branches e.g. as in uterus

**bilateral** pertaining to both sides.

**bile** dark-green secretion from liver cells, stored in gallbladder, passes through bile ducts to intestine, emulsifies fats, activates lipase. *B. pigments* bilirubin, biliverdin. *Adj* biliary.

**bilirubin** yellow/orange bile pigment, results from haemoglobin breakdown; fat soluble, unconjugated until rendered water soluble by liver i.e. conjugated; excreted as stercobilin in faeces. If excess bilirubin in skin and sclera, causes JAUNDICE.

**bilirubinometer** instrument measuring serum bilirubin levels.

**biliverdin** green bile pigment, oxidized bilirubin.

**Billings method** contraceptive method; recognition of cervical mucus changes 3–4 days before ovulation. Cervical mucus increases, becomes thinner around ovulation, to facilitate passage of spermatozoa through cervix; intercourse avoided at that time.

**bimanual** using both hands. *B. examination* assessment of pelvic cavity; one hand on abdomen and finger(s) of other hand in rectum or vagina. *B. compression* of uterus manoeuvre to arrest severe postpartum haemorrhage after placental delivery when uterus atonic. Right hand in vagina presses into anterior vaginal fornix. Left hand, on abdominal wall, pulls uterus forwards so anterior and posterior walls press firmly together, enabling direct pressure to be applied to placental site to stop bleeding.

**Bimanual compression of uterus**

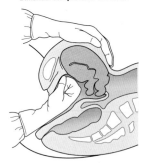

**binovular twin pregnancy** (*dizygotic, dichorionic, fraternal twins*) pregnancy with two fertilized ova; two gestation sacs, each with fetus, placenta, chorion, amnion; gender of babies may be same or different. About five times more common than uniovular twins.

**bioavailability** amount of drug which, after administration, reaches site of physiological activity.

**biochemical screening** tests for conditions or diseases through analysis of biochemical markers; in pregnancy, maternal serum screening for fetal Down syndrome or inherited metabolic disorders; newborn blood-spot screening test relies on biochemical MARKERS to identify babies with conditions such as cystic fibrosis.

**biochemistry** chemistry of living matter.

**biological nurturing** relaxed maternal positioning for breastfeeding, with mother semi-prone, baby on top of mother's abdomen; works on reflexes and innate behaviours.

**biophysical profile** well-being assessment of fetal adaptations to declining placental function in presence of growth restriction or maternal disease; assesses fetal body or limb movements, tone, breathing movements, amniotic fluid volume, cardiotocograph, each with score of 0 or 1; score of 5 indicates healthy fetus.

**biopsy** tissue removal for microscopic examination and diagnosis.

**biorhythm** cyclic biological event affecting daily life, e.g. menstrual cycle, sleep pattern.

**biparietal diameter (BPD)** measurement of distance between parietal eminences of fetal skull. ULTRASOUND assessment aids confirmation of gestational age. Head engages when BPD passes through maternal pelvic brim. CROWNING: when BPD distends vulva during birth, fetal head no longer recedes between contractions. See ENGAGEMENT.

**biparous** giving birth to two infants at same time, i.e. twins.

**bipartite placenta** See PLACENTA.

**bipolar** relating to two poles or ends, in reference to fetus and uterus. *B. disorder* mental illness: elevated and depressive mood states; changes in sleep pattern, activity, cognitive functioning; may be with psychosis; women with disorder have 50% chance of PUERPERAL psychosis.

**Bird vacuum extractor** See VACUUM EXTRACTOR.

**birth canal** bony and soft tissue structures through which fetus passes to be born. See PELVIS.

**birth centre** midwife-led, low-risk birth centre supporting women anticipating normal birth with minimal intervention; freestanding or adjacent to hospital maternity unit (alongside, co-aligned).

**birth certificate** statement issued for any baby born alive, irrespective of gestation, by registrar for births, marriages and deaths for district in which baby is born; certifies parentage, name, sex of baby, date, place of birth. Certificate of Stillbirth issued for babies born after 24 weeks' gestation who did not breathe or show signs of life after complete delivery. See BIRTH, REGISTRATION OF.

**birth control** prevention of conception.

**birth injury** neonatal trauma sustained at birth. See HAEMORRHAGE, CEPHALHAEMATOMA and ERB'S PARALYSIS.

**birth mark** congenital skin blemish or spot, usually visible at birth or soon after. *See also* NAEVUS.

**birth, notification of** form automatically generated by computerized record system in maternity unit, forwarded to registrar of births, deaths and marriages; allows cross-referencing to ensure parents formally register the birth.

**birth plan** plan of woman's preferences for care in labour.

**birth rate** number of births in 1 year per 1000 total estimated mid-year population (crude b. r.), per 1000 estimated mid-year female population (refined b. r.), per 1000 estimated mid-year female population between ages of 15 and 45 (true b. r.).

**birth, registration of** parent must by law register birth within 42 days at registrar's office in district where birth took place (21 days in Scotland). Responsibility rests with midwife if parents default.

**birthweight** baby's weight immediately after birth; provides baseline to assess future development, used for national statistics.

**birthing aids** items used by labouring women to adopt comfortable positions to facilitate progress and normal birth, e.g. balls, stools, ropes, specially designed chairs.

**bisacodyl** oral aperient or suppository used to combat constipation.

**bisacromial diameter** diameter between acromion processes on shoulder blades. Fetal measurement 12 cm.

**bisexual** 1. hermaphrodite. Having gonads of both sexes. 2. sexual preference for intimate contact with others of both sexes.

**Bishop score** pre-labour scoring system to assess cervical favourability for labour induction. *See also* CALDER SCORE.

**bitemporal diameter** distance between widest points of coronal suture; on fetal skull 8.2 cm.

**bitrochanteric diameter** diameter between greater trochanters · of femora that engages in breech presentation; 10 cm on fetus.

**bladder** urinary reservoir in front of uterus and vagina. Pressure on bladder from enlarging uterus, or engaged presenting part towards term, causes micturition frequency. If uterus retroverted incarceration may occur, leads to urinary retention at 12–20 weeks' gestation. Bladder distension in labour may inhibit uterine action, causing delay or haemorrhage.

**Bladder 67 acupuncture point** Chinese pressure point on little toes; used for MOXIBUSTION to convert breech presentation to cephalic.

**blastocyst** fertilized ovum about a week after conception; trophoblastic outer layer becomes placenta, chorion; inner cell mass, projecting into cavity, develops into fetus, amnion.

**blastoderm** germinal cells of embryo consisting of three layers: ectoderm, mesoderm, endoderm.

**bleeding** blood loss from wound or orifice. *B. disorders* coagulation disorders, e.g. DISSEMINATED INTRAVASCULAR COAGULATION. *B. time* time needed for small wound to stop bleeding, normally 3–4 minutes.

**blighted ovum** pregnancy with no visible embryo in gestation sac, as in embryonic death; common cause of miscarriage.

**blinding** practice of keeping investigators and/or subjects of a research study ignorant of group to which subjects are assigned to avoid bias *See also* SINGLE-BLIND TRIAL, DOUBLE-BLIND TRIAL.

# Birthweight: conversion chart

## CONVERSION OF BABIES' WEIGHTS (lb, oz to g)

| OZ→ LB↓ | 0 | 1 | 2 | 3 | 4 | 5 | 6 | 7 | 8 | 9 | 10 | 11 | 12 | 13 | 14 | 15 |
|---|---|---|---|---|---|---|---|---|---|---|---|---|---|---|---|---|
| 0 | | 28 | 57 | 85 | 113 | 142 | 170 | 198 | 227 | 255 | 283 | 312 | 340 | 368 | 397 | 425 |
| 1 | 454 | 482 | 510 | 539 | 567 | 595 | 624 | 652 | 680 | 709 | 737 | 765 | 794 | 822 | 850 | 879 |
| 2 | 907 | 935 | 964 | 992 | 1020 | 1049 | 1077 | 1105 | 1134 | 1162 | 1190 | 1219 | 1247 | 1275 | 1304 | 1332 |
| 3 | 1360 | 1389 | 1418 | 1446 | 1475 | 1503 | 1531 | 1560 | 1588 | 1616 | 1645 | 1673 | 1701 | 1730 | 1758 | 1786 |
| 4 | 1815 | 1843 | 1871 | 1900 | 1928 | 1956 | 1985 | 2013 | 2041 | 2070 | 2098 | 2126 | 2155 | 2183 | 2211 | 2240 |
| 5 | 2268 | 2296 | 2325 | 2353 | 2381 | 2410 | 2438 | 2466 | 2495 | 2523 | 2551 | 2580 | 2608 | 2636 | 2655 | 2683 |
| 6 | 2721 | 2750 | 2778 | 2806 | 2835 | 2863 | 2891 | 2920 | 2948 | 2976 | 3005 | 3033 | 3061 | 3090 | 3118 | 3146 |
| 7 | 3175 | 3203 | 3231 | 3260 | 3288 | 3316 | 3345 | 3373 | 3401 | 3430 | 3458 | 3486 | 3515 | 3543 | 3571 | 3600 |
| 8 | 3628 | 3656 | 3685 | 3713 | 3741 | 3770 | 3798 | 3826 | 3855 | 3883 | 3911 | 3940 | 3968 | 3996 | 4025 | 4053 |
| 9 | 4081 | 4110 | 4138 | 4166 | 4195 | 4223 | 4251 | 4280 | 4308 | 4336 | 4355 | 4383 | 4421 | 4450 | 4468 | 4506 |
| 10 | 4535 | 4563 | 4591 | 4620 | 4648 | 4676 | 4705 | 4733 | 4761 | 4790 | 4818 | 4846 | 4875 | 4903 | 4931 | 4960 |

**Bishop score for assessing favourability of cervix before induction**

| CRITERIA | SCORE | | | |
|---|---|---|---|---|
| | 0 | 1 | 2 | 3 |
| **CERVIX** | | | | |
| Dilatation (cm) | Closed | 1–2 | 3–4 | 5+ |
| Length (cm) | 3 | 2 | 1 | 0 |
| Consistency | Firm | Medium | Soft | |
| Position | Posterior | Central | Anterior | |
| **HEAD** | | | | |
| Station (in cm) above ischial spines | −3 | −2 | −1 | 0 |

Score of 5 or below: unfavourable in primigravida. 6 or more: cervix favourable for induction.

**blinking reflex** primitive neonatal reflex lasting into adulthood; eyes blink when baby is touched or in presence of sudden bright light.

**blister** serum collection between epidermis and true skin. Watery blisters in neonate may indicate PEMPHIGUS NEONATORUM.

**block** 1. obstruction. 2. regional anaesthesia. *See also* EPIDURAL ANALGESIA, PARACERVICAL BLOCK, PUDENDAL NERVE BLOCK.

**blood** fluid circulating through heart and blood vessels; supplies oxygen and nutritive material to body, removes waste products, etc.; essential to maintain fluid balance; comprises 55% fluid plasma, 45% blood cells and platelets suspended in fluid. *Fresh b.* useful for active sepsis or haemolytic disease or to replace blood lost through haemorrhage. *Stored b.* kept for up to 3 weeks at 4°C, for acute haemorrhage. *See also* BLOOD CELLS, PLATELETS, PLASMA.

**blood cells** erythrocytes (red cells) carry oxygen via haemoglobin from lungs to tissues; leucocytes (white cells) act as main defence against infection; platelets (thrombocytes) initiate blood clotting.

**blood clotting** coagulation. *See* CLOTTING.

**blood count** calculated number of white or red blood cells in cubic millimetre of blood.

**blood gas analysis** laboratory analysis of arterial and venous blood; measures oxygen, carbon dioxide, pressure or tension, hydrogen ion concentration (pH); determines $Pao_2$, arterial partial oxygen pressure; percentage of available haemoglobin saturated with oxygen; partial arterial carbon dioxide pressure; pH, blood alkalinity or acidity; level of plasma

27

bicarbonate, indicating metabolic acid–base status.

**blood groups** *See* ABO BLOOD GROUPS.

**blood 'patch'** 10–20 mL of maternal blood injected into epidural space to treat POST-DURAL HEADACHE, sealing puncture from which cerebrospinal fluid is leaking.

**blood pressure** force exerted by blood against arterial walls; determined by heart muscle contraction, arteriolar resistance, elasticity of artery walls, blood and extracellular fluid volume, blood viscosity; measured in brachial artery via sphygmomanometer or electronically. *Diastolic b. p.* lowest pressure in arteries when ventricles are resting. *Systolic b. p.* maximum pressure during contraction of ventricles. Blood pressure assessed at every antenatal appointment; systolic pressure above 130 mm Hg or diastolic pressure above 90 mm Hg or more than 15 mm Hg above first-trimester BASELINE reading constitutes HYPERTENSION.

**blood products** products from blood, e.g. red cells, platelets, fresh frozen plasma; factor VIII concentrate. Units of blood for transfusion issued as packed red cells or plasma containing platelets, white cells, coagulation factors, plasma proteins, immunoglobulin.

**blood sampling** removal of blood sample from mother or baby for investigation. *Fetal b. s.* in labour, blood sample taken intravaginally from scalp to test for blood pH to determine degree of fetal distress. ≤7.25 indicates test be repeated; ≤7.20 indicates birth should be expedited.

**blood sugar** concentration of sugar in blood, commonly glucose; recorded in millimoles per litre (mmol/L). Non-pregnant values 3.3 and 5.3 mmol/L; pregnancy 3.3 and 6.1 mmol/L. Neonatal 2.2–5.3 mmol/L. *See also* HYPOGLYCAEMIA.

**blood tests** in pregnancy, blood taken at booking appointment for ABO BLOOD GROUPS, full BLOOD COUNT, RHESUS FACTOR, HAEMOGLOBIN, RUBELLA immunity, HEPATITIS B and C, sexually transmitted infections, HIV/AIDS, CYTOMEGALOVIRUS, TOXOPLASMOSIS.

**blood transfusion** introduction of blood from donor to recipient.

**blood urea** proportion of urea in blood; non-pregnant 2.5–5.8 mmol/L (15–35 mg/100 mL); pregnancy 2.3–5.0 mmol/L (14–30 mg/100 mL).

**blood volume** total quantity of blood in body; affected by fluid exchange at capillary membranes, hormones, nervous reflexes affecting fluid excretion by kidneys. Rapid fall, as in haemorrhage, reduces cardiac output, causes SHOCK; increase, as in water and salt retention, increases cardiac output, arterial blood pressure. Assessed via intravascular CENTRAL VENOUS PRESSURE catheter.

**'blues', postnatal** physio-psychological maternal adaptation to early postnatal period, usually 3–5 days postnatally; labile emotions due to fluctuating hormones; if condition protracted, serious psychological problems may develop.

**body mass index (BMI)** weight (kilograms) divided by height (metres) squared. Normal BMI 20–25; below 20 underweight; over 25 overweight; 30 kg/m$^2$ or more at booking indicates OBESITY.

**Bolam test** in legal cases of alleged medical negligence, test used to determine standard of care owed to patient by health practitioners; no breach in duty of care if health practitioner acted in accordance with contemporary medical opinion or behaved 'reasonably' or 'logically' regardless of medical opinion.

**bonding, maternal–infant bonding** process of psychological attachment between mother and baby; aided by breastfeeding.

**bone marrow** substance in hollow cavities of bones. *Red b. m.* in trunk, skull bones only; forms all red and white blood cells except some lymphocytes. *Yellow fatty b. m.* in long bones of adults, not normally concerned with blood formation.

**booking** pregnant woman's initial appointment with midwife to introduce maternity services, give information, discuss pregnancy and birth care options; midwife takes full personal, family medical, surgical, obstetric, social, history, baseline observations of weight, urinalysis, blood pressure; blood samples for BLOOD TESTS.

**bottle feeding** See ARTIFICIAL FEEDING.

**bougie** flexible plastic instrument used to dilate stricture, e.g. in oesophagus, urethra, vagina.

**bowel** intestine. *B. sounds* borborygmi; sounds due to propulsion of intestinal contents through lower alimentary tract; absence indicates decreased or absent peristaltic movement, as in paralytic ileus, intestinal obstruction after abdominal surgery.

**Bowman capsule** glomerular capsule; start of kidney nephron, surrounding renal capillaries, glomerulus; filtration from blood into TUBULE.

**brachial** relating to arm. *B. artery* axial artery continuation along inner upper arm. *B. plexus* nerve network above clavicle in root of neck; anterior primary rami of fifth, sixth, seventh and eighth cervical spinal nerves and first thoracic nerve; at birth, forcible neck extension, especially with shoulder dystocia or during breech birth, may cause ERB'S PARALYSIS or KLUMPKE PARALYSIS.

**brachydactylia** abnormally short fingers.

**bradycardia** abnormally slow heartbeat: pulse rate below 60 beats per minute (adult); heart rate below 100 beats per minute (fetus).

**bradykinin** peptide formed by protein degradation by enzymes; powerful vasodilator causing smooth muscle contraction.

**brain** specialized area of central nervous system in cranium. *See also* FALX CEREBRI *and* TENTORIUM CEREBELLI. *B. death* irreversible coma. *B. scan* imaging technique to detect brain abnormalities e.g. neonatal intraventricular haemorrhage.

**brassiere (bra)** garment supporting breasts to prevent ligament overstretching; well-fitting, supportive brassiere with wide shoulder straps needed in pregnancy; front-opening for breastfeeding.

**Braxton Hicks contractions** painless, irregular uterine contractions of pregnancy; improve blood flow to placenta, fetus; intensity, frequency, regularity increase towards term; may be mistaken for labour contractions.

**breast** mammary gland, normally two, on anterior chest wall over second to sixth ribs, layer of loose connective tissue between. *B. abscess* fluctuant swelling in previously inflamed area, usually postnatally; pus may exude from nipple.

Treatment: aspiration or incision, drainage. Breastfeeding on affected side difficult; milk expression continues. **B. changes in pregnancy** tenderness due to increased blood supply; size, weight increase; prominent bluish veins on skin surface; Montgomery tubercles more prominent on darkened areola, sebum secreted to lubricate nipple; colostrum present from 16 weeks' gestation. **B. engorgement** full, hard, painful breasts; occurs around fourth postnatal day when milk supply does not yet equal demand; in severe cases gentle expression with pump may ease tension.

**breastfeeding** optimum method of infant feeding; mother may require help to fix baby to breast, advice on management.

**breast milk** substance secreted from breasts via nipples, initially COLOSTRUM, then foremilk with relatively low-fat

**Cross-section of breast**

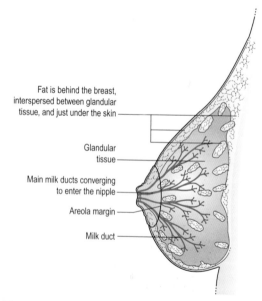

Fat is behind the breast, interspersed between glandular tissue, and just under the skin

Glandular tissue

Main milk ducts converging to enter the nipple

Areola margin

Milk duct

milk, followed by hindmilk with up to five times more fat than foremilk; contains fats, fatty acids, carbohydrates, proteins, vitamins, minerals, trace elements, growth factors, anti-infective immunoglobulins, lysozymes, lactoferrin, bifidus, hormones. **B. m. substitutes** infant formulae, usually from modified cow's milk; formulae may be whey dominant or casein dominant. **B. milk jaundice** physiological jaundice; may be prolonged in breastfed babies. Continue breastfeeding; exclude pathological causes for jaundice.

**breast pump** manual or electrical vacuum suction apparatus to withdraw milk from breast.

**breathing** See RESPIRATION.

**breech** buttocks. **B. presentation** longitudinal lie, fetal buttocks in lower uterine pole due to pelvic, uterine, fetal or incidental causes; incidence at term about 2.5%. Abdominally, fetal head felt in fundus; vaginally, buttocks, anal orifice, genitalia or feet palpated; ultrasound confirms diagnosis; EXTERNAL VERSION or MOXIBUSTION may change presentation to cephalic. **Vaginal b. birth** discouraged if medical or obstetric complications present. Fetal dangers: intracranial haemorrhage, hypoxia, fractures, dislocations, soft tissue injuries. Second-stage episiotomy before anterior buttock born may minimize aftercoming fetal head compression; feet are guided over perineum, loop of cord pulled down to prevent umbilical traction. If arms are flexed, shoulders born with next contraction; extended arms born using LÖVSET'S MANOEUVRE. Once trunk and shoulders born, baby hangs by own weight (BURNS−MARSHALL MANOEUVRE) to aid flexion, descent of head. When hairline appears at vulva, baby is held firmly by ankles, trunk raised in wide arc up and over mother's abdomen. MAURICEAU−SMELLIE−VEIT MANOEUVRE used if head extended, not descending.

**bregma** anterior fontanelle, kite-shaped membranous area in fetal skull at junction of frontal, coronal and sagittal sutures; normally closes about 18 months after birth.

**brim of pelvis** pelvic inlet. See PELVIS.

**British National Formulary** twice-yearly professional publication on medicine prescription, dispensing, administration.

**British Pharmacopoeia** official annual publication of standards for UK medicinal products and pharmaceutical substances.

**broad ligaments** two peritoneal folds, continuous with perimetrium; extend to pelvic sides; contain fallopian tubes, parametrium, ovarian blood and lymph vessels, uterine nerves, ureters.

**bromocriptine mesylate** dopamine agonist, inhibits prolactin secretion; used for female infertility, galactorrhoea, hyperprolactinaemia; may reduce HbA1c in type 2 diabetes mellitus.

**bronchopulmonary dysplasia** chronic neonatal respiratory condition; occurs after prolonged oxygen therapy or ventilation; serious lung growth disruption, patches of collapse, fibrosis. Prolonged ventilation and oxygenation required to maintain arterial oxygen tension above 55 kPa.

**bronchus** one of the main branches of trachea. *Pl* bronchi.

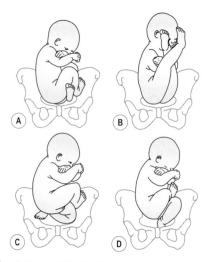

**A,** flexed breech; **B,** extended breech; **C,** knee breech; **D,** footling presentation.

**bronze baby syndrome** brownish or bronze skin discoloration of jaundiced hyperbilirubinaemic babies, complication of PHOTOTHERAPY.

**brow presentation** cephalic presentation, fetal attitude between flexion and extension; mentovertical diameter 13.0–13.75 cm presents, leads to obstructed labour. Causes: android pelvis, large fetal head, e.g. hydrocephaly, anencephaly. Abdominally, fetal head high above pelvic brim; vaginally, head not felt, occasionally bregma and orbital ridges felt. Management: Caesarean section or vaginal manipulation to flex head to vertex presentation or extend it further into face presentation, with forceps then applied. Internal podalic version, breech birth may be attempted.

**brown fat** thermogenic adipose tissue containing dark pigment, arising in embryonic life between shoulder blades, behind sternum, in neck, around kidneys, suprarenal glands; used for neonatal heat production as required.

**Brushfield spots** grey or yellow spots in irises of eyes of children with Down syndrome.

**buccal smear** scrapings from buccal mucosa, examined microscopically to study BARR BODIES.

**buffer** chemical substance; when present in solution, helps resist pH change. *Bicarbonate b.* principal buffering system in blood, involving bicarbonate ions and carbon dioxide.

**bulbocavernosus muscles** two perineal muscles surrounding vaginal introitus with weak sphincter-like action.

**bulbourethral glands** in male, two small bilateral glands, behind and lateral to urethra; discharge a component of seminal fluid into urethra; cf. female Bartholin's glands.

**bulimia nervosa** emotional disorder of distorted body image, obsessive desire to lose weight; overeating, fasting, self-induced vomiting, purging.

**bulla** blister. *Pl* bullae. *Adj* bullous.

**bullous impetigo** neonatal skin condition; erythematic blisters, usually staphylococcal; often in napkin area; may cause umbilical sepsis, breast abscess, conjunctivitis.

**bupivacaine hydrochloride** local analgesic drug for epidural, intrathecal, paracervical analgesia. Acts for 2–4 hours; may cause hypotension; intravenous infusion usually sited to allow rapid fluid replacement to correct hypotension.

**Burns–Marshall manoeuvre** method of delivering fetal head in breech birth. Trunk is delivered, baby hangs by own weight to aid head flexion, descent; when hairline appears at vulva, head is at outlet; born by raising trunk, holding baby's ankles, exerting slight traction, carrying trunk through wide arc up and over mother's abdomen. Perineum retracts, exposing baby's nose and mouth, enables airway clearance, oxygen administration; birth of head completed slowly, usually with forceps applied.

**Burns–Marshall method of delivering after-coming head in breech presentation**

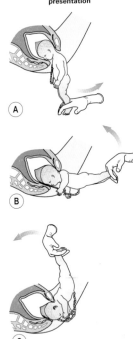

# C

**cabergoline** dopamine receptor agonist, drug for anovulatory hyper-prolactinaemia with fewer side effects than bromocriptine.

**cadmium** chemical element, similar to zinc and mercury; by-product of zinc metabolism; embryotoxic and teratogenic metal; exposure in pregnancy may cause miscarriage, fetal abnormalities.

**caecum** blind pouch, proximal part of large intestine from which extends vermiform appendix.

**Caesarean section** surgical procedure to extract fetus from uterus through incision in abdominal and uterine walls, after 24 weeks of pregnancy. *Classical upper segment C. s.* involves longitudinal incision in upper uterine segment; rarely performed due to risk of scar DEHISCENCE. *Crash C. s.* urgent, in event of cord prolapse, uterine rupture, antepartum haemorrhage. *Elective C. s.* planned antenatally for true cephalopelvic disproportion, major placenta praevia, triplets or higher multiples, serious maternal medical or obstetric conditions. *Emergency C. s.* performed for complications in labour, e.g. fetal distress, failure to progress, malpresentation, malposition, sometimes for pre-term birth. *Lower segment C. s.* involves horizontal incision in lower uterine segment to reduce risk of dehiscence. *Vaginal birth after C. s.* TRIAL LABOUR offered to women with previous C. s. to enable them to attempt vaginal birth.

**calcaneum, calcaneus** bone of foot forming heel.

**calcification** lime deposit in tissue, in mature or postmature placenta.

**calcitonin** thyroid hormone that lowers blood calcium.

**calcium** chemical element; with phosphorus, forms calcium phosphate of bones and teeth. Symbol Ca. *Ca ion* positively charged ion in intracellular and extracellular fluid, aids blood clotting, maintains normal heartbeat, initiates neuromuscular and metabolic activities; vitamin D aids absorption. Tetany from HYPOCALCAEMIA may occur in neonates. *C. channel blockers* drugs that block calcium entry into cardiac and arterial muscle cells, dilate arteries, reduce arterial pressure e.g. nifedipine, antihypertensive; may cause severe hypotension if used with magnesium sulphate; side effects: headache, must exclude fulminating pre-eclampsia.

**calculus** stone in gallbladder, bile duct, kidney, ureter. *Pl* calculi.

**Calder score** modified BISHOP SCORE, method of assessing ease with which mother will commence labour after induction.

**Caldicott guardian** named senior member of NHS authority, responsible for protecting confidentiality of

**Calder score**

| CERVICAL FEATURE | PELVIC SCORE | | | |
|---|---|---|---|---|
| | 0 | 1 | 2 | 3 |
| Dilation of | <1 cm | 1–2 cm | 2–4 cm | >4 cm |
| Length of | 4 cm | 2–4 cm | 1–2 cm | <1 cm |
| Station of presenting part (relative to the ischial spines) | −3 cm | −2 cm | −1/0 cm | +1/+2 cm |
| Consistency of | firm | average | soft | |
| Position of cervix | posterior | mid; anterior | | |

patient and service-user information and facilitating appropriate information sharing.

**calendar calculation** natural family-planning method assessing length of menstrual cycles in previous 6–12 months to determine fertile period.

**callus** 1. tissue that grows around fractured bone end, develops into new bone to repair injury. 2. localized hyperplasia of horny layer of epidermis caused by pressure or friction.

**calorie** the energy needed to raise temperature of 1 kilogram of water through 1 °C, equal to 1000 small calories; used to measure energy value of foods.

**cancer** *See* CARCINOMA.

***Candida albicans*** yeast-like fungus; normal flora of mouth, skin, intestinal tract, vagina. *See also* CANDIDIASIS.

**candidiasis** 'thrush', infection of mucus membrane with *Candida albicans* in vagina, skin, mouth or nails; can become systemic.

**Canesten** *See* CLOTRIMAZOLE.

**cannula** hollow tube for insertion into cavity or blood vessel; TROCAR is used to aid insertion.

**capillary** minute, hair-like vessels connecting arterioles and venules, with semipermeable walls; facilitate interchange of substances between blood and tissue fluid; also occur in lymphatic system. *C. haemangiomata* red, raised skin lesions in neonate, more common in girls, preterm babies; usually disappears by age 5–6.

**caput** head. *C. succedaneum* oedematous fetal head swelling, present at birth, due to pressure of dilating cervical os after forewater rupture, restricting venous return in superficial tissues; pits on pressure can cross suture lines on scalp; may occur on face in face presentation; bruising may also occur; usually disperses within hours. *See also* CEPHALHAEMATOMA.

**Caput succedaneum**

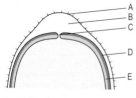

A, skin; B, subcutaneous tissue;
C, aponeurosis; D, periosteum; E, bone.

**carbamazepine** anticonvulsant, mood-stabilizing drug used for epilepsy and bipolar disorder; relatively safe in pregnancy.

**carbimazole** thyrotoxicosis drug; antenatal use may cause fetal hypothyroidism.

**carbetocin** oxytocic drug to control postpartum haemorrhage.

**carbohydrate** food composed of carbon, hydrogen, oxygen; sugar, starch, cellulose foods that provide energy; stored as glycogen for future use or, in excessive amounts, as fat.

**carbon dioxide ($CO_2$)** gas formed in body tissues by carbon oxidation, excreted by lungs; used with oxygen to stimulate respiration; measured as $PaCO_2$.

**carbonate** carbonic acid salt.

**carboprost** synthetic prostaglandin analogue of $PGF_2$ with oxytocic properties; used in uncontrolled POSTPARTUM HAEMORRHAGE. Contraindications: cardiovascular, renal, hepatic, pelvic inflammatory disease; precautions: asthma, anaemia, jaundice, diabetes mellitus, epilepsy, previous Caesarean or uterine surgery. Side effects: sudden onset diarrhoea, nausea.

**carcinogenic** causing carcinoma.

**carcinoma** malignant epithelial tumour; cancer. *Cervical c.* most frequently diagnosed cancer in first or second trimester, from blood-stained discharge or routine screening; may be associated with HUMAN PAPILLOMA VIRUS. Colposcopy, cervical biopsy confirms diagnosis. Treatment: cone biopsy; if advanced, termination of pregnancy offered plus radical treatment.

**cardia** 1. cardiac opening. 2. cardiac part of stomach surrounding oesophagogastric junction.

**cardiac** pertaining to heart. *C. anomalies* congenital defects: TRANSPOSITION OF GREAT VESSELS, pulmonary or tricuspid ATRESIA, TETRALOGY OF FALLOT, total anomalous pulmonary venous drainage, univentricular or complex heart structure. *C. arrest* sudden, often unexpected cessation of heart action requiring emergency cardiopulmonary resuscitation. *See* APPENDICES 2 and 3. *C. disease in pregnancy* congenital heart disease often worsens in pregnancy due to extra stress on heart. Care: careful monitoring; hospital admission if necessary. In labour aim to prevent overexertion, cardiac overload; first stage often short; forceps delivery or Caesarean to avoid active second-stage pushing; third stage most dangerous due to increased blood volume from strong uterine contractions, exacerbated by oxytocics. *C. output* increased in pregnancy due to increased stroke volume, heart rate; may be affected by SUPINE HYPOTENSIVE SYNDROME.

**cardinal ligaments** transverse cervical or Mackenrodt's ligaments; help to support uterus; two thickened bands of parametrium stretching from uterine cervix to lateral walls of pelvis.

**cardiogenic shock** impaired ability of heart to pump blood, sometimes after pulmonary embolism or in mother with cardiac defects.

**cardiogram** graphic representation of heart action on electrocardiograph.

**cardiomegaly** enlarged heart, myocardial inflammation, enlargement.

**cardiomyopathy, postpartum** rare complication of puerperium, 25%–50% mortality; causes left ventricular heart failure, thromboembolic problems; associated with older, multiparous women, obesity, hypertension, diabetes. Management aims: relieve congestive heart failure; heart transplant occasionally needed.

**cardiotocograph** fetal heart activity (*cardio-*), uterine contraction (*-toco-*) recording (*-graph*) to assess fetal well-being in pregnancy or labour via transducers on maternal abdomen; fetal heart rate may be assessed via fetal scalp electrode in labour after membrane rupture. Recording analysed for reduced baseline variability, decelerations, irregularities in fetal heart rate in response to maternal uterine action, aids detection of fetal hypoxia.

**cardiovascular** relating to heart and blood vessels.

**Care of Next Infant scheme** national health visitor-led scheme service for bereaved parents, supporting them before and after birth of new baby.

**Care Quality Commission** independent regulator of all health and social care services in England; ensures care provided by hospitals, dentists, ambulances, care homes, services in people's own homes meets government standards of quality and safety.

**carneous mole** blood or fleshy mole, missed miscarriage; blood clot surrounding dead embryo, retained in utero. *See* TUBAL MOLE.

**carotene** deep yellow pigment converted to vitamin A by liver; found in yellow and orange fruit, vegetables.

**carotid bodies** small neurovascular structures in bifurcation of right and left carotid arteries containing chemoreceptors that monitor oxygen content in blood and help to regulate respiration.

**carpal tunnel syndrome** hand tingling and numbness from pressure of local oedema on median nerve in carpal tunnel in wrist, often worse at night. Treatment: splinting of hands at night; physiotherapy. Usually resolves spontaneously after birth.

**carpopedal spasm** muscular spasm of hands and feet in TETANY.

**carrier** 1. person carrying pathogenic organisms with no disease symptoms; organisms may pass to others. 2. in genetics, apparently normal individual carrying RECESSIVE or sex-linked gene.

**cartilage** fibrous connective tissue in adults; forms most of temporary skeleton in embryo, providing model in which most bones develop; important part of organism's growth mechanism.

**carunculae myrtiformes** small elevations of mucous membrane around vaginal orifice; remnants of ruptured hymen.

**cascade of intervention** iatrogenic consequences of intervening in physiological labour, e.g. induction of labour, artificial membrane rupture, analgesic medication, dorsal position; interfere with oxytocin release, adversely affect woman's ability to labour normally.

**case conference** meeting of all professionals involved in care of person (often a child) to agree on management/treatment options, monitor progress.

**case control study** research study involving group of individuals with same characteristics (e.g. people with a particular disease) compared with control group (e.g. people without the disease).

**casein** milk protein; less digestible, present in larger quantities in cows' than human milk. *C. dominant infant formula* milk formula, same proportion of macronutrients as whey-dominant formulae, but more casein; indigestible curds from casein make baby feel fuller longer, increase metabolic demands.

**caseinogen** precursor of casein; converted to casein by rennin in gastric juice of babies.

**case law** the law as established by the outcome of former similar cases.

**caseload midwifery** group with each midwife responsible for group of women; aims to improve communication, continuity of care.

**case mix database** computerized record system combining all data from patient administration and operational systems; provides comprehensive information on treatments and services received during episodes of care.

**case report/study** detailed report on one patient (case), covering the course of the patient's condition and response to treatment.

**case series** report of several cases of a given condition, including course of condition and response to treatment; method of collating evidence for research without a comparison (control) group.

**caspofungin** antifungal drug, effective against *Candida* and *Aspergillus*; administered intravenously.

**cast** structure moulded in hollow organ, retaining shape of cavity of organ when shed, e.g. decidual cast shed from uterus in tubal pregnancy, casts in urine from renal tubules in kidney disease.

**castor oil** oil sometimes ingested by women to avoid induction of labour; causes abdominal pain, severe diarrhoea, possible dehydration: women should be discouraged from taking it.

**catamania** menstruation.

**cataract** opacity of crystalline lens or its capsule, impairs vision. *Congenital c.* sometimes due to familial condition or maternal RUBELLA in early pregnancy; associated with GALACTOSAEMIA.

**catecholamine** dopamine, adrenaline, noradrenaline in physiologic stress response. Release at sympathetic nerve endings increases cardiac output, constricts peripheral blood vessels, increases blood pressure; hepatic and skeletal muscle glycogenesis increases blood glucose; blood lipids raised by increasing fat catabolism.

**catheter** polythene or rubber tube, perforated near blind end; introduced into various hollow organs, vessels or canals for CATHETERIZATION.

**catheterization** insertion of catheter to introduce or withdraw fluid or to measure fluid pressure, e.g. bladder, umbilicus.

**cathode** negative electrode.

**cation** ion carrying positive electric charge, e.g. sodium, copper.

**cauda equina** nerves into which spinal cord divides at its termination in lumbar region.

**caudal block** regional analgesia via sacral hiatus; less reliable than entering epidural space by lumbar route. *See* EPIDURAL ANALGESIA.

**caul** rare condition; amnion fails to rupture in labour, enveloping baby's head at birth; must be ruptured quickly to clear airway.

**cautery** hot instrument or chemical agent used to destroy tissue by burning it, e.g. cervical erosion.

**cavity of pelvis** *See* PELVIS.

**cefotaxime cephalosporin** broadspectrum antibiotic, effective against numerous gram-positive and gramnegative bacteria.

**ceftazidime cephalosporin** broadspectrum antibiotic

**ceftriaxone cephalosporin** antibiotic for pneumonia, urinary, pelvic infections, gonorrhoea etc., administered intravenously or intramuscularly.

**cefuroxime cephalosporin** antibiotic for urinary, skin, respiratory infections, gonorrhoea etc., administered by mouth.

**-cele** suffix meaning 'tumour', e.g. MENINGOCELE.

**cell** structural unit of all multicellular organisms; consists of nucleus with central nucleolus, CHROMOSOMES with surrounding semifluid cytoplasm containing mitochondria, RIBOSOMES, other bodies, within cell membrane. All living cells arise from other cells, either by division of one cell to make two, as in MITOSIS and MEIOSIS, or by fusion of two cells to make one, e.g.

sperm and ovum become zygote. Cells differentiate during development into specialized types organized into tissues, then into organs.

**cellulitis** diffuse inflammatory process within solid tissues; oedema, redness, pain, functional disturbance; caused by infection with streptococci, staphylococci, etc. Occurs in loose tissues beneath skin, mucous membranes or around muscle bundles or surrounding organs. *See also* PARAMETRITIS.

**cellulose** carbohydrate; fibrous outer covering of vegetable cells, indigestible in alimentary tract; gives bulk, stimulates peristalsis.

**census** enumeration of population, introduced 1801 in England and Wales, repeated every 10 years; records name, address, sex, occupation, marital status, social information of every household.

**centile** *See* PERCENTILE.

**centimetre** one-hundredth of metre.

**central nervous system** brain and spinal cord. In embryo, development commences 18 days after conception. *CNS abnormalities* include SPINA BIFIDA, ANENCEPHALY, HYDROCEPHALUS, MICROCEPHALY.

**central venous pressure** pressure of blood in right atrium; indicating balance between cardiac output and venous return; measured via catheter inserted through median cubital vein to superior vena cava; distal end of catheter attached to manometer, positioned so zero point level with right atrium; each time mother's position changes, zero point on manometer must be reset. Used to assess accurately amount of blood lost during haemorrhage and ensure

**Monitoring central venous pressure**

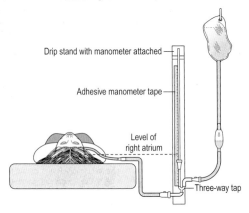

Drip stand with manometer attached

Adhesive manometer tape

Level of right atrium

Three-way tap

adequate fluid replacement without overloading circulation. Normal fluid volume range in right atrium: 15–110 cm of saline when zero point of scale corresponds to mid-axillary line.

**centrifuge** apparatus to rotate test tubes at great speed to precipitate bacteria, cells and other substances.

**cephalexin cephalosporin** antibiotic for respiratory, urinary, skin infections.

**cephalhaematoma** blood collection beneath periosteum of one cranial bone, fluctuant swelling develops on baby's head within 48 hours of birth; distinguishable from CAPUT SUCCEDANEUM that develops after birth, limited to one bone. Takes several weeks to subside; no treatment needed unless severe jaundice occurs.

**Cephalhaematoma**

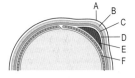

A, skin; B, subcutaneous tissue; C, aponeurosis; D, periosteum; E, blood under periosteum; F, bone.

**cephalic** pertaining to head, usually fetal head. *C. presentation* normal presentation of fetus, i.e. with head in lowest pole of uterus. *C. version* conversion to head presentation. *See* VERSION.

**cephalometry** antenatal head measurement of BIPARIETAL DIAMETER to assess fetal maturity, growth, ULTRA-SOUND SCAN most accurate.

**cephalopelvic** relationship of fetal head to maternal pelvis. *C. disproportion* misfit between fetal head and maternal pelvis, assumed when head will not engage in pelvis after 36 weeks' gestation; may be diagnosed in labour; may cause obstructed labour.

**cephaloridine** antibiotic derived from CEPHALOSPORIN; if given antenatally, orally, intramuscularly or intravenously, crosses placenta, entering fetal circulation.

**cephalosporin** naturally occurring antibiotic, similar to PENICILLIN.

**cerclage** encircling with ring or loop of non-absorbable suture to keep cervix closed in case of incompetent cervix.

**cerebellum** hindbrain, below cerebrum, behind medulla oblongata.

**cerebral** pertaining to cerebral hemispheres. *C. dysrhythmia* brain shows abnormal electrical wave pattern on electroencephalograph tracing, as in epilepsy, eclamptic convulsions. *C. haemorrhage* bleeding from or into one of cerebral hemispheres. *C. palsy* persistent motor disorder due to hypoxia in utero, asphyxia neonatorum, apnoea, cyanosis, as in RESPIRATORY DISTRESS SYNDROME, HYPOGLYCAEMIA, etc.

**cerebrospinal** relating to brain and spinal cord. *C. fluid* fluid in ventricles of brain secreted by choroid plexuses, circulating in subarachnoid space and membranes surrounding spinal cord; protects nerves in brain and spinal cord from jarring and injury. Excess cerebral fluid is found in HYDROCEPHALUS.

**cerebrum** centre of higher functions of brain, occupying large part of cranium and consisting of right and left cerebral hemispheres.

**cervical** pertaining to neck. 1. in obstetrics, uterine cervix. *C. canal* channel starting at internal cervical os, communicates with body of uterus, ends at external os, opens into vagina. *C. cytology* examination of cervical cells to detect abnormal changes. *C. dilatation* opening of cervix in first-stage labour, from closed cervical os to full dilatation, approximately 10 cm; assessed on examination per vaginam. *C. ectropion (eversion)* physiological response by cervical cells to pregnancy hormone changes; cells proliferate, cause cervix to appear eroded. *C. incompetence* failure of cervix to hold pregnancy in uterus; causes second-trimester miscarriage, premature membrane rupture, painless expulsion of fetus; treated by cervical CERCLAGE. *C. intraepithelial neoplasia (CIN)* classification of cervical dysplasia: CIN I – mild, reversible; CIN II – moderate, reversible; CIN III – severe, irreversible carcinoma. *C. polyps* small vascular pedunculated squamous or columnar epithelium covering core of connective tissue and blood vessels in cervical canal or ectocervix; may be asymptomatic or cause bleeding; no treatment in pregnancy unless severe bleeding or malignancy. *C. ripening* physiological or artificially induced cervical softening, making it more susceptible to effects of uterine contractions. *See* BISHOP SCORE. 2. *C. vertebrae* small, joined neck bones.

**cervicitis** mucous membrane infection in uterine cervix. *Acute c.* occurs in gonorrhoea. *Chronic c.* usually low-grade infection after tearing of cervix during birth; inflamed mucous membrane protrudes through external os to vaginal cervix forming erosion, which bleeds readily; cauterization destroys infected tissues.

**cervix** neck *C. uteri* uterine neck, opens into vagina; 2.5 cm long.

**cervicograph** diagrammatic representation of cervical dilatation, charted against hours in labour.

**Chadwick's sign** dark purplish discoloration, congestion of vaginal membrane from increased vascularity; sign of pelvic congestion.

**chancre** initial lesion of SYPHILIS, developing at site of inoculation.

**CHARGE syndrome** genetic condition including eye, heart, ear defects, oesophageal atresia, growth retardation; associated with CHOANAL ATRESIA; cause of congenital deafness, blindness.

**chemical** pertaining to chemistry. *C. compound* substance produced by chemical change, broken up only by chemical means, unlike a mixture, which can be separated mechanically.

**chemoreceptor** collection of cells sensitive to alterations in chemicals in contact with them, found in carotid and aortic bodies; responsive to changes in serum OXYGEN, CARBON DIOXIDE, HYDROGEN ion concentration. If arterial blood OXYGEN concentration falls below normal, chemoreceptors send impulses to stimulate respiratory centre, increasing alveolar ventilation and OXYGEN intake.

**chemotherapy** treatment of illness by chemical means, i.e. with medication. *Adj* chemotherapeutic.

**chest** thoracic cavity containing lungs, heart, trachea, bronchi, oesophagus, large blood vessels and nerves. *C. compression* application

of pressure to chest to help blood flow through heart in emergency situation *See* APPENDICES 2 and 3.

**chickenpox** varicella zoster infectious childhood disease, incubation period 12–20 days; slight fever, transparent skin vesicles erupt, itch, dry up, may leave pits in skin; severe in neonates. Previous disease usually gives lifelong immunity; immunoglobulin given to those in contact with condition who are not immune.

**chignon** large caput succedaneum seen on head of baby delivered by vacuum extraction.

**child abuse** act or omission by individuals, institutions or processes that directly or indirectly harms child or compromises safe, healthy development to adulthood. If child seen to be in danger of significant physical, sexual, emotional or neglectful abuse, his or her name is recorded in Child Protection Register. Midwife with reasonable cause to suspect abuse of a child must take appropriate action to protect child. *See also* CHILDREN ACT 2004.

**child benefit** weekly social security payment for primary carer of child under 16, or up to age 19 if still in full-time education.

**child minder** person approved by and registered with local authority social services department to provide day care for small number of children from birth to 5 years.

**child protection register** confidential list of children at risk of, or suspected of being at risk of, physical, sexual, emotional abuse or neglect; access to register restricted.

**Child Maintenance Group** part of Department for Work and Pensions responsible for implementing Child Support Act via Child Support Agency and Child Maintenance Service.

**childbirth** process of giving birth, parturition. *Natural c.* approach in which mother and partner are prepared and remain in control of labour, allowing it to progress naturally without medical intervention, drugs or other stimuli, if possible.

**Children Act 2004** Act of Parliament that defines children's rights, identifies parental responsibilities, details procedures to protect children. Children's services authorities must establish Local Safeguarding Children Boards to protect children from harm; local authorities must ascertain wishes and feelings of children when making decisions about services for children in need and providing accommodation for children under the act.

**Children's Centres** centres responding to local community needs, providing child and family health services, child care advice, early learning, specialist services, e.g. speech therapy, healthy eating advice, help with managing money, help for parents to find work, stop smoking, dental services, language and translation services.

**chiropractic** statutorily regulated medical system involving joint mobilization and manipulation to realign musculoskeletal system. In pregnancy, useful for backache, pelvic girdle pain etc.; effective for colic in infants, hyperactivity. *See also* OSTEOPATHY.

**chi-squared test** statistical test to determine if two or more groups of observations differ significantly from one another, i.e. more than expected by chance.

**Chlamydia trachomatis** common sexually transmitted bacterial infection, prevalent in those under 25 or those with multiple sexual partners; approximately 50% of men, 75% of women asymptomatic or have non-specific urethritis; may cause subfertility, ectopic pregnancy, preterm labour, membrane rupture. Signs and symptoms: post-coital or intermenstrual bleeding, purulent vaginal discharge, cervicitis, dyspareunia, lower abdominal pain; associated with bartholinitis, perihepatitis, chorioamnionitis, postpartum endometriosis. Babies born to untreated mothers can contract severe conjunctivitis leading to blindness, PNEUMONIA. Free testing is offered to those under 25 through National Chlamydia Screening Programme.

**chloasma** 'pregnancy mask', skin pigmentation on forehead, nose, cheeks.

**chloramphenicol** broad-spectrum antibiotic against gram-positive and gram-negative bacteria, including most anaerobic organisms. Not used in developed countries but still used in low-income countries as inexpensive and readily available. Most serious adverse effects: bone marrow toxicity, aplastic anaemia, usually fatal.

**chlordiazepoxide** benzodiazepine anti-anxiety drug for short-term use; may cause congenital anomalies if taken in pregnancy.

**chlorhexidine (Hibitane)** liquid antibacterial action skin cleanser for surgical scrub, preoperative skin preparation, cleansing wounds.

**chloride** chlorine salt; electrolyte maintains normal blood balance.

**chlorphenindione** long-acting oral anti-coagulant drug.

**chlorothiazide** diuretic and antihypertensive drug, not generally used in pregnancy.

**chlorphenamine (chlorpheniramine) maleate (Piriton)** drug to relieve allergy and for emergency treatment of anaphylactic reactions.

**chlorpromazine (Largactil)** antipsychotic agent and antiemetic phenothiazine drug sometimes used for HYPEREMESIS GRAVIDARUM; side effects include drowsiness, hypotension.

**chlorpropamide** anti-diabetic drug, contraindicated in pregnancy; may cause neonatal hypoglycaemia.

**choanal atresia** membranous or bony obstruction of posterior nares, causes neonatal respiratory difficulty at or shortly after birth, leading to cyanosis.

**cholecystitis** inflammation of gall-bladder.

**cholestasis of pregnancy** See INTRAHEPATIC CHOLESTASIS OF PREGNANCY.

**chondroblast** embryonic cell that forms cartilage.

**chondrocranium** primitive cartilaginous skeletal structure of fetal skull; grows to envelop rapidly growing embryonic brain.

**chordee** downward curvature of penis caused by congenital anomaly such as HYPOSPADIAS.

**chorditis** inflammation of spermatic (or vocal) cords.

**chorea** St Vitus' dance, Sydenham's chorea. Disease related to rheumatism, probably bacterial, affects nervous system; characterized by irregular involuntary muscular movements. *C. gravidarum* occasionally seen in primigravidae with history of childhood rheumatism or chorea; puts additional strain on already impaired heart.

**chorioamnionitis** intra-amniotic bacterial inflammation due to ascending bacteria from vagina; associated with prolonged labour.

**chorioangioma** fetal blood vessel collection in WHARTON'S JELLY; forms tumour on placenta; little clinical significance but may be associated with POLYHYDRAMNIOS.

**choriocarcinoma** highly malignant neoplasm, may occur with HYDATIDIFORM MOLE; detected by raised serum or urinary chorionic gonadotropin, radioimmunoassay; treated with cytotoxic chemotherapy, hysterectomy.

**chorion** outer membrane enclosing fetus in utero, derived from TROPHOBLAST; opaque, friable, sometimes retained after delivery. *C. biopsy* removal of tissue from gestational sac to identify inherited disorders, performed from 8 weeks' gestation, facilitating termination before 12 weeks. *C. frondosum* part of chorion covered by villi in early weeks of embryonic development before placenta is formed. *C. laeve* non-villous, membranous part of trophoblast, which develops into chorion.

**chorionic** pertaining to chorion. *C. gonadotropin* See human CHORIONIC GONADOTROPIN. *C. villi* tiny finger-like projections arising from TROPHOBLAST, persist in chorion frondosum, outer SYNCYTIOTROPHOBLAST, inner CYTOTROPHOBLAST layer. Fetal capillaries embedded in mesoderm; oxygenated maternal blood cascades over villi in intervillous spaces;

oxygen, nutrients, pass into fetal circulation, CARBON DIOXIDE passes out; after 24 weeks' gestation cytotrophoblastic cell layer remains only in isolated areas. *C. villus sampling* antenatal placental biopsy after 11 weeks' gestation to obtain chorion frondosum sample; needle or fine cannula inserted into uterus transabdominally or transvaginally under ultrasound guidance; to determine fetal KARYOTYPE, obtain fetal DNA; procedure-induced, operator-dependent risk of miscarriage 1%–2%.

**chorionicity** placental formation in MULTIPLE PREGNANCY; monochorionic twins connected to single placenta with increased risk of TWIN-TO-TWIN TRANSFUSION SYNDROME; dichorionic twins have two separate placentae (may fuse), lower risk of complications.

**choroid plexus** vascular fringe-like folds in PIA MATER in third, fourth and lateral ventricles of brain; concerned with formation of cerebrospinal fluid.

**Christmas disease** haemophilia B; hereditary haemorrhagic disease, deficiency of clotting factor IX.

**chromatin** chromosome substance composed of DNA and basic proteins; stains with basic dyes. *Sex c.* Barr body; mass of condensed, inactive X chromosome found in cells of normal females.

**chromatography** technique to separate components of substance dependent on differences in absorbency of each component when passed through medium such as paper; used for investigations, e.g. newborn blood-spot screening for SICKLE CELL DISEASE.

**chromosome** tiny thread-like structures in cell nucleus, composed of DEOXYRIBONUCLEIC ACID and protein, carrying genes transmitting inherited characteristics. Human cells carry 46 chromosomes, 22 pairs of autosomes, 2 sex chromosomes (XX or XY). *C. abnormalities* include Down, Edward, Patau, Potter, Turner syndrome. *C. analysis* test to analyse fetal cells; cells are cultured, cell division is arrested mid-stage by colchicine (drug); chromosomes are stained to produce distinct pattern of light and dark bands, each one recognized by its size and banding pattern. Individual's chromosomal characteristics are referred to as KARYOTYPE. *See also* GENE.

**chronic** prolonged or permanent, e.g. chronic disease. *cf.* acute.

**cilia** fine hair-like processes growing on free border of certain epithelial cells. In fallopian tubes, epithelial; cilia propel ovum from ovarian end of fallopian tube to uterus. *Sing* cilium. *Adj* ciliated.

**ciprofloxacin** antimicrobial drug, active against gram-negative organisms, particularly *Chlamydia*; use with caution during pregnancy, breastfeeding.

**circulation** movement in circular course, e.g. blood. *Fetal c.* circulation of blood in fetus; foramen ovale and ductus arteriosus bypass lungs, blood is carried to and from placenta by umbilical vessels and ductus venosus.

**circumcision** in male, excision of prepuce of penis; may be necessary if urinary meatus obstructed, or performed routinely for religious reasons. *Female c.* excision of labia, clitoris, narrowing of vaginal introitus. *See* FEMALE GENITAL MUTILATION.

**circumvallate placenta** placenta with distinct ridge on fetal surface, caused by peripheral double fold of chorion, liable to separate partially, causing antepartum haemorrhage.

**citalopram** antidepressant selective serotonin reuptake inhibitor; can be taken under medical supervision in pregnancy.

**clamp** surgical instrument to compress part of body, e.g. to prevent or arrest haemorrhage. *Hollister c.* plastic device to occlude umbilical cord vessels, applied at birth about 1–2 cm from umbilicus for 48 hours, then removed.

**clary sage** aromatherapy oil; contra-indicated in pregnancy until term; sedative, hypotensive, may accelerate uterine contractions. Early, prolonged or inappropriate use causes fetal hypoxia, distress, uterine hypertonia, hypotension. Contraindications at term: uterine scar, multiple pregnancy, medical or obstetric complications. Midwives must be trained to use AROMATHERAPY oils.

**clavicle** collar bone, articulating with sternum and acromion process of scapula. *Fractured c.* uncommon birth injury, may occur with traumatic breech delivery, shoulder dystocia or spontaneously due to congenital OSTEOGENESIS IMPERFECTA.

**cleft** split, divided into two. *C. lip* congenital unilateral or bilateral split in lip from embryonic failed fusion of median nasal and maxillary processes; usually operable in infancy. *C. palate* congenital central or unilateral split in upper palate of mouth; interferes with sucking and speech; requires corrective surgery, Most severe form is complete cleft palate with bilateral CLEFT LIP.

**cleidotomy** surgical division of clavicles to allow birth of fetus in shoulder dystocia.

**climacteric** physiological changes occurring around MENOPAUSE.

**clinical** pertaining to observation and treatment of patients. *C. trial* assessment of effectiveness of treatment by following responses to therapy in defined patient groups. *Controlled c. trial* study involving comparisons of one or more active treatments with each other and/or with placebo. *C. governance* framework through which NHS organizations are accountable for continuous improvement of service quality and care standards by creating environment that excellence flourishes. *Double-blind c. trial* comparison of different treatments (active and placebo) in which neither participants nor observers know who is receiving treatment until after study is completed in an attempt to remove bias. *C. Negligence Scheme for Trusts* organization handling all clinical negligence claims against member trusts; all NHS trusts in England belong to scheme.

**clinical risk index for babies** professional scoring tool to assess initial neonatal risks and compare performance of one neonatal intensive care unit with another.

**clinical risk management** systematic review of adverse events, usually related to delivery of patient care, in order to prevent further incidents.

**clitoridectomy** excision of clitoris. *See* FEMALE GENITAL MUTILATION.

**clitoris** small sensitive erectile organ at anterior junction of labia minora; homologue of penis.

**clomiphene citrate (Clomid)** GONADO-TROPHIC drug used to stimulate ovulation in anovulatory women undergoing infertility treatment.

**clonazepam** anti-epileptic drug, only used in pregnancy if benefits outweigh risks; baby born to mother taking it may suffer withdrawal.

**clone** cells descended by asexual reproduction from parent cell, genetically identical to each other and to parent cell.

**clonic** convulsive stage of a fit.

***Clostridium welchii*** anaerobic, gram-positive, spore-bearing bacillus, e.g. tetanus or gas gangrene.

**clotrimazole (Canesten)** antifungal agent administered vaginally as pessary or cream to treat vaginal 'thrush'.

**clotting** formation of jelly-like substance from blood shed at site of injury to blood vessel. Occasionally clots form in blood vessels, causing arteriosclerosis, thrombosis, varicose veins. *See also* COAGULATION. *C. factors* several factors in blood plasma involved in clotting process.

**cloxacillin** semi-synthetic penicillin used to treat staphylococcal infections caused by penicillinase-producing organisms.

**clozapine** sedative drug used in schizophrenia.

**clubfoot** *See* TALIPES.

**coagulase** substance produced by certain strains of staphylococci; causes clotting in plasma; coagulase-positive staphylococci, e.g. *Staphylococcus aureus*, more dangerous to neonates, than coagulase negative, e.g. *S. albus.*

**coagulation** clot formation. *C. disorder* condition occurring in severe placental abruption, intrauterine death, endotoxic shock, amniotic fluid embolism; signified by reduced clotting factors, low fibrinogen, THROMBO-CYTOPENIA; profuse bleeding occurs, blood fails to clot, fibrinogen is redirected, leading to DISSEMINATED INTRAVASCULAR COAGULATION. Investigations: cross-matching, full blood count, prothrombin time, clotting time, platelet counts, fibrinogen, fibrinogen degradation products; treatment dependent on results.

**coagulopathy** impaired blood clotting, causes prolonged or excessive bleeding.

**coarctation of aorta** stricture of aorta at, or just below, ductus arteriosus; often diagnosed by absence of femoral pulses.

**cobalamin** vitamin $B_{12}$.

**cocaine hydrochloride** topical anaesthetic applied to mucous membranes; common recreational drug, leads to psychological dependence in long-term users; absorbed through mucosal surfaces or smoked, e.g. highly addictive 'crack'. In pregnancy causes miscarriage, maternal hypertension, arterial thrombosis, placental abruption, stillbirth, small for gestational age babies. Maternal death results from cardiac arrhythmias, coronary ischaemia, intracranial aneurysm, cerebral haemorrhage, hypertensive convulsions; fetal malformations include intestinal atresia, limb defects, genitourinary disorders, neurological problems.

**coccus** spherical micro-organism. *See* BACTERIA.

**coccydynia** persistent pain in COCCYX.

**coccygeus, ischiococcygeus** two muscles arising from ischial spines, inserted into lateral borders of sacrum and COCCYX; form part of PELVIC FLOOR.

**coccyx** terminal bone of spinal column, fusion of four rudimentary vertebrae.

**Cochrane database** international multidisciplinary collaboration, database of systematic reviews of published clinical research, notably randomized controlled clinical trials.

**co-codamol** oral analgesic, paracetamol and codeine, avoid in pregnancy.

**Code: Standards of Professional Conduct, Performance and Ethics** Nursing and Midwifery Council document informs registrants, public and employers of standards required in professional practice.

**codeine** phosphate oral analgesic, probably safe in pregnancy although may depress neonatal respiration and cause withdrawal effects.

**coeliac plexus** network of sympathetic nerve ganglia in abdomen; nerve supply to abdominal organs below diaphragm.

**cohort** group of people possessing common characteristics, used in research to make generalizations derived from quantitative data. *C. study* observational research study following progress of cohort of patients with same condition to measure outcomes and make comparisons according to treatments or interventions given; may be prospective or retrospective.

**coitus** sexual intercourse, copulation. *C. interruptus* contraceptive method; penis is withdrawn from vagina before semen ejaculation.

**colic** severe spasmodic abdominal pain, common in infants; baby pulls up legs, cries loudly, becomes red faced, expels flatus or burps. *Biliary c. spasm* from passage of gallstone through bile ducts. *Renal c. spasm* from passage of stone along ureter.

**coliform** resembling *Escherichia coli*. *See* BACTERIA.

**collapse** prostration due to circulatory failure. *See also* SHOCK.

**colloidal solution** suspension in water, other fluid, of molecules that do not readily pass through cell membranes, e.g. blood, plasma, plasma substitutes; retained in circulation so used to treat shock.

**coloboma** absence or defect of tissue in eye, causing pupil to appear keyhole shaped; associated with CHARGE SYNDROME.

**colon** section of large intestine from caecum to rectum.

**colostrum** thin, yellow, milky fluid secreted from breasts from 16 weeks' gestation and for 3–4 days after birth until lactation initiated; high protein, initially low lactose content, with fat content equivalent to breast milk; important source of passive antibodies.

**colour index** measure of proportion of haemoglobin in erythrocytes; normally 1; iron deficiency anaemia $<1$, megaloblastic anaemia $>1$.

**colpo-** pertaining to vagina.

**colpocele** herniation of bladder or rectum into vagina.

**colpohysterectomy** removal of uterus via vagina.

**colpoperineorrhaphy** repair of pelvic floor, vagina and perineal body; usually undertaken for PROLAPSE.

**colporrhaphy** repair of vagina.

**colposcope** device for examining vagina and cervix by means of magnifying lens; used for early detection of malignant changes.

**colposcopy** examination of vaginal and cervical tissue with colposcope;

usually performed after abnormal cervical smear result to detect abnormal epithelium or benign tumours.

**colpotomy** vaginal wall incision. *Posterior c.* incision through posterior vaginal fornix to pouch of Douglas to drain pelvic abscess.

**columnar epithelium** type of epithelium containing cylindrical cells.

**coma** deep unconsciousness due to cerebrovascular accident, diabetes mellitus, alcoholism, eclampsia. *Adj* comatose.

**combined test** first-trimester Down syndrome screening test; NUCHAL TRANSLUCENCY (NT) ultrasound scan; blood test for PREGNANCY-ASSOCIATED PLASMA PROTEIN-A; results combined with maternal age-related Down syndrome risk for overall result.

**combined oral contraceptive pill** contraceptive method; oestrogen (oestrodiol) and progestogen (progestin) prevents ovulation; suppresses follicle-stimulating hormone, luteinizing hormone. Given orally, via skin patch or slow-release injectable.

**commensal** organism that lives on another without harming it.

**commissure** connection. *Posterior c.* fold of skin connecting labia minora posteriorly.

**Common Assessment Framework** interagency assessment; basis for identifying early children's additional needs; information shared between organizations aids coordination of service provision.

**Community Health Council** organization representing consumers' interests at district level of NHS.

**compaction** 1. in breech vaginal birth, fetal descent occurs with increasing compaction due to increased limb flexion. 2. pre-embryonic zygote divides to become morula by 8 days after fertilization, with the cells becoming tightly bound together.

**compatibility** mixing together of two substances without chemical change or loss of power.

**compensation** in heart disease, ability of weakened heart to function adequately.

**complement** 1. factor that adds to something or makes up deficiency. 2. thermo-labile group of proteins in normal blood serum and plasma that, in combination with antibodies, causes destruction of particular antigens (bacteria, foreign blood corpuscles).

**complementary** making up deficiency, completing. *C. feed* artificial infant feed to make up deficient amount of breastfeed, not recommended for normal healthy babies. *C. medicine, therapies* therapeutic strategies used in conjunction with conventional care, e.g. acupuncture, herbal, homeopathic remedies, massage, aromatherapy, reflexology, hypnotherapy, shiatsu etc.

**complete breech presentation** breech presentation with flexion of fetal hips and knees, feet tucked beside buttocks. See BREECH.

**compound presentation** rare labour complication; more than one part of fetus presents, e.g. head and hand or foot; breech, hand, cord.

**compression** 1. pressing together. See BIMANUAL COMPRESSION of uterus. 2. in embryology, shortening or omission of certain developmental stages. *C. stockings* See THROMBOEMBOLITIC D STOCKINGS. *C. sutures* absorbable sutures inserted through thickness of both uterine walls to compress uterus in case of massive bleeding.

**computed (axial) tomography** radiological computerized examination of internal organs producing series of images in cross-section; can show different types of tissue in detail, e.g. lung, bone, soft tissue, blood vessels; assists with diagnosis of infectious diseases, musculoskeletal disorders, cancers; contrast dye may be injected into bloodstream to improve image quality.

**computerized records** health records held on computer systems, legally required to be secure and maintain confidentiality, usually achieved by limiting access. *See also* DATA PROTECTION ACT.

**conception** fusion of spermatozoon and ovum to form viable zygote, onset of pregnancy.

**conceptus** embryo in utero in early pregnancy.

**condom** sheath covering penis used in sexual intercourse for contraception and to prevent sexually acquired infections. *Female c.* sheath inserted into vagina.

**condyloma** wart-like growth near external genitalia or anus, occasionally syphilitic.

**cone biopsy** removal of cone-shaped section from cervix to confirm diagnosis if cervical smear indicates precancerous cells present.

**confidence interval** means of expressing certainty about findings from research study using statistical techniques.

**confidential enquiry** Centre for Maternal and Child Health Enquiries audit: case notes are scrutinized by relevant professionals to identify substandard care and make recommendations for future practice; includes enquiries into maternal deaths, stillbirths, deaths in infancy, perioperative deaths.

**confidentiality** ethical principle in which information about individuals is made available only to those who need it; midwives must maintain confidentiality about all mothers and babies in their care.

**confounding variable** a factor that influences a research study, possibly contributing to misleading findings.

**congenital** born with, describes malformations present at birth, infection acquired in utero. *C. Disabilities (Civil Liabilities) Act 1976* Act in England, Wales, Northern Ireland; entitles child to recover damages if proven that she or he suffered due to breach in duty of care, except where breach occurred before conception with knowledge of one or both parents. *C. hip dislocation* condition resulting from abnormal development of acetabulum, femoral head or surrounding tissues; more common if family history, in breech presentation and in girls. 1%–2% of neonates have dislocated or dislocatable hips, usually found on routine examination in first 24 hours of life, confirmed on ultrasound. Treatment aims to stabilize hip in abduction and flexion using PAVLIK HARNESS; many dislocatable hips resolve spontaneously, but some children need surgery. *C. infection* infection acquired in utero, e.g. rubella, cytomegalovirus, herpes simplex, HUMAN IMMUNODEFICIENCY VIRUS, toxoplasmosis. *C. heart disease* pre-existing heart disease: atrial-septal defect, patent ductus arteriosus, pulmonary or aortic stenosis, Fallot's tetralogy; if uncorrected in childhood, pregnancy at high risk of pulmonary hypertension, left ventricular failure, fetal complications or loss, preterm birth. Affects 1% of babies, usually asymptomatic in neonatal period; baby may be breathless, cyanotic, but with no rib recession or grunting; cardiac failure may occur rapidly, sometimes resembling septicaemia, pneumonia or meningitis.

**congestive heart disease** condition in which heart's pumping capability is impaired.

**conjoined twins** Siamese twins; rare congenital abnormality; MONOZYGOTIC (identical) twins are fused together; due to incomplete embryonic cell mass division, or embryos become joined again after they have split. *See also* TWINS.

**conjugate** 1. to join together, e.g. in liver, bilirubin is combined with albumin by activity of GLUCURONYL TRANSFERASE to render it water soluble to be excreted via gut. *See also* ICTERUS *and* JAUNDICE. 2. conjugate diameter of pelvis. *See* PELVIS.

**conjunctiva** mucous membrane lining inner surface of eyelids, covering anterior aspect of eye.

**conjunctivitis** conjunctival inflammation. *See* OPHTHALMIA NEONATORUM.

**connective tissue** tissue that binds together or supports body structures, e.g. adipose, fibrous, areolar tissue, bone, cartilage, fat, blood.

**consanguinity** blood relationship; close relatives, e.g. first cousins have greater risk of chromosomal abnormalities in baby.

**consent** in law, voluntary agreement of action proposed by another; person giving consent must be of sufficient mental capacity, in possession of all essential information to give informed consent. Written consent generally required before invasive clinical procedures; midwives must record when verbal consent is given. Failure to gain consent may constitute assault.

**constipation** decreased frequency of defaecation, difficulty in defaecating, change in bowel habits from norm; common in pregnancy due to smooth muscle relaxation by progesterone. Exacerbated by poor fluid intake, low-fibre diet, iron supplementation.

**constriction ring** localized spasm of uterine muscle, often near junction of upper and lower segments. In first- and second-stage labour may form round fetal neck; in third stage forms HOURGLASS CONSTRICTION of uterus, causing retained placenta; may result from oxytocic drug use in uterus with uncoordinated function following early membrane rupture, especially if intrauterine manipulation performed.

**consultant** professional who gives advice to others. *C. midwife* senior midwife, responsible for improving midwifery care, through research, audit, education, professional development of staff; spends 50% of time in direct clinical contact; usually has remit to enhance overall care of women, e.g. facilitating normal birth, dealing with public health issues.

**contagion** communication of disease from one person to another by direct contact. *Adj* contagious.

**contingency screening** antenatal Down syndrome screening method: first-trimester BIOCHEMICAL SCREENING (hCG, PAPP-A); may be combined with NUCHAL TRANSLUCENCY scan. High-risk women offered more precise diagnostic investigations; those at low risk exit screening programme; those with mid-range risks proceed to second-trimester biochemical screening to obtain results combining first- and second-trimester values, improving DETECTION RATE and reducing FALSE-POSITIVE RATE.

**continuing professional development** further study after achieving basic qualifications; all midwives must undergo periodic updating to ensure contemporary, research-based practice.

**continuity of care** care of woman from booking to transfer to health visitor: communication from one appointment to next and between all professionals prevents omissions or duplications in care; verbal and written communication between professionals to avoid errors. See CASELOAD MIDWIFERY, TEAM MIDWIFERY.

**continuous nasal end expiratory pressure** neonatal ventilation method using principles similar to mechanics of iron lung; may require transfer of baby to specialist unit; unsuitable for newly birthed preterm babies, as tight fixation of tubing around neck increases risk of INTRAVENTRICULAR HAEMORRHAGE.

**continuous positive airway pressure** technique to prevent total alveolar collapse on expiration in baby with RESPIRATORY DISTRESS SYNDROME who is able to breathe spontaneously. Positive pressure of 2–5 cm $H_2O$ is applied to respiratory tract by nasal or endotracheal route or face mask.

**contraception** prevention of conception. *Barrier c.* include occlusive diaphragm, vault cap, vimule; usually combined with spermicidal cream, foam or jelly for extra protection. Men use CONDOM. *Chemical c.* oestrogen and/or progesterone; administered orally, by injection or as intrauterine device. *'Natural' c.* includes rhythm method ('safe period'), temperature method, Billings method, coitus interruptus or withdrawal. Most reliable method: sterilization, of woman by laparoscopy or laparotomy, of male by vasectomy. *Adj* contraceptive.

**contracted pelvis** pelvis in which any diameter of brim, cavity or outlet is reduced to extent that it interferes with labour progress.

**contraction** temporary shortening of muscle fibre, which returns to its original length during relaxation. During labour contractions are accompanied by RETRACTION. *Braxton Hicks c.* painless uterine contractions during pregnancy, improve placental blood flow.

**control group** group of patients recruited to research study who receive no treatment in order to provide a comparison for a group receiving experimental treatment.

**Control of Substances Hazardous to Health Regulations** states requirements for employers to protect employees and others from hazards of substances used at work, with risk assessments, control of exposure, health surveillance, incident planning.

**controlled clinical trial (CCT)** research method with two or more groups of patients with same condition; experimental group receives treatment being investigated, control group receives different or no treatment or placebo, to decrease risk of error, increase possibility that results accurately reflect reality. *Randomized CCT* research study with participants randomly allocated to receive experimental, alternative or placebo treatment.

**controlled cord traction** method of delivering placenta and membranes. When placenta separates, midwife places ulnar border of left hand in suprapubic region, pushes contracted uterus upwards (guarding); with right hand gains firm hold on cord, exerts gentle traction, following curve of Carus. Membranes eased out slowly to avoid tearing, retained products. If oxytocic given to facilitate separation, it is not necessary to await signs of separation and descent before attempting controlled cord traction; if physiological separation is encouraged, it is imperative to await signs to avoid risks of haemorrhage or uterine inversion.

**controlled drugs** preparations subject to Misuse of Drugs Act, regulating prescription and dispensing of narcotics, hallucinogens, depressants, stimulants. Midwives must follow locally agreed procedures and policies for administration in hospital. In community, Midwives Exemptions apply; midwife remains responsible for drugs; if not required, midwife must return drugs to pharmacy. Destruction must be in presence of accountable officer. For home birth, pethidine is individually prescribed; mother collects it, legally owns it; midwives cannot collect on mothers' behalf.

**conventional mechanical ventilation** standard positive pressure ventilation for preterm and ill neonates, using techniques which mimic individual's natural breathing rate and pressure to minimize associated lung trauma, although during critical phase of illness, preset rates and pressures are used.

**convulsions** violent involuntary contractions of voluntary muscle, e.g. in mother, due to eclampsia, epilepsy or hysteria, e.g. in neonate, due to HYPOXIA, cerebral birth injury, HYPOGLYCAEMIA.

**Cooley's anaemia** rare fatal form of THALASSAEMIA inherited from both parents; characterized by no haemoglobin; skeletal deformities; heart, spleen, liver enlargement.

**Coombs' test** blood test to determine presence of red cell antibodies, enables detection of HAEMOLYTIC DISEASE OF NEWBORN; if mother rhesus negative, cord blood is taken at birth to check ABO and rhesus typing. *Direct C. t.* direct antiglobulin test detects maternal antiglobulin antibodies coating baby's red cells; if positive, haemolytic disease may develop; baby's serum bilirubin levels should be checked. *Indirect C. t.* indirect antiglobulin test used to match blood products before transfusion.

**copper** cuprum, element; trace amounts essential to health. Symbol Cu.

**copulation** sexual intercourse, coitus.

**cord** *See also* UMBILICAL CORD. *C. blood sampling* blood sample taken from cord at delivery; if mother's blood rhesus negative or rhesus factor unknown, when atypical antibodies detected on routine antenatal screening, or if haemoglobinopathy suspected. *C. presentation* umbilical cord lies in front of presenting part, membranes intact. *Occult c. presentation* cord lies alongside but not in front of presenting part, membranes have ruptured. *C. prolapse* umbilical cord lies in front of presenting part, membranes have ruptured. Predisposing factors: high parity, preterm labour, high or ill-fitting presenting part, multiparity, malpresentation, POLYHYDRAMNIOS. Perform examination per vaginam immediately; membranes rupture if risk factors present. Diagnosis: cord felt below or beside presenting part, in vagina or cervical os; cord loop may be visible externally. Compression of cord may cause fetal bradycardia or prolonged fetal heart decelerations. *See* APPENDIX 5.

**cordocentesis** blood sampling from umbilical cord or intrahepatic vein under ultrasound after 18 weeks' gestation to check fetal blood indices or perform in utero blood transfusion for haemolytic disease. Risks: miscarriage, fetal haemorrhage, infection.

**cornea** transparent anterior part of eyeball in front of lens, covered by conjunctiva. *See also* OPHTHALMIA NEONATORUM.

**cornu** junction of uterus and fallopian tube. *Pl* cornua.

**corona radiata** follicular cell layer attached to outer protective layer of oocyte (zona pellucida) as it passes through ruptured follicular wall on its way to fallopian tube infundibulum. For fertilization to occur, sperm must break through layer by secreting hyaluronidase.

**coronal suture** skull suture between two frontal and two parietal bones. *See* FETAL SKULL.

**coronary** encircling. *C. arteries* those that supply heart. *C. thrombosis see* THROMBOSIS.

**corpus** body. *C. albicans* white scar left on ovarian surface after retrogression of corpus luteum. *C. luteum* literally, yellow body; structure, first greyish, later yellow, developing from Graafian follicle after ovulation, lasts 12 days before degenerating; if conception occurs, lasts 14–16 weeks until placenta fully functioning. *C. uteri* body of uterus.

**corpuscle** small body or cell, e.g. blood cell.

**cortex** outer layers of organ, e.g. cortex of cerebral hemispheres, kidney, suprarenal gland or ovary.

**cortical necrosis of kidneys** irreparable renal cortex damage due to severe arterial vasospasm after severe shock.

**corticoids** group of hormones secreted by adrenal cortex.

**corticosteroids** adrenocortical steroid hormones produced by adrenal cortex and synthetic equivalents; divided into glucocorticoids (cortisol, hydrocortisone, cortisone, corticosterone), mineralocorticoids (aldosterone, corticosterone), androgens. Prednisolone may be given antenatally for pre-existing asthma, rheumatoid arthritis, other inflammatory diseases. Risk of maternal adrenal suppression, failure of normal endogenous corticosteroid increase in labour; requires intravenous hydrocortisone. Betamethasone, dexamethasone may be used to aid fetal lung maturation in preterm labour, reducing respiratory distress syndrome, intraventricular haemorrhage, perinatal mortality.

**corticotrophin-releasing hormone**  peptide hormone and neurotransmitter involved in stress response.

**cortisol**  steroid hormone produced by adrenal gland in response to stress, low blood glucocorticoids; increases blood sugar through gluconeogenesis; suppresses immune system; aids fat, protein, carbohydrate metabolism; decreases bone formation. In pregnancy, increased production at 30–32 weeks' gestation initiates fetal lung surfactant production to promote lung maturation. Synthetic cortisol used to treat various diseases.

**cortisone**  STEROID hormone produced by adrenal cortex; anti-allergic, anti-inflammatory used in allergic states, e.g. asthma, rheumatoid arthritis, severe skin conditions, ulcerative colitis. Hydrocortisone is similar; prednisone and prednisolone are synthetic forms of cortisone and hydrocortisone, respectively.

**costal**  pertaining to ribs.

**cost–benefit analysis**  economic evaluation of costs and benefits of healthcare treatment measure; where benefits exceed costs, the evaluation would recommend providing treatment.

**cot death**  *See* SUDDEN INFANT DEATH SYNDROME.

**cotyledon**  placental division or lobe.

**Council for Healthcare Regulatory Excellence**  UK statutory overarching body; promotes best practice and regulatory consistency in all healthcare professions, i.e. doctors, dentists, nurses, midwives, health visitors, opticians, osteopaths, pharmacists and other professions supplementary to medicine.

**counselling**  consultation and discussion process in which counsellor listens and facilitates client to solve problems, constructively, ma decisions so that be approached more and more constructively.

**couvade**  psychosomatic pregn symptoms experienced by the fathe

**Couvelaire uterus**  uterine apoplexy. Deep purplish-blue bruised uterine appearance in severe concealed placental abruption due to high uterine tension forcing blood between myometrial fibres.

**coxa**  hip joint. *C. valga* hip deformity with increased angle between neck and shaft of femur. *C. vara* deformity with decreased angle between neck and shaft of femur.

**cracked nipple**  nipple damage occurring during breastfeeding, usually due to incorrect fixing of baby on breast; causes soreness and bleeding; prevented by teaching mother how to position baby at breast correctly. If nipple too sore to continue feeding, mechanical milk expression maintains lactation. Creams or application of colostrum may ease discomfort and aid healing.

**cramp**  painful spasmodic muscular contraction, usually in calf; may be associated with vitamin B, calcium or salt deficiency; relieved by eating appropriate foods; ischaemia of leg muscles may cause night cramps, eased by elevating foot of bed.

**cranial**  relating to cranium. *C. nerves* 12 pairs of nerves arising directly from brain.

**craniosacral therapy**  very gentle manipulation of cranium to release tensions within skull, successfully used to treat fractious babies after difficult forceps delivery, colic, hyperactivity in older infants.

**stenosis** premature closure of anial suture lines, requiring surgery o relieve raised intracranial pressure.

**anium** skull.

**cravings in pregnancy** unusual or excessive desire, commonly for food, often due to nutritional deficiency. *See also* PICA.

**C-reactive protein** plasma protein produced by liver in response to inflammation; serum marker for inflammation; can give indication of underlying disease or effectiveness of treatment.

**creatine** non-protein substance synthesized from amino acids (arginine, glycine, methionine); readily combines with phosphate, stored as high-energy phosphate, needed for muscle contraction.

**creatinine** nitrogenous compound end product of creatine metabolism, formed in muscle, passed into blood and excreted in urine. Raised serum creatinine levels indicate impaired kidney function or abnormal muscle wasting. 24-hour urine collection and venous blood sampling to determine creatinine clearance allows rate of creatinine excretion per minute to be calculated; may be undertaken in pregnant women with severe hypertension.

**cretinism** severely stunted physical and mental growth due to untreated congenital thyroid hormone deficiency (congenital hypothyroidism), usually due to maternal hypothyroidism.

**cri du chat syndrome** hereditary congenital syndrome: wide-set eyes, microcephaly, severe learning disability, plaintive cat-like cry; results from deletion of part of short arm of chromosome 5.

**cricoid** ring shaped. *C. cartilage* ring-like cartilage forming lower and back of larynx. *C. pressure* manual pressure applied to cricoid cartilage during general anaesthesia induction to occlude oesophagus, preventing acid reflux from stomach and pulmonary aspiration (MENDELSON SYNDROME). Pressure applied to whole ring of tracheal cricoid cartilage, maintained by assistant until endotracheal tube is in position and anaesthetist has checked that seal provided by cuff is effective.

**Crigler-Najjar syndrome** rare, autosomal-recessive inherited disorder affecting bilirubin metabolism; jaundice at birth or in infancy leads to KERNICTERUS, encephalopathy.

**critical incident** incidents occurring in course of midwife's work, usually related to clinical practice, requiring intervention to resolve and sufficiently serious to raise concerns about actions required in future similar circumstances. Midwives involved in critical incidents must write a report and engage in debriefing and formulation of action plan, e.g. remedial work.

**critique** objective, critical assessment and evaluation, often used in academic research to determine extent to which research methodology is valid.

**cross-infection** *See* INFECTION.

**cross-matching** vital procedure to ensure compatibility between donor and recipient blood in transfusion and organ transplantation; donor's erythrocytes or leucocytes are placed in recipient's serum and vice versa; absence of agglutination, haemolysis and cytotoxicity indicates that donor and recipient are compatible.

**Cricoid pressure, showing oesophageal occlusion by pressure applied to cricoid cartilage**

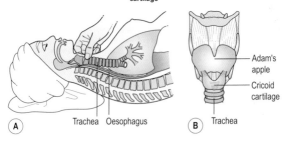

A  Trachea  Oesophagus

B  Adam's apple — Cricoid cartilage — Trachea

**crossover study** research study comparing two or more interventions; on completion of the course of one treatment, participants are switched to receive the other treatment.

**cross-sectional study** observation of defined set of people at a single point in time or time period—a snapshot. *See also* LONGITUDINAL STUDY.

**crown–heel length** distance from crown of head to heel in embryo, fetus, baby, equivalent to standing height.

**crowning** fetal movement during birth; suboccipitobregmatic and biparietal diameters of head distend vulva, head no longer recedes between contractions.

**crown–rump length** distance from crown of head to breech in embryo, fetus, baby, equivalent to sitting height; measured by ultrasound in first 14 weeks of pregnancy to assess fetal maturity.

**cryoprecipitate** extract rich in blood-clotting factor residue obtained from frozen blood plasma.

**cryosurgery** operation using refrigerated probe to remove abnormal tissue, e.g. cervical erosion.

**cryptomenorrhoea** subjective menstruation symptoms without blood flow.

**culture** 1. propagation of micro-organisms or cells in culture medium to obtain sufficient sample for analysis; increased availability of molecular techniques, e.g. POLYMERASE CHAIN REACTION reduces need to culture cells. 2. learned set of values, beliefs, attitudes common to group of individuals; may relate to society, organization or profession.

**curettage** operation using curette commonly performed to remove uterine endometrium in cases of incomplete MISCARRIAGE.

**curette** blunt or sharp metal loop used to remove unhealthy tissues by scraping or to obtain biopsy material.

**curve of Carus** arc corresponding to pelvic axis, route taken by fetus on passage through birth canal.

**Cushing syndrome** adrenal cortex overactivity causes excess glucocorticoids governing carbohydrate metabolism; leads to obesity, especially face and trunk, amenorrhoea, hirsutism, weakness.

**customized fetal growth chart** individually adjusted standard for fundal height, estimated fetal weight and birthweight taking into consideration maternal characteristics, e.g. height, country of family origin, smoking, presence of diabetes, etc. *See also* GROW CHART.

**cutaneous** concerning skin.

**cyanocobalamin** vitamin $B_{12}$, found in liver, eggs and fish, essential for formation of erythrocytes and prevention of anaemia; administered intramuscularly for pernicious anaemia.

**cyanosis** blueness of skin and mucous membranes due to oxygen deficiency.

**cyclizine** antihistamine drug to treat nausea, vomiting, dizziness, motion sickness; useful for gestational and post-operative sickness.

**cyesis** pregnancy. *Pseudocyesis* false pregnancy.

**cyst** fluid-filled tumour with membranous capsule. *Chocolate c.* ovarian cyst associated with endometriosis. *Corpus luteum or luteal c.* cyst developing from corpus luteum in hydatidiform mole. *Dermoid c.* cyst containing skin, hair, teeth, etc., caused by abnormal development of embryonic tissue. *Multilocular c.* ovarian cyst divided into compartments. *Papilliferous c.* ovarian cyst lined with papillae growing through cyst wall into peritoneal cavity, causes ascites. *Pseudomucinous c.* ovarian cyst containing mucin-like fluid.

In pregnancy, early diagnosis essential; cysts may be removed to avoid labour complications and risk of malignancy.

**cystic** pertaining to cysts. *C. fibrosis* fibrocystic, autosomal-recessive, inherited pancreatic disease; body's mucus-secreting glands secrete thick tenacious mucus, causing neonatal pancreatic fibrosis, MECONIUM ileus, repeated chest infections. Diagnosis is by serum immune-reactive trypsin test; sweat test shows raised sodium chloride; raised albumin may be detected in meconium.

**cystic hygroma** multilocated cystic collection of lymphatic fluid, commonly at back of neck, resulting from abnormal lymphatic development. Fetal cystic hygromas seen on ultrasound from 10–11 weeks' gestation, differentiated from enlarged NUCHAL TRANSLUCENCY as septated; associated with chromosomal abnormalities, e.g. TURNER SYNDROME, EDWARD SYNDROME; CHORIONIC VILLUS SAMPLING or AMNIOCENTESIS offered if seen on ultrasound. Fetal prognosis usually poor, although cystic hygromas occasionally disappear when KARYOTYPE is normal.

**cystitis** inflammation of bladder.

**cysto-** prefix relating to bladder.

**cystocele** herniation of bladder into vagina due to pelvic floor damage during childbirth. See COLPORRHAPHY.

**cystoscope** instrument for inspecting interior of bladder.

**cystoscopy** inspection of interior of bladder with cystoscope.

**cystotomy** incision of bladder, e.g. for removal of calculi.

**cyto-** pertaining to cells.

**cytogenetics** branch of genetics involving study of CHROMOSOMES.

**cytokines** small proteins released by cells; have specific effects on cell behaviour and communication between cells; includes interleukins, lymphokines, cell signal molecules and interferons, which trigger inflammation and respond to infections.

**cytology** science of structure and functions of cells to detect abnormalities. *Cervical c.* test to detect very early genital tract malignancy; routine in antenatal, postnatal and family planning clinics and for women over 35. *Vaginal c.* antenatal examination of desquamated cells from vaginal wall for hormone changes suggesting placental insufficiency and fetal risk.

**cytomegalic inclusion disease** infection caused by cytomegalovirus, marked by nuclear inclusion bodies in large infected cells; may be congenital, with HEPATOSPLENOMEGALY, cirrhosis, microcephaly; acquired infection presents similarly to infectious mononucleosis.

**cytomegalovirus** common infection, may cause severe fetal anomaly through damage to fetal cells, resulting in loss of function; incidence in primary infection approximately 7%; adverse effects more severe with first-trimester infection; may be indicated by early-onset INTRAUTERINE GROWTH RESTRICTION, bright (echogenic) bowel or cerebral ventriculomegaly. Up to 60% of women in developed countries immune due to previous asymptomatic infection or mild infection presenting as general malaise, fever and lymphadenopathy.

**cytoplasm** protoplasm of cell, excluding nucleus.

**cytotrophoblast** cellular layer of trophoblast; Langhans cell layer, less obvious after 19–20 weeks' gestation. *See also* CHORIONIC VILLI.

**dactyl** finger or toe.

**danazol** anterior pituitary suppressant drug.

**Data Protection Act 1998** Act defining UK law on data processing, giving people control over use of information about themselves. Organizations holding personal data, e.g. patient records, legally obliged to maintain privacy, not disclose information without consent, facilitate access of individuals to own records.

**database** information collected, stored, reviewed, updated; used for evaluation and audit or as research resource.

**D-dimer test** blood test to detect cross-linked fibrin degradation fragment, D-dimer, indicator of coagulopathy.

**deafness** complete or partial loss of hearing. *Congenital d.* deafness present at birth, often due to antenatal infection e.g. rubella.

**death** cessation of all physical and chemical processes in all organs or cellular components. *Cot d.* sudden infant death syndrome. *D. certificate* statement issued by Registrar for Deaths on receipt of preliminary signed certificate from attending doctor, indicating date and probable cause of death; burial/cremation cannot take place until this is issued. *D. rate* number of deaths per stated number of persons (100, 10,000 or 100,000) in certain region in certain time period.

**deceleration** decreased speed; in obstetrics, refers to fetal heart rate.

*Early d.* begins at, or after, contraction onset, returns to baseline rate by end of contraction; normally no fetal difficulty. *Late d.* transitory heart rate decrease due to compromised fetal blood flow, insufficient oxygen to withstand labour stress. *Prolonged d.* fetal heart decrease of $\geq 15$ beats per minute measured from most recent baseline rate; lasts 2–10 minutes. *Variable d.* abrupt FHR decrease of $\geq 15$ beats per minute measured from most recent baseline rate; lasts 15 seconds–2 minutes.

**decidua** pregnant endometrium in which fertilized ovum embeds; thicker, more vascular than non-pregnant endometrium. *D. basalis* part on which ovum rests, covering maternal placental surface. *D. capsularis* part covering ovum as it projects into uterine cavity. *D. vera* true uterine lining, not in contact with ovum for first trimester.

**decidual cast** expulsion of decidua intact, in shape of uterine cavity, following death of ovum in ECTOPIC PREGNANCY.

**decompensation** inability of heart to maintain adequate circulation, marked by dyspnoea, venous engorgement, cyanosis, oedema.

**deep transverse arrest** fetal head obstruction during second-stage labour due to occipitoposterior position; fetus attempts to turn anteriorly (long rotation), head becomes caught between ischial spines of pelvic outlet,

http://dx.doi.org/10.1016/B978-0-7020-6906-2.00004-8

especially if prominent. FORCEPS delivery is required to release obstructed head. Baby may have excessive moulding, leading to possible intracranial damage.

**deep vein thrombosis** blood clot in vessel, may be life threatening if completely occluding vessel, e.g. coronary arteries causing heart attack. Thrombosis may migrate, causing problems elsewhere, e.g. pulmonary embolism. Newly birthed mothers are at risk of deep vein thrombosis due to clotting factor changes occurring at term. Signs: red, tender, hot area on calf.

**defaecation** evacuation of bowels.

**defibrillation** electrical termination of atrial or ventricular fibrillation.

**deficiency** lack of. *D. disease* condition caused by dietary or metabolic deficiency.

**deflexion** fetal attitude; head is not flexed, or only partially flexed, e.g. occipitoposterior position.

**degeneration** structural change, lowering vitality of tissue in which it takes place. *Red d. See* NECROBIOSIS.

**dehiscence** bursting open or rupture, e.g. abdominal wound rupture after surgery, e.g. of Caesarean section scar; rupture of Graafian follicle at ovulation.

**dehydration** excessive body fluid loss, or inadequate fluid intake, often with ketoacidosis; occurs in severe vomiting, prolonged labour, excessive haemorrhage. Signs: dry, inelastic skin; dry tongue; sunken eyes; ketotic breath odour; oliguria; ketonuria; electrolyte imbalance; abnormal blood reactions. Maternal dehydration with ketoacidosis can be life threatening to fetus; intravenous dextrose is administered, with saline if urinary chlorides are severely diminished. *D. fever* neonatal condition due to insufficient fluid intake; severe dehydration from diarrhoea, depressed fontanelle, poor skin turgor, weight loss; corrected orally if mild or intravenously if severe.

**delay in labour** unusually prolonged labour; most common in first stage—cervical dilatation is slower than expected; delay over 2 hours may require AUGMENTATION OF LABOUR. Second-stage delay—technically, more than 2 hours in nullipara and 1 hour in multipara, but if fetomaternal condition remains satisfactory and gradual progressive descent of presenting part is made, no action is taken. Third stage: physiologically managed over 2 hours; actively managed over 30 minutes; delay in placental separation and/or expulsion may require manual removal of placenta.

**delayed cord clamping** clamping and cutting of umbilical cord delayed until cord stops pulsating or expelled; provides baby with 30% more feto-placental blood volume than with early clamping, with full complement of red blood cells, stem cells and immune cells.

**deletion** in genetics, loss of genetic material from chromosome.

**delivery** birth, expulsion or extraction of baby, placenta and membranes. *Abdominal d.* CAESAREAN SECTION. *Instrumental d.* facilitated by use of forceps or vacuum cup. *Spontaneous d.* birth occurring without mechanical aid. *Vaginal d.* complete birth via birth canal, cephalic or breech presentation.

**Delphi technique** method to facilitate agreement on an issue; participants do not meet or interact directly, but are sent questionnaires to record their views, repeated in light of initial group feedback.

**demand feeding** feeding when baby appears hungry, not according to fixed timetable; 'on demand' feeding, baby-led feeding.

**demography** statistical science dealing with populations, including health, disease, births and mortality.

**denaturation test** Singer's test; blood test to distinguish fetal from maternal blood.

**denidation** degeneration and expulsion of uterine lining during menstruation.

**Denis Browne splint** special boot designed to correct TALIPES.

**denominator** point on presenting part of fetus used to indicate its position in relation to particular part of mother's pelvis, e.g. occiput in vertex presentation, sacrum in BREECH presentation, mentum (chin) in face presentation.

**dental** pertaining to teeth. *D. care* dental care is free during pregnancy and up to 1 year after delivery. *D. caries* tooth decay.

**dentition** teething. *Primary d.* eruption of temporary (milk) teeth, from 6 or 7 months of age until end of second year; eight incisors, four canines, four premolars, four molars. *Secondary d.* appearance of 32 permanent teeth (8 incisors, 4 canines, 8 premolars, 12 molars), between 6–7 years and 12–15 years; posterior molars may not appear until early adulthood.

**deoxygenated** deprived of oxygen. *D. blood* blood that has lost oxygen in tissues, returning to lungs for fresh supply.

**deoxyribonucleic acid** nucleic acid of complex molecular structure occurring in cell nuclei as basic structure of GENES; present in all living cells.

**Department of Health** government body responsible for policy and administration of National Health Service.

**Department for Work and Pensions** largest UK government body, deals with incapacity benefit, income support, bereavement benefits, maternity allowance, jobseeker's allowance, industrial injury benefits, social fund, pension, disability, carer service.

**Depo-Provera** *See* MEDROXYPROGESTERONE ACETATE.

**depression** 1. lowering of spirits; mood change, sadness; may occur postnatally, within 2 weeks of birth, develops gradually. Treatment: support, psychotherapy and/or antidepressants in mild cases; hospital admission, antidepressants, electroconvulsive therapy if severe. *Endogenous d.* occurs in bipolar disorder; slowing of thoughts and action, guilt feelings. *Reactive d.* in response to event. 2. dip, felt on palpation.

**dermatocranium** roof of skull covering brain and eyes.

**dermoid cyst** tumour with fibrous wall lined with stratified epithelium, contains pulpy material with epithelial elements, e.g. hair.

**descent** downward movement, e.g. of fetus in labour, through pelvic brim, cavity, outlet; assessed by abdominal examination, may be measured in fifths. *See* diagram.

**desquamation** shedding of superficial epithelial cells from body.

**detection rate** sensitivity of screening test's performance; proportion of people found to be positive (or high risk).

**Descent of fetal head estimated in fifths palpable above brim**

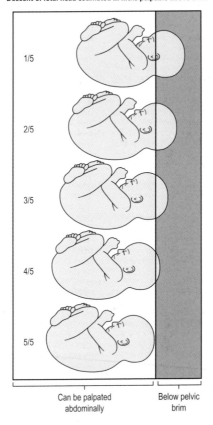

1/5

2/5

3/5

4/5

5/5

Can be palpated
abdominally

Below pelvic
brim

**detoxication** neutralization of toxic substances, a function of liver.

**detrusor** body part that pushes downwards, e.g. *d. muscle.*

**developmental** pertaining to development. *D. anomaly* absence, deformity or excess of body parts due to faulty embryological development. *D. milestones* significant behaviour, marking child development process, e.g. sitting, walking, talking, etc.

**dexamethasone** synthetic glucocorticoid, anti-inflammatory agent used for diseases, allergic states and in screening test to diagnose CUSHING SYNDROME. If preterm birth imminent, may accelerate fetal lung maturity.

**dextran** polysaccharide preparation, plasma substitute to treat shock; restores circulatory volume; does not leak out of blood vessels, unlike physiological saline; can be used when blood grouping not possible; carries no risk of viral infections, unlike plasma.

**dextrose** glucose, monosaccharide, simplest carbohydrate.

**diabetes insipidus** rare disease, deficiency of antidiuretic hormone secretion from posterior pituitary gland, characterized by polyuria, thirst, dehydration; treated with vasopressin.

**diabetes mellitus** familial deficiency of insulin secretion from pancreatic islet cells, or increased resistance to action of insulin; symptoms: polyuria, weight loss, thirst, lassitude, hyperglycaemia, ketosis, possibly coma. Abnormal glucose tolerance test with signs and symptoms usually insulin dependent; abnormal results without signs and symptoms: non-insulin-dependent. *Gestational d. m.* temporary diabetic state due to increased metabolic workload and pregnancy insulin resistance. Predisposing factors: previous baby over 4.5 kg, unexplained stillbirth, neonatal death. Complications: infection, hypertension, polyhydramnios, ketoacidosis, fetal abnormality, death, hypoxia, cephalopelvic disproportion, birth trauma, neonatal hypoglycaemia, respiratory distress; clinical diabetes in later life. Care shared between obstetrician and physician; blood sugar assessments required in labour and postnatally when insulin requirements fall sharply; extra carbohydrate needed if breastfeeding. *Type 1 d. m.* due to autoimmune destruction of beta cells in pancreas; insulin-dependent. *Type 2 d. m.* long-term metabolic disorder; high blood sugar, insulin resistance, lack of insulin.

**diabetic** pertaining to diabetes. *D. coma* loss of consciousness occurring due to severe diabetic ketosis.

**diabetogenic** inducing diabetes. In pregnancy, susceptible women may become temporarily diabetic; condition may recur in subsequent pregnancies and later life.

**diacetic acid** acetoacetic acid, colourless compound present in minute quantities in normal urine and in abnormal amounts in urine of diabetic women and those with hyperemesis.

**diagnosis** determination of nature of disease. *Clinical d.* diagnosis made by studying actual signs and symptoms. *Differential d.* symptoms compared and contrasted with those of other diseases.

**diagnostic study** research study to assess effectiveness of a test or measurement in terms of accuracy in detecting or excluding a specific condition.

**diagonal conjugate** internal pelvic measurement between sacral promontory and lower border of symphysis pubis, usually 12.5 cm in normal pelvis; true conjugate estimated as 1.3 cm less than this. In vaginal examination, examining finger cannot normally reach sacral promontory, unless pelvis is unusually small, so true conjugate is inferred as average.

**dialysis** passage of salts, water and metabolites through semipermeable membrane. Renal d. use of artificial kidney; patient's blood is separated from dialyzing fluid by membrane, retaining blood cells and plasma proteins and losing toxic substances normally excreted by kidneys.

**diameter** straight line passing through centre of circle or sphere. See FETAL SKULL, PELVIS.

**diamorphine hydrochloride** powerful analgesic sometimes used for pain relief in labour, effective for up to 4 hours, more rapidly eliminated from maternal and neonatal plasma than PETHIDINE. Less used in obstetrics than pethidine or MEPTAZINOL.

**diaphragm** 1. Muscular d. dome-shaped partition separating thorax from abdomen, muscle of respiration; convex when relaxed, flattens as contracts during inhalation, enlarging chest cavity, allowing lung expansion. 2. Contraceptive d. rubber or soft plastic device placed over uterine cervix to prevent entrance of spermatozoa.

**diaphragmatic hernia** protrusion of abdominal organ through diaphragm into thoracic cavity.

**diaphysis** shaft of long bone.

**diarrhoea** frequent passage of loose stools, usually due to infection; in neonate, leads to rapid dehydration and disturbed electrolyte balance. Baby isolated to avoid transmission to others.

**diastasis** separation, usually of muscle, e.g. abdominal diastasis recti, or cartilage, e.g. symphysis pubis diastasis.

**diastole** cyclical relaxation of cardiac muscle after atrial and ventricular SYSTOLE.

**diastolic** pertaining to diastole. D. murmur abnormal sound produced during diastole occurs in valvular heart disease. D. blood pressure pressure of blood in arteries during resting stage of cardiac cycle. See BLOOD PRESSURE.

**diathermy** high-frequency electrical currents to cauterize blood vessels, preventing excessive bleeding, or to treat cervical erosions, neoplasms, warts. See also CRYOSURGERY.

**diazepam** oral, intramuscular or intravenous benzodiazepine tranquillizer, preoperative anti-anxiety agent, skeletal muscle relaxant, anticonvulsant, e.g. in eclampsia.

**dicephalus** fetus with two heads.

**dichorial, dichorionic** having two distinct chorions, dizygotic twins.

**didactylism** presence of only two digits on hand or foot.

**didelphia** double uterus.

**didymitis** inflammation of testicle; orchitis.

**didymus** 1. testis. 2. fetus with duplication of parts, or one consisting of conjoined symmetrical twins.

**diembryonic** production of two embryos from single egg.

**dietetics** branch of therapeutics concerned with diet for maintenance of health and dietary treatment of disease.

**differential** making a difference. *D. blood count* comparison of numbers of different white cells present in blood. *D. diagnosis. See* DIAGNOSIS.

**diffusion** passage of substances in solution into area of weaker concentration through semipermeable membrane, e.g. OXYGEN, CARBON DIOXIDE; minerals, urea across placental CHORIONIC VILLI.

**DiGeorge syndrome** congenital deletion of part of chromosome 22, incidence 1:4000. Features: heart, palate, kidney, neuromuscular defects, learning disability, feeding problems, facial disfigurement, recurrent infections: immune system impairment from absent or hypoplastic thymus. Early signs: heart defects, convulsions from hypocalcaemia; later, autoimmune disorders may develop.

**digestion** process by which ingested food is changed and rendered suitable for absorption into blood.

**digit** finger or toe.

**digital** pertaining to finger (or toe). *D. examination* examination carried out with one or more fingers.

**digoxin** drug obtained from leaves of *Digitalis lanata*; used in treatment of congestive heart failure; used in pregnancy only when benefits outweigh risks.

**dilatation** stretching of orifice or hollow organ, e.g. cervix during labour. *D. and curettage* gynaecological operation; cervical os surgically dilated to allow scraping and evacuation of uterine lining or contents, e.g. after spontaneous miscarriage.

**dilator** instrument used to effect dilatation, e.g. HEGAR DILATORS.

**dimenhydrinate** over-the-counter anti-histaminic anti-emetic used in HYPEREMESIS GRAVIDARUM; used in pregnancy, breastfeeding only when benefits outweigh risks.

**dimetria** double uterus.

**dimorphism** existing in two distinct forms. *Sexual d.* 1. physical or behavioural differences associated with sex. 2. having some properties of both sexes, e.g. early embryo, some hermaphrodites.

**dinoprostone** prostaglandin E2; slow-release drug for induction of labour, termination of pregnancy, usually administered as pessary.

**diphtheria** acute, contagious upper respiratory tract infection caused by *Corynebacterium diphtheriae* (Klebs–Löffler bacillus largely eradicated). *See* IMMUNIZATION.

**diphtheroids** non-pathogenic corynebacteria resembling diphtheria bacilli; COMMENSALS of throat, nose, ear, conjunctiva, skin.

**diplococci** cocci in pairs; may be encapsulated, e.g. pneumococci, or intracellular, e.g. gonococci. *See* GONOCOCCUS.

**diploid** having two sets of chromosomes within cells; in humans diploid number is 46, i.e. 23 pairs.

**diplosomatia** condition in which complete twins are joined at some of their body parts.

**direct antiglobulin test** test used to detect HAEMOLYTIC DISEASE OF NEWBORN. *See* COOMBS' TEST.

**direct latex agglutination tests** laboratory pregnancy diagnostic tests.

**disability** restriction or lack of ability to perform activity in manner or within range considered normal for humans. *Developmental d.* substantial disability of indefinite duration; onset before age 18 years, attributable to learning disability, autism, cerebral palsy, epilepsy or other neuropathy.

**disaccharide** carbohydrate; two simple sugar units, e.g. lactose in milk, sucrose; readily broken down into MONOSACCHARIDES.

**disc** circular or rounded flat plate. *Embryonic d.* flattish area in cleaved ovum in which first traces of embryo are seen. *Intervertebral d.* layer of fibrocartilage between bodies of adjoining vertebrae. *Prolapsed intervertebral d.* rupture of intervertebral disc, commonly in lower back or neck.

**discharge** flow of substances from body. *Vaginal d. in pregnancy* hormonal changes increase discharge, normally white, mucoid, non-irritating; if profuse, offensive, irritating, requires investigation.

**Disclosure and Barring Service** government department; helps employers recruit safely, prevents appointment of people unsuitable to work with vulnerable members of society, including children.

**discus proligerus** compact mass of follicular cells surrounding ovum before expulsion from Graafian follicle.

**disease** abnormal condition causing local or general disturbance in body structure or function.

**disinfect** destruction of microorganisms so not harmful to health.

**dislocation** displacement of bone from natural position; may be congenital, resulting from faulty construction of joint, e.g. hip.

**displacement** movement to unusual position, e.g. retroversion or PROLAPSE of non-gravid uterus.

**disproportion** lack of harmonious relationship between two objects.

*Cephalopelvic d.* disparity between fetal head and maternal pelvis; head may be too large or abnormally positioned, or pelvis too small or abnormally shaped; suspected if fetal head fails to engage towards term. If severe, Caesarean section is needed; in mild disproportion labour contractions help mould fetal head through pelvis, often with increased flexion. See TRIAL LABOUR.

**disseminated intravascular coagulation** widespread thromboses in circulation, mainly capillaries; complication of placental abruption, retained dead fetus, amniotic fluid embolism, infections, due to introduction of coagulation-promoting factors into circulation. Intravascular clotting ultimately triggers haemorrhage due to rapid consumption of fibrinogen, platelets, prothrombin, clotting factors V, VIII and X. Treatment: replacement of relevant blood products. If primary condition cannot be treated, intravenous heparin may inhibit clotting process and raise level of depleted clotting factors.

**distal** sited away from centre of body or point of origin. *cf.* proximal.

**diuresis** increased urinary secretion.

**diuretic** drug that increases excretion of urine, e.g. furosemide.

**diurnal** pertaining to or occurring during daytime or period of light.

**dizygotic** pertaining to or derived from two separate zygotes. *D. twins* binovular twins from two ova and two spermatozoa; separate placentae, chorions and amnions, of same or different sexes, more common than MONOZYGOTIC twins. See MULTIPLE PREGNANCY.

**docosahexanoic acid** long-chain polyunsaturated fatty acid in breast milk; may affect retina and visual cortex development in newborn.

**docusate sodium** stool softener, increases amount of water absorbed by stool in gut, making it easier to pass; used to avoid straining at stool.

**Döderlein bacillus** non-pathogenic lactobacillus occurring normally in vaginal secretions; metabolism of glycogen within vaginal squamous epithelium lining produces lactic acid and pH of 4.5, which counteracts alkalinity of cervical mucus and is hostile to pathogenic organisms.

**Doering rule** first fertile day of female menstrual cycle, determined by calculation based on earliest previous temperature shift; enables determination of onset of fertile phase to facilitate conception/contraception.

**dolichocephalic** long head; increased anteroposterior diameter.

**domiciliary** within or at home.

**DOMINO scheme** antenatal/postnatal care provided by community midwife; birth in hospital, with community midwife in attendance.

**dopamine** intermediate noradrenaline synthesis product; central nervous system neurotransmitter. Synthetic intravenous drug to correct haemodynamic imbalance in shock syndrome.

**Doppler ultrasound** procedure using series of pulses to detect blood flow, e.g. in fetal umbilical artery (to assess placental function), middle cerebral artery (to assess placental failure and fetal anaemia), ductus venosus (to detect hypoxia).

**dorsal** concerning the back. *D. position* mother lies on back with head and shoulders slightly elevated.

**double-blind trial** test for real effect of new drug or treatment in clinical practice; neither patients receiving nor staff administering treatment know which of two apparently identical treatments is being tested.

**double uterus** abnormal uterine development due to failed fusion of Müllerian ducts; produces two uterine bodies with or without duplication of cervix and vagina; may cause repeated miscarriages; very occasionally, two independent conceptions occur and implant into two sections of uterus; preterm labour common.

**douche** 1. stream or jet of fluid applied to body. *Vaginal d.* procedure in which warm saline is used to produce hydrostatic pressure to distend vagina, causing INVERSION OF UTERUS to revert to its normal position. 2. apparatus used for douching.

**doula** lay person providing emotional and practical support, during pregnancy, labour and postnatally.

**Down syndrome** chromosome 21 abnormality; commonly due to extra chromosome (*trisomy 21*), associated with older mothers. Also caused by TRANSLOCATION between chromosomes 14 and 21; 10% chance of subsequent pregnancy being affected. Baby has obliquely slanting, wide-set eyes; broad, flat nose; thick, rough tongue; brachycephaly; small head with flat occiput; short neck with loose skin; HYPOTONIA; single palmar crease; third fontanelle; BRUSHFIELD SPOTS in iris. Risk of learning disability, cardiac anomalies, cataracts, hearing loss, leukaemia, hypothyroidism.

**doxepin** tricyclic antidepressant.

**doxycycline hyclate** broad-spectrum antibiotic in tetracycline group; avoid in pregnancy.

**drepanocyte** sickle cell.

**drepanocytosis** occurrence of drepanocytes (sickle cells) in blood.

**dressing** covering applied to wound surface.

**droplet infection** passage of pathogenic bacteria in minute droplets from respiratory tract during talking, coughing, sneezing, etc.

**drospirenone** progestin steroid used in contraceptive pills and hormone replacement therapy for menopausal symptoms.

**drug** medicinal substance. *D. abuse* drug used for recreational purposes. *D. addiction* periodic or chronic intoxication from repeated drug use; psychological and physical dependence, leads to addiction, often in increasing doses. *D. interaction* modification of potency of one drug by others taken concurrently or sequentially, producing either harmful or therapeutic effects.

**Dubowitz score** method to assess gestational age in low-birthweight baby.

**Duchenne muscular dystrophy** hereditary X-linked muscular dystrophy, usually in boys.

**Ducrey's bacillus** organism causing soft chancre (*Haemophilus ducreyi*).

**duct (ductus)** tube or channel for conveying secretions of glands.

**ductus arteriosus** fetal blood vessel bypassing pulmonary circulation by connecting pulmonary artery and descending aorta, normally closes at birth.

**Duffy blood group** type of red blood cell containing rare antigen.

**duodenum** first part of small intestine, from pylorus to jejunum. *Duodenal atresia* incomplete canalization of duodenum; causes projectile vomiting with bile when baby starts feeding.

**duplication** in genetics, repetition of part of chromosome.

**dura mater** tough, fibrous membrane lining skull; outermost covering of brain and spinal cord. Double fold of inner dura mater, falx cerebri, dips between cerebral hemispheres; horizontal fold, tentorium cerebelli, separates cerebellum from cerebral hemispheres above; both membranes carry large venous sinuses draining blood from skull; may be stretched and torn during delivery, causing intracranial haemorrhage.

**dural tap** occurs occasionally during siting of epidural anaesthesia; needle being introduced between vertebrae progresses beyond epidural space, puncturing dura mater, causing cerebrospinal fluid to leak from around brain and spine. Severe POST-DURAL HEADACHE develops due to reduced cerebrospinal pressure.

**duration of pregnancy** pregnancy averages 266 days from conception to birth, 280 days (40 weeks) from first day of last menstrual period to labour onset. Estimated due date can be calculated by adding 9 months and 7 days for average 28-day menstrual cycle to first day of last normal menstrual period, adjusted accordingly for long or short cycle. Normal labour commences any time after 37 weeks' gestation; pre-term labour occurs before 37 weeks; induction of labour may be advised if pregnancy persists beyond 42 weeks.

**duty of care** legal term denoting responsibility to patient/client of skilled professional midwife, nurse or doctor, irrespective of contractual agreement existing between parties; based on rules regarding expected care standards determining whether the professional has neglected her/his duty of care, based on standards prevailing at time of legal case.

**dydrogesterone** orally effective, synthetic progestin for diagnosis and treatment of primary amenorrhoea; may be used for infertility and spontaneous miscarriage.

**dys-** prefix: 'difficult', 'disordered' or 'painful'.

**dysentery** notifiable intestinal infection; severe diarrhoea with blood, mucus, pus; usually caused by *Shigella* species or *Entamoeba histolytica*.

**dyslexia** impairment of ability to comprehend written language due to central lesion. *Adj* dyslexic.

**dysmature** small for gestational age baby.

**dysmenorrhoea** difficult, painful menstruation.

**dyspareunia** difficult or painful coitus.

**dyspepsia** indigestion.

**dyspnoea** difficult or laboured breathing.

**dyspraxia** impaired movement due to immaturity in brain's processing of information, associated with problems of perception, language and thought; more common in males; may be familial.

**dystocia** difficult or abnormal labour.

**dystrophia** difficult or abnormal growth. *Dystocia d. syndrome* rare obstetric sequence to which some short, heavily built, subfertile, hirsute women with android pelves may be prone; pre-eclampsia and occipitoposterior fetal position may occur.

**dysuria** difficult or painful micturition.

**Ebstein anomaly** congenital heart defect; opening of tricuspid valve displaced towards apex of right ventricle; often associated with other abnormalities. Enlarged aorta increases risk of abnormality in infant if taken by mother during first trimester.

**ecbolic** oxytocic, i.e. causes uterine muscles to contract.

**ecchymosis** skin discoloration from bleeding beneath skin; bruising.

**echogenic bowel** on ultrasound scan, bright bowel appearance; associated with intra-amniotic bleeding, fetus swallowing blood-stained amniotic fluid.

**echovirus** group of viruses (enteroviruses) causing aseptic meningitis, diarrhoea, respiratory diseases, etc.

**eclampsia** rare, serious, sometimes fatal complication of PRE-ECLAMPSIA; peripartum epileptiform fits can cause maternal cerebral haemorrhage, pulmonary oedema, renal or hepatic failure, inhalation pneumonia, fetal hypoxia and death. Midwife should summon medical aid, position mother on left side and prevent her from harming self; insert airway; administer oxygen; check reflexes regularly; monitor fetal condition. Intravenous magnesium sulphate may control fits. Labour may start spontaneously; distress from contraction pain may mask additional fits. *Adj* eclamptic.

**'ecstasy'** methylenedioxymethamphetamine, 'E'; illicit synthetic hallucinogenic amphetamine; may contain other substances, e.g. caffeine, paracetamol, ketamine. Inhibits serotonin reabsorption, reduces brain reserves, affects mood, initially boundless energy; prolonged use leads to appetite loss, sweats, palpitations, insomnia, jaw stiffness, teeth grinding, micturition frequency, cardiac arrhythmia, hepatotoxicity, neurological, psychiatric damage. Hyperthermia can be lethal, often with disseminated intravascular coagulation, metabolic acidosis, hyperkalaemia, renal failure.

**ecto-** prefix meaning 'outside'.

**ectoblast** *See* ECTODERM.

**ectocervix** part of cervix protruding into vagina.

**ectoderm** outer germinal layer of developing embryo from which skin, external sense organs, mucous membrane of mouth, anus and nervous system are derived.

**-ectomy** suffix: 'cutting out', e.g. appendicectomy, hysterectomy.

**ectopia** abnormal position of any structure. *E. vesicae* uncommon congenital abdominal wall defect, interior of bladder is exposed.

**ectopic pregnancy** embedding of fertilized ovum, usually in fallopian tube, occasionally in ovary, abdominal cavity or uterine cornu (interstitial or angular pregnancy). Separation of gestational sac from fallopian tube lining causes pregnancy loss; peristaltic

http://dx.doi.org/10.1016/B978-0-7020-6906-2.00005-X

action of tube moves fertilized ovum into peritoneal cavity; slight vaginal bleeding occurs as decidua shed. Alternatively, tubal rupture occurs when trophoblast has penetrated fallopian tube more deeply, causes severe pain, intraperitoneal or intraligamentary haemorrhage, profound shock; requires immediate blood transfusion and laparotomy. Very occasionally, abdominal pregnancy progresses almost to term with live baby being born by laparotomy; placenta, usually adherent to major abdominal organ such as liver, is left *in situ* to reabsorb slowly over period of months.

**ectro-** prefix meaning 'miscarriage', 'congenital absence'.

**ectrodactyly** congenital absence of all or part of digit.

**ectromelia** gross long bone hypoplasia or aplasia (limbs).

**ectrosyndactyly** condition in which some digits are absent; remaining ones are webbed.

**eczema** allergic skin condition, often hereditary; in infancy, may be precipitated by cows' milk. If family history of eczema, hay fever, asthma, mother should be encouraged to breastfeed exclusively.

**Edinburgh Postnatal Depression Scale** 10-item questionnaire to identify women with postnatal depression.

**Edward syndrome (trisomy 18)** congenital additional chromosome 18; second most common TRISOMY after DOWN SYNDROME (trisomy 21), occurs in 1:3000 conceptions, risk increases with maternal age. Baby has small head, low-set ears, small jaw and mouth, clenched fist with overlapping fingers, 'rocker bottom' feet, cardiovascular and gastrointestinal defects, significant developmental delay. 50% die *in utero*; of those born alive, 50% die within 1 week, 90% within 5 months. Occasionally, less severe mosaic trisomy 18 occurs (see MOSAICISM); not all cells have extra chromosome.

**effacement** 'taking up' of cervix; internal os dilates, opening out cervical canal, leaving circular external os; occurs in first-stage labour, before cervical dilatation in primigravidae but simultaneously in multiparous women.

**efferent** carrying outward, i.e. from centre to periphery. *E. nerves* motor nerves that obey impulses from nerve centres of brain.

**effleurage** light, circular, stroking massage; in labour reduces pain perception, as touch impulses reach brain before pain impulses.

**effusion** escape of blood or serum into surrounding tissues or cavities.

**egg** ovum, female gamete, oocyte. *E. donor* woman who gives eggs to infertile recipient; multiple ovulation is pharmacologically induced, ova removed by laparoscopy, fertilized *in vitro*, transferred to uterus of recipient.

**Eisenmenger syndrome** large ventricular septal defect, overriding of aorta, right ventricular hypertrophy, high maternal mortality.

**ejaculation** forcible, sudden expulsion, especially of semen from male urethra, reflex action occurring from sexual stimulation.

**elective** planned. *E. Caesarean section* operative delivery planned when considered safest for maternal or fetal condition.

**electrocardiogram** tracing of heart action shown by electrical waves, used in diagnosis of heart disease.

**electrode** conductor through which electricity leaves its source to enter another medium. *Fetal scalp e.* applied to fetal scalp in labour to record electrocardiogram.

**electroencephalogram** tracing of electrical brain waves.

**electrolyte** substance dissociating into electrically charged particles in solution (ions), e.g. sodium bicarbonate, potassium chloride. *E. imbalance* disturbance of electrolyte levels, usually resulting from severe vomiting or renal failure; diagnosed by blood tests.

**electronic fetal heart monitoring** measurement of fetal heart with handheld Doppler device or CARDIOTOCOGRAPH. *See also* TELEMETRY, BASELINE, VARIABLE, DECELERATION, ACCELERATION.

**electrophoresis** technique involving electrically charged particles moving under influence of applied electrical field, enabling substances to be separated into constituent parts; used for serum protein analysis and to analyse neonatal haemoglobin for sickle cell disease and other haemoglobinopathies.

**elimination** expulsion of waste substances from body, e.g. urea from kidneys, food products from bowel, carbon dioxide from lungs.

**embolism** blocking of blood vessel by solid or foreign substance introduced into circulation; causes immediate death if large; smaller embolus causes collapse, chest pain, dyspnoea, cyanosis. *Air e.* air bubbles enter circulation, possibly during vaginal or intrauterine douching in pregnancy. *Amniotic fluid e.* amniotic fluid enters maternal circulation, via placental or uterine site, causing immediate collapse and rapidly progressive complications;

can be fatal. *Pulmonary e.* often consequence of pelvic or leg vein thrombosis, occasionally occurs after labour; part of clot detaches and travels in bloodstream until arrested in branch of pulmonary artery.

**embolus** foreign substance circulating in blood, e.g. detached thrombus, bacterial mass, air bubble, amniotic fluid. *Pl* emboli.

**embryo** developing baby, first 8 weeks after conception, thereafter termed fetus. *E. reduction* medical or surgical intervention to reduce number of viable fetuses/embryos if there are a high number of fertilized ova, usually from fertility treatment.

**embryology** science of embryo development.

**embryonic plate** part of inner cell mass of blastocyst from which embryo is formed.

**emergency** condition requiring immediate attention. *E. protection order* court order by which child can be arbitrarily removed from parents in interests of his or her safety. *E. contraception* hormonal treatment to prevent unwanted pregnancy, normally taken within 24 hours; 'morning after' pill.

**emetic** substance that induces vomiting.

**emmenagogue** substance that induces vaginal bleeding. *Adj* emmenagogic.

**empowerment** capacity to give power or authority; philosophy that women should be empowered to take control over own care and work in partnership with maternity care providers.

**emulsion** mixture of minute particles of fatty or oily substance suspended in fluid.

**encephalins, enkephalins** two naturally occurring pentapeptides isolated from brain, with potent opiate-like effects, neurotransmitters; ENDORPHINS.

**encephalitis** inflammation of brain caused by viral infections.

**encephalocele** hernia of brain through congenital or traumatic opening of skull.

**encephalopathy** diffuse disease or damage of brain. *Wernicke e.* inflammatory haemorrhagic encephalopathy due to thiamine deficiency; rare complication of HYPEREMESIS GRAVIDARUM.

**encopresis** faecal incontinence not due to organic defect or illness.

**endemic** pertaining to infectious disease always present in locality.

**endo-** prefix meaning 'inside' or 'within'.

**endocarditis** inflammation of endocardium lining heart.

**endocervicitis** inflammation of membrane lining uterine cervix; CERVICITIS.

**endocervix** mucous membrane lining cervical canal.

**endocrine** glands whose secretions (hormones) pass directly into bloodstream.

**endogenous** originating inside body.

**endometrioma** cyst formed when endometrial tissue grows in ovaries; may cause dysmenorrhoea.

**endometriosis** tissue resembling and functioning similarly to endometrium but outside uterus; dark "chocolate" cysts of ovary contain endometrial material.

**endometritis** inflammation of endometrium.

**endometrium** mucous membrane lining body of uterus.

**endorphins** opiate-like peptides produced naturally at neural synapses at various points in central nervous system pathway, where they modulate transmission of pain perceptions, producing sedation and euphoria; effects are blocked by naloxone, a narcotic antagonist.

**endoscope** instrument fitted with light to inspect hollow organs and structures, e.g. cystoscope, laparoscope.

**endotoxic shock** *See* BACTERAEMIC SHOCK.

**endotracheal** within trachea. *E. tube* catheter inserted into trachea during intubation for upper airway and removal of secretions. *E. intubation* resuscitative process, sometimes with cardiac massage; also performed during general anaesthesia.

**enema** injection of fluid into rectum.

**energy (calorie) requirement** body processes require energy from food; pregnant woman requires 2500 cal (625 kJ) per day. Excess is stored as fat, gives extra energy if diet inadequate.

**engagement** entry of presenting fetal part into true pelvis. In cephalic presentation head is engaged when BIPARIETAL DIAMETER passes plane of pelvic brim, about 36 weeks' gestation in primigravida but possibly at onset of labour in multipara.

**engorgement of breasts** painful accumulation of secretion in breasts, often with oedema, lymphatic and venous stasis at onset of lactation; can be avoided by early on-demand breastfeeding, baby correctly positioned. Firm supporting bra or breast binder may help; avoid pressure on oedematous tissue.

**ensiform cartilage** lowest part of sternum, xiphisternum, used as marker for antenatal abdominal examination to estimate gestation.

**enteritis** intestinal infection. *See* DYSENTERY.

**entoderm** cells in inner cell mass lining yolk sac; later developing into epithelium of fetal alimentary tract, trachea, bronchi, bladder, urethra.

**Entonox** gas, 50% NITROUS OXIDE, 50% OXYGEN, premixed in blue cylinder with white collar, administered via face mask or nasal catheter; approved by Nursing and Midwifery Council for use by midwives for labour pain relief.

**enuresis** involuntary micturition; bed wetting due to psychological, neurological or pathological causes.

**environmental health** concept that health of individuals can be affected by environment, e.g. pollution, housing. *E. h. practitioner* local authority employee responsible for improving and regulating environment, enforcing statutory regulations related to housing, food hygiene, refuse collection, infestation, air pollutants, noise, etc.

**enzyme** biological catalyst; substance present in small amounts producing chemical reaction, e.g. milk sugar (lactose) broken down by lactase enzyme in small intestine to form GLUCOSE and GALACTOSE.

**eosin** red stain used in identification of cells and bacteria.

**eosinophil** white blood cell; granules can be stained red with eosin.

**ephedrine** adrenergic alkaloid, bronchodilator, anti-allergen, central nervous system stimulant, pressor agent.

**epicanthic folds** vertical folds of skin either side of nose, sometimes covering inner canthus (junction of eyelids), prominent in certain races and Down syndrome babies.

**epidemic** situation when disease attacks large number of people at one time.

**epidemiology** study of distribution of factors determining health and disease in human populations for disease prevention and control.

**epidermis** non-vascular outer layer or cuticle of skin.

**epidermolysis bullosa** severe, usually fatal, autosomally RECESSIVE skin disorder characterized by profusion of fluid-filled blisters resembling PEMPHIGUS NEONATORUM.

**epididymis** elongated, cord-like structure along posterior border of testis; coiled duct allows storage, transport and maturation of spermatozoa.

**epidural analgesia** injection of local analgesic, e.g. BUPIVACAINE HYDROCHLORIDE, into epidural space to block spinal nerves. Injection may be caudal, through sacrococcygeal membrane covering sacral hiatus; or lumbar, through intervertebral space and ligamentum flavum. Used for pain relief in labour, instrumental delivery, Caesarean section. Risks: sudden hypotension and fetal hypoxia, instrumental delivery due to poor head flexion because of relaxed pelvic floor. Rare but serious complications: spinal or dural tap; toxic drug reactions; neurological sequelae from injury or haematoma; infection. Intravenous cannula is sited to allow immediate fluid supplementation in event of hypotension. Midwife monitors maternal blood pressure and fetal heart rate frequently, after first dose of bupivacaine, given by anaesthetist and after each 'top up', by appropriately trained midwives. *See also* MOBILE EPIDURAL, SPINAL ANAESTHESIA.

**epigastrium** upper, middle abdominal region within sternal angle. *Adj* epigastric. Epigastric pain in pre-eclamptic women may indicate ECLAMPSIA due to hepatic oedema and/or haemorrhage.

**Sagittal section of lumbar spine with Tuohy needle in position**

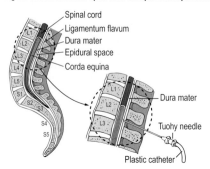

**epigenetics** study of changes in organisms caused by modification of gene expression rather than alteration of genetic code itself.

**epiglottis** cartilaginous structure overhanging entrance to larynx.

**epilepsy** paroxysmal transient nervous system disturbance due to abnormal brain electrical activity; anticonvulsive drugs prevent maternal seizures that can cause intrauterine hypoxia, but may have teratogenic effect, causing lip, palate, heart defects in fetus.

**epileptiform** resembling epileptic fit, as in eclampsia.

**epiphysis** end of long bone, shaft is separated by cartilage in children; ossification in fetus, seen on ultrasound, provides guide to fetal maturity. *Pl* epiphyses.

**episiorrhaphy** repair of EPISIOTOMY.

**episiotomy** mediolateral or midline incision in thinned-out perineal body to enlarge vaginal orifice during birth, under local anaesthetic; expedites birth if fetal distress; performed before forceps or ventouse delivery; reduces intracranial damage risk in preterm or breech birth; midwives permitted to infiltrate perineum, perform episiotomy, repair perineal trauma.

**Episiotomy**

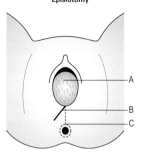

**A,** fetal head; **B,** mediolateral incision; **C,** midline incision.

**epispadias** abnormal urethral opening on dorsal surface of penis.

**epistaxis** nose bleed.

**epithelial tissue** *See* EPITHELIUM.

**epithelium** layer of cells covering all outer surfaces and lining all inner surfaces, including cavities, glands and vessels.

**epsilon-aminocaproic acid** antifibrinolytic drug, prevents breakdown of FIBRIN by plasmin, used in severe placental abruption.

**Epstein pearls** small, whitish-yellow epithelial spots forming on gums and roof of mouth in neonate.

**Equality Act 2010** consolidation of several UK parliamentary anti-discrimination acts, including Equal Pay Act 1970, Sex Discrimination Act 1975, Race Relations Act 1976, Disability Discrimination Act 1995 and directives protecting employment discrimination on grounds of religion or belief, sexual orientation and age.

**equinovarus** congenital foot deformity; combined talipes equinus and talipes varus; child walks on toes and outer side of soles.

**Erb's paralysis, palsy** upper arm muscle paralysis due to brachial nerve plexus injury as nerves leave spinal cord in cervical region; arm hangs medially rotated with elbow extended, wrist and fingers flexed; due to traction on fetal neck, e.g. in breech birth or in SHOULDER PRESENTATION.

**erectile** having power to become erect. *E. tissue* vascular tissue that becomes congested and swollen under stimulus, causing erection of part, e.g. female nipple, male penis.

**ergometrine** active alkaloid principle of ergot; constricts smooth muscle, used to prevent or control postpartum haemorrhage, often used in conjunction with oxytocin (Syntometrine).

Administered intravenously, acts within 45 seconds; intramuscularly within 7 minutes; produces sustained uterine contraction of 2–3 hours. Side effects: nausea, vomiting, hypertension. Contraindicated in pre-eclampsia. Oral ergometrine is used to treat secondary postpartum haemorrhage due to retained products of conception.

**ergonomics** scientific study of humans in relation to their work and effective use of human energy.

**ergot** drug obtained from fungus grown on rye; causes strong sustained contraction of smooth muscle, especially uterus.

**erosion of cervix during pregnancy** reddened columnar epithelium near external cervical os due to hormonal changes, causing softening and increased HYGROSCOPIC qualities of collagen connective tissue; usually resolves spontaneously after delivery.

**erythema** skin redness.

**erythroblast** immature, nucleated red blood cell.

**erythroblastosis fetalis** haemolytic disease of newborn, with ERYTHROBLASTS in neonatal circulation.

**erythrocyte** red blood cell; contains haemoglobin, carries oxygen. *E. sedimentation rate* speed at which red blood cells settle at bottom of tube of blood, normally below 10 mm per hour, increased in pregnancy and infection, average 78 mm per hour.

**erythromycin** antibiotic similar to penicillin.

**erythropoiesis** formation of red blood cells.

*Escherichia coli* gram-negative bacillus normally in intestines; may cause urinary tract infection, epidemic diarrhoeal diseases, especially in babies, endotoxic shock if enters circulation.

**essential hypertension** persistently high blood pressure; unknown cause, often hereditary; diagnosed if first-trimester blood pressure above 140/90 mm Hg; may worsen, remain static or improve. Dangers: pre-eclampsia, ECLAMPSIA, placental abruption, subarachnoid haemorrhage, cardiac or renal failure, placental insufficiency, small-for-gestational-age baby, stillbirth.

**essential oils** concentrated plant oils used in aromatherapy; chemicals can be harnessed for therapeutic purposes, but may also cause side effects and complications; many oils contraindicated in pregnancy, labour, breastfeeding. Midwives must be appropriately trained to use AROMATHERAPY oils in their practice.

**estimated date of delivery, estimated due date** approximate date around which labour can be expected; calculated by adding 9 months and 7 days to date of first day of the last normal menstrual period, adjusted according to length of menstrual cycle.

**estradiol** See OESTRADIOL.

**estriol** See OESTRIOL.

**estrogen** See OESTROGEN.

**estrone** See OESTRONE.

**ethambutol** tuberculostatic agent.

**ethics** rules or principles governing correct conduct, personal and social values.

**ethinyloestradiol** See OESTRADIOL. Contraceptive pills containing oestrogen and progesterone; commenced 3–4 weeks postpartum, contraindicated during breastfeeding.

**ethmoid bone** square bone at root of nose, part of cranium; has many perforations through which olfactory nerves pass to nose.

**ethnic, ethnicity** pertaining to a social group sharing cultural bonds or physical (racial) characteristics. *E. minority* social group of people sharing cultural or racial factors but who constitute a minority within the wider culture or society.

**ethnography** study of culture of a single race; data are collected through observation, usually whilst living with group being studied.

**ethyl chloride** local anaesthetic applied topically to intact skin.

**etiology** See AETIOLOGY.

**eu-** word prefix meaning normal, good, pleasant.

**eugenics** study of measures taken to improve future generations.

**eutocia** normal labour or birth.

**evacuation** emptying. *E. of retained products of conception* surgical emptying of uterus, removing blood clots and placental tissue to prevent or control postpartum haemorrhage.

**eversion** turning inside out; to turn outward.

**evidence-based practice** systematic appraisal of clinical situations; use of contemporary research findings as justification for clinical decision making.

**evolution** natural development; process of unfolding or opening out. *Spontaneous e.* rare spontaneous delivery of fetus in transverse lie; shoulder escapes first, then thorax, pelvis, limbs and finally head. *cf.* spontaneous EXPULSION.

**EVRA** combined hormonal contraceptive patch, suitable for women unable to tolerate oral medications, thus improving compliance.

**ex-** prefix meaning 'out of', 'outside', 'away from'.

**exacerbation** increase in severity of disease symptoms.

**examination under anaesthetic** procedure undertaken in theatre; woman with PLACENTA PRAEVIA is lightly anaesthetized, manual examination *per vaginam* is performed to determine whether vaginal birth possible; full preparations are made to proceed immediately to Caesarean section in the event of torrential haemorrhage or worsening of maternal or fetal condition.

**exchange transfusion** method of replacement transfusion in which blood sample is withdrawn from patient, replaced by same volume of donor blood; used in neonates to treat severe hyperbilirubinaemia and anaemia, usually resulting from rhesus incompatibility.

**exclusion criteria** in research, characteristics that exclude potential subjects from entering a study, e.g. age, presence of medical condition.

**excreta** waste matter excreted from body: faeces, urine, sweat, sputum, etc.

**excretion** expulsion or elimination of waste matter, e.g. via kidneys as urine, intestines as faeces, sweat glands as sweat.

**exfoliation** falling off in scales or layers. *Adj* exfoliative. *Lamellar e. of newborn* ichthyosis congenita, ichthyosis fetalis, lamellar ichthyosis; congenital hereditary disorder, baby is completely covered with parchment-like membrane, peels off within 24 hours; healing may occur or scales reform and process is repeated. In severe form, baby (harlequin fetus) is completely covered with thick, armour-like scales, usually stillborn or dies shortly after birth.

**exocoelomic cavity** yolk sac.

**exocrine** 1. secreting externally via duct. 2. denoting gland or its secretion.

**exogenous** of external origin.

**exomphalos** rare herniation via umbilicus of abdominal contents covered with peritoneum; in unanticipated cases, midwife should cover area with sterile non-adhesive dressing and cotton wool to avoid damage from infection and call doctor.

**exotoxin** potent toxin formed and excreted by bacterial cells into surrounding medium, most commonly due to *Clostridium*; diphtheria, botulism, tetanus are caused by bacterial toxins.

**experimental study** research study designed to test if a treatment or intervention has an effect on the course or outcome of a condition, where the conditions of testing are controlled by the researcher *See also* CONTROLLED CLINICAL TRIAL.

**expression** pressing out, e.g. mechanical or digital pressure on areola to compress lacteal sinuses to remove milk from breast.

**expulsion** forcible driving out, e.g. of fetus from uterus. *Spontaneous e.* manner in which very small macerated fetus can be forced through pelvis with shoulder presenting so that head and trunk are born together. *E. of placenta See* SCHULTZE EXPULSION *and* MATTHEWS DUNCAN EXPULSION.

**exsanguinate** to deprive of blood, as after severe haemorrhage.

**extension** drawing out, lengthening, opposite of flexion; e.g. in normal labour, occiput escapes under pubic arch, forced downwards by uterine contractions and forwards by pelvic floor muscles; head extends, pivoting under symphysis pubis.

**external genitalia** parts of reproductive system seen externally; vulva in women; penis and scrotum in men.

**external version** manoeuvre designed to convert breech presentation to cephalic or transverse/oblique lie to longitudinal lie. Complications: true cord knots, placental abruption, fetal distress.

**external os** opening from cervical canal into vagina.

**extra-** prefix meaning 'outside'.

**extracellular fluid** fluid outside cells.

**extracorporeal membrane oxygenation** neonatal ventilation method; oxygenation of blood supply outside body, similar to cardiac bypass support, allowing lungs to rest and recover; baby must be at least 34 weeks' gestation and weigh over 1.8 kg.

**extrauterine pregnancy** *See* ECTOPIC PREGNANCY.

**extravasation** discharge or leaking of fluid from its normal channel into surrounding tissue, e.g. escape of blood or lymph from vessel.

**extrinsic** of external origin. *E. factor* vitamin $B_{12}$, cyanocobalamin; haematopoietic vitamin that combines with intrinsic factor for absorption; needed for erythrocyte maturation.

**extubation** removal of tube used in intubation.

**exudation** outward flow of liquid or semi-liquid substance, e.g. sebum from sebaceous glands.

**face** 14 fused bones from mentum (chin) to supraorbital ridges.

**face presentation** cephalic presentation with fetal spine and head extended, face lowest in pelvis; incidence about 1:500–600 births; due to poor flexion in occipitoposterior position, biparietal diameter caught in sacrocotyloid diameter of pelvis extends head. Denominator: mentum; if mentoanterior birth, may be spontaneous but unlikely if mentoposterior unless chin rotates anteriorly; persistent, mentoposterior position causes obstructed labour; Caesarean section required. Baby's face bruised and oedematous at birth.

**Abdominal palpation of head in face presentation; position right mentoanterior**

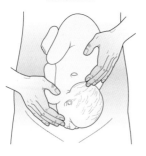

**face-to-pubes** persistent occipitoposterior position; attitude of head is military, neither flexed nor extended; sinciput, meeting pelvic floor first, rotates forwards, bringing occiput to hollow of sacrum; first- and second-stage delay is common. Maternal squatting may enlarge pelvic outlet to facilitate vaginal delivery; severe stretching and laceration of pelvic floor often occurs. Forceps delivery is sometimes necessary. See PERSISTENT OCCIPITOPOSTERIOR.

**Face to pubes delivery**

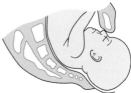

**facial** pertaining to face. *F. paralysis* paralysis of facial muscles, usually unilateral, due to seventh cranial (facial) nerve injury, sometimes after forceps delivery; usually resolves spontaneously within a few days.

**factor** agent or element contributing to production of particular result. *Anti-haemophilic f.* factor VIII, one of the CLOTTING factors. *Anti-haemorrhagic f.* vitamin K. *Coagulation f.* 12 or more factors essential for blood clotting; absence, deficiency or excess may lead to abnormal clotting.

http://dx.doi.org/10.1016/B978-0-7020-6906-2.00006-1

*Extrinsic f.* See EXTRINSIC. *Intrinsic f.* glycoprotein secreted by parietal cells of gastric glands, necessary for VITAMIN B$_{12}$ absorption; deficiency causes pernicious anaemia. *F. V Leiden mutation* inherited coagulation disorder; risk of thrombosis and stroke in presence of other factors, e.g. obesity, surgery; associated with poor placentation, fetal loss, pre-eclampsia; screened for during THROMBOPHILIA SCREEN. *Releasing f.* factor produced in one structure that triggers release of hormones from another structure. *Rhesus f.* See RHESUS FACTOR.

**faeces** food residue, other waste products excreted from bowels. *Adj* faecal.

**failure to progress** prolonged labour of more than 24 hours, inadequate contractions and cervical dilatation; may be identified from observations recorded on PARTOGRAM. Risk of obstructed labour and uterine rupture if not diagnosed and managed correctly.

**faint** temporary loss of consciousness due to generalized cerebral ischaemia; syncope.

**falciform** sickle-shaped.

**fallopian tubes** uterine tubes, oviducts; two narrow canals, each 10 cm long, leading from uterine cornua to ovaries.

**Fallot tetralogy** See TETRALOGY.

**false labour** painful uterine contractions simulating labour, without cervical dilatation or uterine FUNDAL DOMINANCE.

**false-negative rate** proportion of affected pregnancies that would not be identified as high risk; tests with low false-negative rate have low sensitivity.

**false pelvis** region between brim of true pelvis and iliac crests. See PELVIS.

**false-positive rate** measure of screening test's performance; proportion of people who have positive screening result but do not have condition.

**falx** sickle, or sickle-shaped structure.

**falx cerebri** sickle-shaped fold of dura mater separating two cerebral hemispheres of brain.

**familial** occurring in families, inherited conditions, e.g. haemophilia.

**family** group of people residing together, usually related by blood or marriage. *Extended f.* nuclear family and close relatives. *Nuclear f.* couple and their children by birth or adoption living together. *Single-parent f.* lone parent and offspring living as family unit. *F. planning* See CONTRACEPTION.

**fascia** sheet or band of fibrous connective tissue, arranged loosely around organs and blood vessels, or in dense strong sheets, often between muscles. *Pelvic f.* in pelvic cavity, with parietal layer lines walls, covers pelvic floor; visceral layer supports pelvic organs.

**fat** 1. adipose or fatty tissue. 2. neutral fat; triglyceride (or triacylglycerol), compound of fatty acids and glycerol.

**fat soluble** capable of being dissolved in fats, e.g. vitamins.

**fatty acids** long-chain lipid carboxylic acid molecules found in fats and oils, and in cell membranes as component of phospholipids and glycolipids.

**favism** acute haemolytic anaemia caused by ingestion of fava beans. See GLUCOSE-6-PHOSPHATE DEHYDROGENASE.

**febrile** feverish; pyrexial.

**fecundation** fertilization.

**fecundity** ability to produce offspring.

**feet to foot** supine position for sleeping baby, with feet at foot of cot; an attempt to prevent airway obstruction.

**female genital mutilation** circumcision; excision of labia majora and minora, clitoris, sometimes partial closure of introitus; prevalent in areas such as Sudan; illegal in UK. Complications: difficulty with micturition and intercourse. Excision and separation of tissues may be required in labour; Caesarean section may be necessary.

**feminization** 1. normal development of female sexual characteristics. 2. development of female sexual characteristics in male. *Testicular f.* individual is phenotypically female but lacks nuclear sex chromatin, genetically male (one X, one Y chromosome).

**femoral** pertaining to femur. *F. artery* principal artery in thigh, continuation of external iliac artery. *F. vein* main vein in thigh, continuation of popliteal vein, passing up leg through groin, continuing as external iliac vein.

**femur** thigh bone, from hip to knee, articulating with innominate bone at acetabulum.

**fenestrated** window-like opening e.g. blades of midwifery forceps. *F. placenta or placenta fenestrata* See PLACENTA.

**fentanyl** intravenous or intramuscular intra- and postoperative analgesic drug.

**Ferguson reflex** surge of oxytocin, resulting in increased uterine contractions, due to stimulation of cervix and upper part of vagina.

**ferment** to induce chemical changes as result of enzymes with specific actions.

**fern test** cytology to assess amount of oestrogen in cervical mucus; oestrogen in dried cervical mucus has fern-like appearance on low-power microscopy.

**ferritin** iron–apoferritin complex; one form in which iron is stored in body.

**ferrous** containing iron in its plus-two oxidation state. *F. fumarate* anhydrous salt, combination of ferrous iron and fumaric acid; used as haematinic. *F. gluconate* haematinic, less irritating to gastrointestinal tract than others, used when ferrous sulphate not tolerated. *F. sulphate* most widely used haematinic for iron-deficiency anaemia, less irritating than ferric salts, more effective.

**fertile** capable of producing offspring. *F. period* 5 days before and 3 days after ovulation when fertilization of ovum is possible; method of CONTRACEPTION.

**fertility** ability to produce young. See also SUBFERTILITY, INFERTILITY.

**fertilization** impregnation, conception; union of spermatozoon and ovum to create new human. *In vitro f.* artificial fertilization of ovum in laboratory conditions. *In vivo f.* artificial fertilization within reproductive tract.

**fetal** pertaining to fetus. *F. abnormality* See MALFORMATION. *F. alcohol syndrome* condition due to heavy maternal alcohol consumption; small-for-gestational-age baby with facial abnormalities and mental retardation. *F. blood sampling* See CORDOCENTESIS. *F. death* See INTRAUTERINE DEATH. *F. haemoglobin* has greater affinity and higher capacity for oxygen than adult haemoglobin; forms 85% of haemoglobin of full-term baby at birth. *F. heart sounds* fetal heart beat, auscultated and counted via abdominal wall, may be continuously recorded electronically. *F. maturity* assessment of developmental stage of fetus by ultrasound, including measurement of long bones of femurs and size of head.

**fetal distress** clinical manifestation of fetal hypoxia. Maternal causes: eclampsia or epilepsy; inadequate circulation, e.g. cardiac failure, severe anaemia, hypertension or hypotension; diabetes mellitus; infection. Uterine causes: hypertonicity, excessive retraction in obstructed labour; placental separation or insufficiency. Fetal causes: intracranial birth trauma; severe rhesus incompatibility with gross anaemia; congenital abnormality; intrauterine infections; multiple pregnancy; malpresentation, malposition; cord prolapse; true knots; cord traction. Diagnosis: abnormal fetal heart rate and regularity, meconium-stained amniotic fluid, excessive fetal movements; birth is expedited by instrumental or operative delivery. *See also* CARDIOTOCOGRAPH.

**fetal movement chart** mother subjectively records fetal movements over given period; usually used in conjunction with other fetal well-being tests; may wear fetal kick counter bracelet.

**fetal skull** fetal bony head structure; vault has two frontal bones divided by frontal suture, two parietal bones divided by sagittal suture, separated from frontal bones by coronal suture; one occipital bone separated from parietal bones by lambdoidal suture. Membranous junction of three or more sutures forms anterior

fontanelle (BREGMA) and posterior fontanelle (LAMBDA). Sutures and fontanelles felt on vaginal examination help to determine position of head in cephalic presentation. Base of skull has two temporal bones, one ethmoid bone, one sphenoid bone, part of occipital bone; contains foramen magnum through which spinal cord passes. Face is composed of 14 fused bones. In labour, diameters and circumferences of skull are assessed to estimate progress. Within skull are brain, intracranial membranes, FALX CEREBRI and TENTORIUM CEREBELLI, carrying venous sinuses by which blood is drained from head: SUPERIOR and INFERIOR LONGITUDINAL SINUSES, STRAIGHT SINUS, TRANSVERSE SINUS and GREAT VEIN OF GALEN. If MOULDING is excessive, membranes and sinuses may tear, causing intracranial haemorrhage.

**Vault of fetal skull**

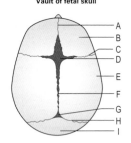

**A,** frontal suture; **B,** frontal bone; **C,** coronal suture; **D,** anterior: fontanelle or bregma; **E,** parietal bone; **F,** sagittal suture; **G,** posterior: fontanelle or lambda; **H,** lambdoid suture; **I,** occipital bone.

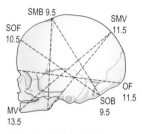

**Longitudinal diameters (in centimetres)**

SMB 9.5
SMV 11.5
SOF 10.5
OF 11.5
SOB 9.5
MV 13.5

**SOF,** suboccipitofrontal; **SMB,** submen-tobregm; **MV,** mentovertical; **SOB,** suboccipitobregmatic; **OF,** occipitofrontal; **SMV,** submentovertical.

**fetal warfarin syndrome** adverse effect of maternal warfarin intake in pregnancy; women on long-term warfarin should preferably seek pre-conception care and consult doctor immediately if they become pregnant. Characteristics: nasal hypoplasia, epiphyseal abnormalities, eye defects, shortening of extremities, deafness, developmental retardation, congenital heart disease, scoliosis, intracerebral haemorrhage.

**feticide** injection to dispose of fetus affected by serious abnormality in twin pregnancy, enables normal growth and development of other twin.

**feto-fetal transfusion syndrome** twin-to-twin transfusion syndrome in which blood from one fetus transfuses into other via placental blood vessels.

**fetoscopy** endoscopic antenatal procedure allowing access to fetus, amniotic cavity, umbilical cord, fetal side of placenta. Incision made in abdomen, endoscope inserted through abdominal wall and uterus into amniotic cavity.

**fetus** human embryo from 8 weeks of pregnancy until birth. *F. in fetu* in monozygotic twin pregnancy, parts of one fetus develop within the other. *F. papyraceus* in twin pregnancy, one fetus dies in early pregnancy, becoming flattened against uterine wall, usually expelled with placenta, resembles parchment.

**fever** pyrexia, high body temperature.

**fibre** thread-like structure; muscle cell. *Dietary f.* ingested foodstuff not broken down by intestinal enzymes, pass through small intestine and colon undigested, assists in preventing constipation.

**fibrin** insoluble protein formed by action of thrombin upon fibrinogen; needed for blood clotting: network of minute long strands in which blood cells are trapped. *F. degradation products* blood components produced by clot degeneration, produced by action of plasmin on deposited fibrin; levels rise after any thrombotic event; used to test for DISSEMINATED INTRAVASCULAR COAGULATION.

**fibrinogen** protein formed in liver, circulates in plasma; activated by THROMBIN when tissue injury occurs, forms FIBRIN, arresting haemorrhage by clotting. Preparations containing human fibrinogen, e.g. fresh frozen plasma, cryoprecipitate, used to restore blood fibrinogen levels after extensive surgery or to treat diseases or haemorrhagic conditions complicated by AFIBRINOGENAEMIA.

**fibrinolysin** 1. plasmin. 2. proteolytic enzyme formed from profibrinolysin (plasminogen) by action of physical agents or by specific bacterial kinases; used to promote dissolution of thrombi.

**fibrinolysis** dissolution of fibrin by enzymatic action. *Adj* fibrinolytic.

**fibrocystic disease** *See* CYSTIC FIBROSIS.

**fibroid** 1. composed of fibrous tissue. 2. leiomyoma; submucosal, interstitial, subserous or intracervical benign uterine tumour. In pregnancy, red degeneration or miscarriage occurs; labour difficulties unlikely, but if near placental site may interfere with contractions, causing postpartum haemorrhage; usually reduce spontaneously in puerperium.

**fibromyomata** fibroids.

**fibronectin, fetal** component of extracellular matrix, secreted by anchoring trophoblastic villi; present in vaginal secretions in early pregnancy, and in blood and amniotic fluid; high levels after 22 weeks' gestation suggest chorio-decidual disruption causing leakage of fetal fibronectin, possibly indicative of impending preterm labour, although false-positive results may occur.

**fibroplasia** fibrous tissue formation as in wound healing. *Retrolental f.* retinal vascular proliferation and tortuosity, presence of fibrous tissue behind lens; leads to retinal detachment and poor eye growth; often due to excessive oxygen concentration use in preterm babies.

**fibrosis** formation of fibrous tissue; fibroid degeneration. *Adj* fibrotic. *Cystic f. See* CYSTIC FIBROSIS.

**fibula** lateral and smaller of two bones of leg.

**fimbria** finger-like fringe, extremity of fallopian tube. *Pl* fimbriae. *Adj* fimbriated.

**first-degree perineal laceration** *See* PERINEAL LACERATION.

**first-pass effect** drugs given orally are absorbed in small intestine, transported to liver via hepatic portal vein, metabolized prior to systemic circulation. Oral administration leads to lower levels of drug reaching target tissue than other administration routes.

**first-stage labour** from onset of painful regular uterine contractions and dilatation of cervix until full dilatation of cervix.

**fish consumption in pregnancy** fish is rich in omega-3 fatty acids; some contains high mercury levels, may harm developing fetus; women should avoid eating shark, marlin, swordfish; limit tuna to two fresh or four tinned portions per week. Shellfish should be thoroughly cooked; raw fish avoided, e.g. sushi, oysters; raw smoked fish, including smoked mackerel or salmon, is safe to eat.

**fission** cleavage or splitting; reproduction by division of cell into two equal parts. *Nuclear f.* splitting of nucleus of atom.

**fissure** cleft; either normal, as in cerebral fissure, or due to disease, e.g. anal fissure.

**fistula** abnormal passage between two cavities or between cavity and surface of body. *Rectovaginal f.* opening between vagina and rectum, usually due to severe perineal body laceration. *Vesicovaginal f.* opening between bladder and vagina, may be due to prolonged pressure in obstructed labour.

**fit** seizure; convulsion, e.g. eclampsia, epilepsy.

**5HT3 receptor antagonists** group of drugs used in treatment of HYPEREM-ESIS GRAVIDARUM.

**flaccid** limp; without tone, e.g. muscles of severe asphyxiated baby.

**flagellum** whip-like protoplasmic filament aids bacterial movement, e.g. *Trichomonas vaginalis* flagellated protozoon. *Pl* flagella.

**flat pelvis** pelvis with anteroposterior diameter of brim shorter than transverse diameter; platypelloid or rachitic pelvis. *See* PELVIS.

**flatulence** gas or air in stomach or intestine, causing discomfort, passage of flatus (wind).

**fleshy mole** CARNEOUS MOLE; mass of clotted blood surrounding dead embryo retained in uterus.

**flexion** bending; normal attitude of fetus in utero. *See* ANTEFLEXION *and* RETROFLEXION.

**floppy baby syndrome** neonatal cyanosis and hypotonia.

**flora** *Intestinal f.* bacteria normally residing in lumen of intestine.

**flucloxacillin** antibiotic active against most staphylococci and streptococci; given orally, intramuscularly or intravenously.

**fluconazole** anti-fungal drug used to treat vaginal candidiasis.

**fluid** liquid. *Amniotic f.* fluid within amnion, bathes developing fetus, protects it from mechanical injury. *Body f.* fluid within body, composed of water and solutes: electrolytes, non-electrolytes. *Intracellular f.* fluid within cell, about two-thirds of total body fluid. *Extracellular f.* fluid outside cell, about one third of total body fluid. *Cerebrospinal f.* fluid within ventricles of brain, subarachnoid space and central canal of spinal cord. *F. balance* normal volume of body water and its solutes, normal distribution of fluids intracellularly and extracellularly; total volume of body fluids normally about 60% of body weight. *F. balance chart* recording of fluid intake and output.

**fluorescent in situ hybridization (FISH)** diagnostic chromosome test to identify trisomy and sex chromosome ANEUPLOIDY (but not whole KARYOTYPE), performed after CHORIONIC VILLUS SAMPLING or AMNIOCENTESIS on uncultured cells to obtain results within 24–48 hours. *See also* QUANTITATIVE FLUORESCENCE POLYMERASE CHAIN REACTION (QF-PCR).

**fluorescent treponemal antibody-absorbed test** specific treponemal antibody test to confirm diagnosis of syphilis when initial VENEREAL DISEASE RESEARCH LABORATORY TEST is positive; sensitive to early stages of infection.

**fluoxetine** selective serotonin reuptake inhibitor anti-depressant drugs (SSRIs); e.g. Prozac.

**folates** compounds derived from FOLIC ACID, necessary for biochemical reactions, especially DNA synthesis. Serum and erythrocyte folate levels used to assess body stores; low levels occur in megaloblastic anaemia secondary to folate deficiency.

**folic acid** constituent of vitamin B complex, needed for normal red blood cell development; found in green vegetables, liver, yeast. Preconception deficiency may lead to fetal neural tube defects: women advised to take folic acid supplements, 400 µg daily for 3–6 months prior to conception. If at risk of neural tube defects or on carbamazepine or valproate, dose is 5 mg daily. Inability of body to absorb or utilize vitamin B causes megaloblastic anaemia, as rapidly dividing fetal cells compete for folic acid to form cell nuclei.

**follicle** very small sac or gland. *Graafian f.* small vesicle containing ovum, formed in ovary. *See* GONADOTROPHIC.

**follicle-stimulating hormone** hormone released from anterior pituitary gland, stimulating one or more GRAAFIAN FOLLICLES to mature during each menstrual cycle.

**fomites** substances or objects that transmit infectious organisms by contamination.

**fontanelle** membranous space where two or more sutures meet between cranial bones of skull. *Anterior f.* bregma. *Posterior f.* lambda. *See* FETAL SKULL.

**footling breech presentation** breech presentation with one or both feet presenting before buttocks. *See also* BREECH PRESENTATION.

**foramen** opening or hole. *F. magnum* occipital bone opening through which medulla oblongata becomes continuous with spinal cord. *Obturator f.* large hole in pelvic innominate bone. *F. ovale* opening between two atria of fetal heart.

**forceps** surgical instrument with two blades used for lifting or compressing object, e.g. *dissecting f. Artery f.* compress bleeding points during operation. *Obstetric f.* used in second-stage labour to deliver fetal head, e.g. KIELLANDS, NEVILLE BARNES and WRIGLEY'S forceps. *Vulsellum f.* with claw-like ends.

**foremilk** thin watery milk at start of breast feed; high in lactose, low in fat and calories.

**foreskin** prepuce; skin covering glans penis.

**forewaters** amniotic fluid in part of bag of membranes lying below presenting part of fetus. *See also* HINDWATERS.

**formula** 1. prescription, recipe, especially for infant's feed. 2. group of symbols making certain statement, as in chemical symbols.

**fornix** arch; four fornices in vault of vagina, in front of (*anterior f.*), behind (*posterior f.*) and at sides (*lateral f.*) of cervix. *Pl* fornices.

**fossa** pit or hollow, e.g. iliac fossa, depression on inner surface of iliac bone.

**foster parents** responsible adults who, under Children Act 2004, are paid to care for children unrelated to them.

**fostering** provision of parental care and nurturing of children who are not related through blood or legal ties.

**Fothergill operation** Manchester repair; operation for uterovaginal prolapse by fixation of cardinal ligaments.

**foundation trusts** NHS organizations with significant managerial and financial freedom compared with other NHS hospital trusts; devolved decision making from centralized NHS so local communities more responsive to local needs.

**fourchette** skin fold between posterior extremities of labia minora.

**fracture** break, usually of bone; occurs occasionally in difficult births, e.g. depressed fracture of skull, or in breech birth, e.g. fracture of clavicle, humerus or femur.

**fragilitas ossium** OSTEOGENESIS IMPERFECTA; fragile brittle bones.

**Frankenhauser plexus** ganglion near uterine cervix from which sympathetic and parasympathetic nerves supply vagina, uterus and other pelvic viscera.

**fraternal    twins** dizygotic—non-identical—twins.

**freebirthing** *See* UNASSISTED BIRTH.

**frenulotomy,      frenotomy** surgery to correct congenital tongue tie; frenulum connecting bottom of mouth to underside of tongue is too short, causing restricted tongue movement (ankyloglossia).

**frenulum** small ligament that checks movement of organ, e.g. *f. linguae* membranous connection between floor of mouth and lower surface of tongue. *See* TONGUE TIE.

**friable** easily torn, broken or crumbled, e.g. placental chorion is friable, may be partially retained in uterus after delivery.

**frontal** pertaining to forehead. *F. bones* two bones forming forehead in fetus. *F. suture* membranous channel between two frontal bones. *F. headache* serious symptom of severe PRE-ECLAMPSIA or impending ECLAMPSIA caused by cerebral oedema.

**fulminating** bursting forth, violently explosive; applied to conditions appearing suddenly and severely, e.g. pre-eclampsia.

**fundal** pertaining to fundus. *F. dominance* normal uterine contractions originate from pacemaker in fundus; wave of contraction gradually weakens as it passes over upper and lower uterine segments. *F. height* distance between fundus and upper border of symphysis pubis, measured abdominally to assess size of uterus in pregnancy and involution in early puerperium.

**fundus** part of organ farthest from opening. *Uterine f.* top of uterus farthest from cervix.

**fungus** group of eukaryotic organisms (mushrooms, yeasts, moulds, etc.); thrush is fungal condition.

**funic** pertaining to umbilical cord. *F. souffle* soft whispering sound from umbilical cord synchronizing with fetal heart sounds.

**funis** umbilical cord. *Adj* funic.

**funnel pelvis** pelvis that narrows from above downwards, e.g. ANDROID PELVIS, outlet is smaller than brim.

**furosemide (frusemide)** diuretic that blocks reabsorption of sodium and chloride in ascending loop of Henle; used in pregnancy for pulmonary oedema, occasionally for oliguria and acute renal failure when benefits outweigh risks; may inhibit lactation.

**gag** 1. instrument for holding open jaws. 2. to retch, or strive to vomit. *G. reflex* elevation of soft palate and retching, elicited by touching back of tongue or wall of pharynx; pharyngeal reflex.

**gait** walk or carriage; abnormal gait may indicate pelvic deformity.

**galact-, galacto-** word element meaning 'milk'.

**galactischia** suppression of milk secretion.

**galactogogue** agent that increases milk secretion.

**galactopoiesis** maintenance of lactation; requires prolactin and oxytocin for let-down reflex in response to suckling.

**galactorrhoea** excessive flow of breast milk.

**galactosaemia** genetically determined biochemical disorder; lack of enzyme necessary for galactose metabolism leads to high levels of galactose in blood and tissues; causes failure to thrive, hepatomegaly, jaundice; mental retardation and death if untreated; treatment: exclusion of galactose- or lactose-containing foods from diet.

**galactose** MONOSACCHARIDE resulting from digestion of LACTOSE, converted to glucose by liver.

**galactose-1-phosphate uridyltransferase** enzyme that converts galactose to glucose; deficiency causes galactosaemia.

**galea aponeurotica** occipitofrontalis muscle tendon, forms scalp layer.

**Galen, vein of** *See* GREAT VEIN OF GALEN.

**gall bladder** sac on underpart of liver, holds and concentrates bile secreted by liver. *G. b. changes in pregnancy* dilatation of gall bladder slows rate of emptying, thickened bile, increased chance of OBSTETRIC CHOLESTASIS; incomplete emptying may lead to gallstones, relatively common in asymptomatic women.

**gamete** female (oocyte) or male (spermatazoon) reproductive cell. *G. intrafallopian transfer* fertility treatment; involves retrieval of oocytes from ovary at laparoscopy and placing sequentially with sperm into fallopian tubes; suitable for women with unexplained infertility and those with one patent, healthy fallopian tube when male sperm parameters are near normal. *See also* ZYGOTE INTRAFALLOPIAN TRANSFER.

**gamgee tissue** absorbent gauze-covered wool for dressing wounds.

**gamma globulin** plasma proteins composed of IgG, IMMUNOGLOBULIN protein; contains most antibody activity and provides almost all known antibodies' circulation. Commercial preparations derived from blood serum prevent, modify and treat various infectious diseases, providing passive immunity against infections to which most of the population has antibodies. Gamma globulin with high anti-rhesus antibody activity is given to

http://dx.doi.org/10.1016/B978-0-7020-6906-2.00007-3

rhesus-negative mothers within 72 hours of delivery to prevent natural formation of antibody.

**ganglion** nerve centre from which nerve fibres proceed.

**gangrene** death of tissue, usually of large area or definite organ. *Dry g.* due to failure of arterial blood supply, e.g. drying and separating of cord from umbilicus. *Moist g.* caused by putrefactive changes, e.g. infection in moist umbilical cord delaying separation.

**Gardnerella** See BACTERIAL VAGINOSIS.

**gargoylism** type of MUCOPOLYSACCHARIDOSIS.

**gas** vaporous matter, neither solid nor liquid; molecules are in constant movement; air is mixture of several gases: oxygen, nitrogen, traces of carbon dioxide, argon and helium.

**'gas and oxygen' analgesia** See INHALATION ANALGESIA, ENTONOX.

**gas gangrene** infection of damaged tissues by anaerobic organism *Clostridium welchii.*

**Gaskin manoeuvre** all-fours position, sometimes required for management of SHOULDER DYSTOCIA. See APPENDIX 4.

**gastric** pertaining to stomach.

**gastritis** inflammation of stomach lining.

**gastro-** prefix relating to stomach.

**gastroenteritis** stomach and intestinal lining inflammation; acute diarrhoea, vomiting causes rapid, severe dehydration; can be fatal in babies. Treatment: immediate isolation; oral or intravenous fluids to combat dehydration, correct electrolyte balance, treat infection.

**gastrointestinal** pertaining to stomach and intestines. *G. tract* alimentary tract.

**gastrojejunostomy** surgical anastomosis of stomach to jejunum, performed to bypass obstruction in babies with duodenal atresia.

**gastro-oesophageal reflux in pregnancy** common physiological disorder due to relaxation of cardiac sphincter at stomach entrance, causing regurgitation of acid stomach contents; antacids may be given to relieve oesophageal burning.

**gastroschisis** congenital fissure of abdominal wall.

**gastrostomy** creation of opening into stomach to allow administration of food and liquids when oesophageal stricture makes swallowing impossible.

**gate control theory of pain** theory of neural mechanism in dorsal horns of spinal cord that acts like gate, increasing or decreasing nerve impulse flow from peripheral fibres to central nervous system, influencing pain perception.

**Geiger counter** instrument used to detect radioactive substances.

**gelofusine** succinylated gelatine solution used as intravenous colloid to increase blood volume, blood flow, cardiac output and oxygen transportation.

**gemellology** scientific study of twins and twinning.

**gemeprost** prostaglandin analogue, pessaries used to soften and dilate cervix, facilitate first-trimester transcervical procedures or mid-trimester pregnancy termination.

**gender** category to which individual is assigned on basis of sex.

**gene** single unit of hereditary factors located in defined position on CHROMOSOME; composed of DEOXYRIBONUCLEIC ACID (DNA) with complex molecular double chain carrying individual genetic codes and controlling functions and reproduction of all body cells. Replicates by mitosis; each daughter cell carries exact replica of genes of parent cell, carrying hereditary traits through successive generations without change. Occasionally, abnormal or mutant genes occur, e.g. as in PHE-NYLKETONURIA in which there are two abnormal RECESSIVE genes. **G. expression** process by which information from genes is used in synthesis of functional gene product. **G. therapy** introduction of normal genes into cells, in place of missing or defective ones in order to correct genetic disorders.

**general anaesthesia** inhibition of sensory, motor and sympathetic nerve transmission at level of brain; causes unconsciousness and lack of sensation; rarely used in obstetrics; significant cause of maternal death, notably due to MENDELSON SYNDROME.

**general sale drugs** drugs that can be sold over the counter with no pharmacy training; generally considered safe for most people when taken correctly. Examples: paracetamol, ibuprofen, anti-allergy medication, laxatives, skin creams. *See also* PRESCRIPTION-ONLY MEDICINES.

**generic** 1. pertaining to genus. 2. general, non-proprietary; e.g. drug name not protected by trademark.

**genetic** pertaining to genetics. *G. counselling* consultation at which geneticist explains chances of recurrence of hereditary diseases, advising couples on risks to future children. *G. fingerprinting* DNA profiling, technique using individuality of DNA molecules to distinguish between organisms or show relationship between them.

**genetics** study of heredity. *See also* EPIGENETICS.

**genital** relating to organs of reproduction. *G. herpes* sexually transmitted herpes simplex virus infection with painful genital blisters *G. warts* condyloma acuminatum, due to HUMAN PAPILLOMA VIRUS; primarily sexually transmitted; neonate may develop laryngeal papilloma after contact during birth; commonest in women aged 16–24. Usually asymptomatic, mostly benign, resolve spontaneously. In pregnancy, multiply quickly, seen as cauliflower-like masses. Investigations: exclude other sexually transmitted infections; colposcopy to exclude flat warts on cervix. Treatment: normally not recommended, but possibly trichloroacetic acid, cryotherapy, diathermy, laser therapy or surgery. Cervical epithelial neoplasia strongly associated with HPV; annual cervical smear tests offered.

**genitalia** organs of reproduction. *Ambiguous g.* rare condition in which baby's external genitalia not clearly either male or female; may be malformed or have characteristics of both sexes.

**genitourinary** pertaining to genital and urinary organs.

**genome** entire genetic complement of a cell or organism; the human genome is thought to have approximately 30,000 genes.

**genomics** specialist discipline in genetics; study of genomes, including determining entire DNA sequence of organisms.

**genotype** classification of genetic makeup of individual. *See* GENE.

**gentamicin** antibiotic complex, effective against gram-negative bacteria, e.g. *Pseudomonas* and gram-positive bacteria, e.g. *Staphylococcus aureus*. Use in pregnancy risks fetal eighth cranial nerve damage, should be avoided.

**genu** knee.

**genupectoral position** knee–chest position, i.e. face downwards, resting on knees and chest. *See* POSITION.

**genus** classificatory group of animals or plants comprising one or more species.

**German measles** *See* RUBELLA.

**germicide** agent that destroys micro-organisms.

**gestagen** hormones with progestational activity.

**gestation** pregnancy. *G. period* in human pregnancy, about 40 weeks from first day of last normal menstrual period. *G. sac* placenta and membranes containing amniotic fluid and fetus during pregnancy. *See also* BALLARD SCORE, DUBOWITZ SCORE.

**gestational** pertaining to gestation. *G. hypertension* raised blood pressure in pregnancy; may progress to pre-eclampsia/eclampsia. *G. diabetes* impaired glucose tolerance in pregnancy, reverts to normal after birth; increased risk of diabetes mellitus in later life.

**giardiasis** beaver fever; tropical parasitic intestinal infection; transmitted by sexual contact; also water-borne, particularly if inadequate sanitation. Symptoms: abdominal cramps; watery diarrhoea; watery, greasy, malodorous stools; no blood or pus; offensive flatus; alternating soft stools and constipation; nausea, vomiting, bloating, halitosis, indigestion, fever lasting 3–4 days. Treatment: metronidazole,

tinidazole but avoid in pregnancy, as adverse fetal effects. Paromomycin best in pregnancy: poorly absorbed by mother, excreted almost 100% in faeces and little crosses placenta.

**gigantism** abnormal overgrowth of whole or part of body due to overactivity of anterior pituitary growth hormone.

**Gigli operation** pubiotomy. *See* SYMPHYSIOTOMY.

**Gigli saw** fine wire instrument for sawing through bone.

**Gilbert syndrome** inherited genetic mutation in which liver fails to process bilirubin properly; requires no treatment.

**ginger** herbal remedy from root, used to treat sickness. Strong anticoagulant: avoid if on anticoagulants, aspirin, similar medication; do not use for prolonged periods. Midwives must be adequately trained to advise on herbal remedies.

**gingivitis** inflammation and bleeding of gums; common in pregnancy due to increased vascularity.

**girdle** belt. *Pelvic g.* bony ring of pelvis formed by two innominate bones and sacrum.

**glabella** area on frontal bone above nose and between eyebrows.

**gland** collection of cells that secrete or excrete materials not related to their own metabolic needs. *Endocrine g.* secretes hormones into bloodstream, e.g. thyroid gland secretes thyroxine.

**glans** acorn-shaped body, e.g. rounded end of penis and clitoris.

**glibenclamide** drug for diabetes mellitus; avoid in pregnancy due to adverse fetal effects.

**gliclazide** drug for diabetes mellitus; avoid in pregnancy due to adverse fetal effects.

**globin** protein constituent of haemoglobin; also, any of group of proteins similar to typical globin.

**globulins** class of plasma proteins, further subdivided into alpha (α), beta (β) and gamma (γ) globulins. *See also* GAMMA GLOBULIN *and* IMMUNOGLOBULIN.

**glomerular filtration rate** quantity of glomerular filtrate formed each minute in kidney nephrons, measured as creatinine clearance rate. In pregnancy, rises 50% by second trimester.

**glomerulus** tuft of capillaries invaginated in kidney tubule at commencement of renal cortex. *Pl* glomeruli.

**glossal** pertaining to tongue.

**glossoptosis** abnormality of downward tongue displacement or retraction.

**glottis** vocal apparatus of larynx; true vocal cords and the opening between them.

**glucagon** polypeptide hormone secreted by islets of Langerhans in response to hypoglycaemia or to stimulation by growth hormone; increases blood glucose concentration by stimulating glycogenolysis in liver; administered to reverse hypoglycaemic coma, especially caused by hyperinsulinism.

**glucocorticoid** any corticoid substance that increases gluconeogenesis, raising concentration of liver glycogen and blood sugar, i.e. cortisol (hydrocortisone), cortisone and corticosterone.

**glucose** dextrose in fruit and honey; monosaccharide to which carbohydrates reduce in digestion, producing energy for cells; controlled by insulin.

Surplus glucose is stored as glycogen in liver and muscle for use when needed. Normal fasting glucose levels 70–90 mg per 100 mL (3.9–5.6 mmol/L); excessive glucose (hyperglycaemia) may indicate DIABETES MELLITUS, HYPERTHYROIDISM, hyperpituitarism; GLUCOSE TOLERANCE TEST assesses glucose metabolism. Found in urine in untreated diabetes mellitus.

**glucose-6-phosphate dehydrogenase** important enzyme in red blood cells. G6PD deficiency: inherited X-linked RECESSIVE trait common in black races, Mediterranean people; causes HAEMOLYSIS, severe or fatal anaemia after fava bean intake (favism).

**glucose tolerance test** test to diagnose gestational DIABETES MELLITUS; mother's blood glucose levels monitored before and after ingesting glucose; fasting blood glucose 5.5–7.0 mmol/L and glucose 7.8–11.1 mmol/L 2 hours after ingestion suggests impaired tolerance; higher levels indicate gestational diabetes. Indications: previous gestational diabetes, previous MACROSOMIA, close relative with diabetes, POLYHYDRAMNIOS, maternal obesity.

**glucuronyl transferase** liver enzyme; converts fat-soluble toxic bilirubin to water-soluble non-toxic type.

**glutaraldehyde** antiseptic used to treat viral warts.

**gluteal** pertaining to buttocks.

**glycerol suppositories** rectally administered medication to stimulate rectal activity.

**glycogen** carbohydrate polysaccharide stored in liver and muscles.

**glycosuria** glucose in urine due to inability to store carbohydrate ingested; lowered renal threshold for sugar; DIABETES MELLITUS.

**glycosylated haemoglobin**  *See* HBA$_{1c}$.

**gnathic**  pertaining to jaw or cheeks.

**goblet cell**  goblet-shaped cell in cubical epithelium of fallopian tubes, producing glycogen secretion to nourish ovum.

**goitre**  thyroid gland enlargement; swelling in front of neck, may cause tracheal pressure.

**gonad**  organ producing ova or spermatozoa; female ovary, male testis.

**gonadotrophic**  stimulating gonads. *G. hormones* those of anterior pituitary lobe or placenta.

**gonadotrophin**  hormone that stimulates gonads, e.g. follicle-stimulating hormone, luteinizing hormone from anterior pituitary. *Chorionic g.* gonad-stimulating hormone produced by chorionic cytotrophoblast cells; female urine is tested for human chorionic gonadotrophin to confirm pregnancy.

**gonococcal**  pertaining to or caused by gonococci. *G. ophthalmia* acute gonococcal conjunctivitis; in newborn babies, may lead to corneal ulceration. *See* OPHTHALMIA NEONATORUM.

**gonococcus**  *Neisseria gonorrhoeae*; gram-negative intracellular diplococcus, causative agent of gonorrhoea.

**gonorrhoea**  sexually transmitted disease due to gonococcal infection; infects mucous membranes of cervix, urethra, Bartholin's glands; may lead to salpingitis, septicaemia; vaginal infection in pregnancy should be treated early. Incubation period 1–16 days; may cause purulent vaginal or urethral discharge, burning pain on micturition but usually symptomless; diagnosis confirmed by smear and cultures. Treatment:

penicillin, tetracycline or quinolone drugs, but resistance may require ciprofloxacin, ofloxacin, probenecid.

**Goodell's sign**  Hegar's sign, softening of uterine cervix and vagina; sign of pregnancy.

**Graafian follicle**  oestrogenic hormone-secreting cystic structure, develops in ovarian cortex during menstrual cycle until ripe; follicle ruptures, discharges ovum (ovulation), becomes CORPUS LUTEUM.

**gram (g)**  metric unit of weight.

**Gram stain**  bacteriology stain; microorganisms retaining it are gram-positive; those that lose it are gram-negative.

**grand mal**  major epileptic seizure with loss of consciousness and convulsive movements, as distinguished from PETIT MAL.

**grande multigravida**  woman in fourth or subsequent pregnancy; has not necessarily delivered live babies in previous pregnancies.

**grande multipara**  woman of high parity, who has delivered four or more babies; high parity increases risk of complications.

**granulation**  process of wound healing; granulations seen as small red projections on wound surface, brings rich blood supply to healing surface.

**granulosa cells**  oestradiol-secreting cells lining Graafian follicle.

**granulosa lutein cells**  granulosa cells after ovulation, which secrete oestradiol and progesterone.

**Graves' disease**  overactive thyroid, causing neck swelling and eye protrusion; in pregnancy may cause miscarriage, pre-eclampsia.

**gravid**  pregnant.

**gravida**  pregnant woman. *See* PRIMIGRAVIDA *and* MULTIGRAVIDA.

**gravity** 1. weight. *Specific g.* weight compared with that of equal volume of water. Specific gravity of water 1.000 g/mL; of normal urine 1.010–1.020 g/mL, increased if solids are dissolved in it, e.g. sugar; decreased when inadequate urea excreted, e.g. in chronic nephritis. 2. pertaining to GRAVID.

**great vein of Galen** large cerebral vein; passes from midbrain, enters junction of inferior longitudinal and straight sinuses; extreme, abnormal or rapid fetal skull moulding at birth may cause cerebral membranes and cerebral vein tears and intracranial haemorrhage.

**grey syndrome** potentially fatal condition in preterm babies, caused by reaction to chloramphenicol; characterized by ashen grey cyanosis, vomiting, abdominal distension, hypothermia, shock.

**grief** sorrow, usually due to death; normal grieving process takes 2 or 3 years, following pattern of numbness and denial, anger, guilt, bargaining and depression, finally acceptance and readjustment.

**groin** junction of front of thigh with trunk.

**group B streptococcus** gram-positive bacterium; vaginal or rectal COMMENSAL found in 20%–25% of pregnant women; not sexually transmitted but infection increases with sexual activity; many babies colonized at birth with no ill effects, but 1:16,000 develop infection in first week of life; 1:10 affected babies die. Risk factors: preterm labour/birth, prolonged membrane rupture >18 hours, chorioamnionitis; previous baby with early-onset GBS infection, GBS in maternal swabs or urine, intrapartum pyrexia >38°C; prophylactic antibiotics may reduce severity of effects.

**group practice** team of healthcare professionals working together, e.g. general practitioners, NHS or independent midwives.

**GROW chart** gestation-related optimal weight measurements and fundal height.

**growth hormone** substance stimulating growth; anterior PITUITARY GLAND secretion directly influences protein, carbohydrate, lipid metabolism; controls skeletal and visceral growth rate; increased production occurs in babies of poorly controlled diabetic mothers.

**grunting** abnormal expiratory sound made by baby with compromised respiration; may be heard audibly or with stethoscope as baby forcibly exhales against closed glottis to prevent alveolar collapse; may require intubation of CONTINUOUS POSITIVE AIRWAY PRESSURE ventilation.

**Guedel airway** oropharyngeal airway device to open or maintain airway; prevents tongue from covering epiglottis.

**guardian ad litem** someone from local authority social services department appointed by court to look after interests of child before full adoption order is granted.

**gum gingiva** enlarged, spongy, fluid-retaining gums caused by oestrogen.

**gumma** syphilitic lesion of tertiary syphilis, any part of body.

**Guthrie test** blood-spot heel-prick test for PHENYLKETONURIA, part of NEWBORN BLOOD-SPOT SCREENING PROGRAMME; taken on day 4–6 after birth, or 48 hours after any blood transfusion. *See also* CYSTIC FIBROSIS, HYPOTHYROIDISM *and* SICKLE CELL DISEASE.

**gynae-** prefix meaning 'woman'.

**gynaecoid** woman-like, feminine characteristics. *G. pelvis* typically female pelvis.

**gynaecologist** doctor specializing in female reproductive tract conditions.

**gynaecology** branch of medicine concerned with diseases of female genital tract.

**gynandroid** hermaphrodite or female pseudohermaphrodite.

**gynandromorphism** presence of chromosomes of both sexes in different tissues of body, producing mosaic of male and female sexual characteristics. *Adj* gynandromorphons.

**gypsies** *See* TRAVELLERS.

**Haberman feeders** special feeding device used to give expressed breast milk to babies with cleft lip and cleft palate before surgery.

**habitual miscarriage** *See* MISCARRIAGE.

**HbA1c (glycosylated haemoglobin)** measure of diabetic glycaemic control; raised blood glucose binds with haemoglobin, produces glycosylated haemoglobin; below 7% in well-controlled diabetes.

**haem** insoluble non-protein iron protoporphyrin constituent of haemoglobin, other respiratory pigments, many cells; enables haemoglobin molecule to transport oxygen.

**haema-, haemo-, haemato-** prefixes denoting or relating to blood.

**haemagglutination** agglutination of erythrocytes.

**haemagglutinin** antibody that causes agglutination of erythrocytes.

**haemangioma** tumour, cluster of blood vessels; may be present at birth, seen as small, blood-filled capillary network near skin surface, forms flat red or purple birthmark ('strawberry' or 'raspberry' mark); most disappear in childhood, 'port-wine' stain may persist.

**haematemesis** vomiting of blood; in neonates may be due to HAEMORRHAGIC DISEASE OF NEWBORN or swallowed maternal blood; fetal and maternal blood are differentiated by SINGER'S TEST.

**haematinic** 1. improving quality of blood. 2. agent that improves blood quality, increases haemoglobin and erythrocyte concentration, e.g. iron, vitamin B complex.

**haematocele** collection of blood in cavity. *Pelvic h.* collection of blood in pouch of Douglas, usually due to tubal abortion or rupture.

**haematocolpos** accumulation of blood in vagina.

**haematocrit** *See* PACKED CELL VOLUME.

**haematology** science of nature, functions and diseases of blood.

**haematoma** local extravasated blood collection in organ, space or tissue; may occur in vagina, vulva or perineum from labour trauma. *See also* CEPHALHAEMATOMA.

**haematometra** accumulation of blood in uterus.

**haematopoiesis** blood cell formation in bone marrow, spleen, liver, lymph nodes (extramedullary haematopoiesis).

**haematoporphyrin** iron-free derivative of haem, produced during haemoglobin decomposition.

**haematosalpinx** accumulation of blood in fallopian tube.

**haematuria** blood in urine, due to bladder injury, infection or disease.

**haemoconcentration** loss of fluid from blood into tissues, as in shock or dehydration.

**haemodialysis** procedure to remove toxic waste from blood in cases of acute or chronic renal failure. *See* PERITONEAL *and* DIALYSIS.

**haemodilution** increased blood plasma in proportion to cells; normal in

http://dx.doi.org/10.1016/B978-0-7020-6906-2.00008-5

pregnancy as blood volume increases (*see* HYDRAEMIA), or in haemorrhage, as fluid is drawn from tissues into blood to maintain circulating blood volume.

**haemoglobin** red blood cell pigment aids oxygen transport; compound of ferrous iron-containing pigment haem with protein globin. Oxygenated haemoglobin is bright red; deoxygenated haemoglobin is darker. In utero fetal haemoglobin (HbF), formed in liver and spleen, has increased oxygen affinity; later, erythropoiesis moves to bone marrow, adult haemoglobin HbA and HbA$_2$ produced.

**haemoglobinopathies** inherited haemoglobin disorders; baby has abnormal quantity (thalassaemia) or quality (e.g. SICKLE CELL DISEASE) of globin chains in haemoglobin.

**haemolysin** ANTIBODY with complement that releases haemoglobin from red blood cells.

**haemolysis** liberation of haemoglobin from erythrocytes; in excess causes ANAEMIA and JAUNDICE; some microbes, e.g. beta-haemolytic streptococcus, form haemolysins which destroy red blood corpuscles. In transfusion reaction or newborn HAEMOLYTIC DISEASE, incompatibility causes red blood cells to clump together; agglutinated cells disintegrate, releasing haemoglobin into plasma; kidney damage may result as haemoglobin crystallizes, obstructing renal tubules, with renal shutdown and uraemia.

**haemolytic** pertaining to, characterized by or producing HAEMOLYSIS. *H. disease of newborn* erythroblastosis fetalis; neonatal blood dyscrasia;

erythrocyte haemolysis; incompatibility between infant and maternal blood. *See* RHESUS INCOMPATIBILITY.

**haemophilia** inherited delayed blood-clotting disease carried by mother as sex-linked recessive gene; occurs only in males; 80% have haemophilia A, deficiency of clotting factor VIII; 15% have haemophilia B (Christmas disease), deficiency of factor IX. Treatment aims to raise and maintain deficient factor to stop bleeding.

**Haemophilus influenza serotype B (Hib)** bacterial infection carried in nasopharynx of 75% of children; spread by coughing, sneezing; causes bacteraemia, bacterial meningitis, otitis media, sinusitis, pneumonia, cellulitis, joint and muscle pain, osteomyelitis. Treatment: cephalosporins or sulphur drugs; erythromycin ineffective. Babies offered immunization at 8, 12 and 16 weeks of age.

**haemopoiesis** *See* HAEMATOPOIESIS.

**haemoptysis** coughing up blood from lungs, distinguishable from vomited blood by bright colour and frothy character.

**haemorrhage** bleeding, either external or internal. *Antepartum h.* bleeding *per vaginam* after 24 weeks' gestation; may be due to PLACENTAL ABRUPTION, PLACENTA PRAEVIA or incidental causes. *Cerebral h.* bleeding from cerebral blood vessel rupture, as in eclampsia, essential hypertension. *Concealed h.* bleeding for which clinical signs, e.g. shock, do not equate to measured blood loss. *Intracranial h.* neonatal bleeding in brain due to difficult birth; causes blood vessel tearing at TENTORIUM CEREBELLI and FALX CEREBRI junction. *Intraventricular h.* bleeding between brain ventricles in small and preterm babies. **Petechial h.** subcutaneous haemorrhage in minute spots; occurs in baby if cord tightly round neck or after difficult birth. *See also* POSTPARTUM HAEMORRHAGE.

**haemorrhagic** characterized by haemorrhage. **H. disease of newborn** bleeding in first week of life; haematemesis, melaena, haematuria, or from umbilicus or puncture sites, with very low blood prothrombin. Treatment: vitamin K and blood transfusion; must be differentiated from HAEMOLYTIC DISEASE OF NEWBORN.

**haemorrhoids** piles; varicose veins of rectum, anal canal (internal), anal orifice (external). In pregnancy, may enlarge, become painful due to smooth muscle relaxation, constipation and congestion. Exacerbated by vaginal birth, direct pressure from fetal head or forceps. Treatment: local analgesic ointment or suppositories. Usually resolve spontaneously after birth but surgery sometimes required; may recur in subsequent pregnancy.

**haemostasis** arrest of bleeding.

**haemostatic** astringent drug or agent capable of arresting bleeding.

**Haig-Ferguson forceps** mid-cavity forceps to deliver fetus when head is engaged but above ischial spines.

**hallucination** false perception or psychosis; false beliefs of seeing, smelling, hearing, tasting or feeling objects or people; may be due to bacterial toxins, drugs, thyrotoxicosis, stress e.g. birth. *See also* PUERPERAL PSYCHOSIS.

**hand presentation** occurs in labour due to uncorrected oblique lie, shoulder presentation with arm prolapse or

in COMPOUND PRESENTATION; on vaginal examination thumb abducts unlike toes, no prominent heel, digits longer than toes.

**haploid** half-number of chromosomes characteristically found in somatic (diploid) cells of organism.

**hard chancre** contagious syphilitic ulcer; may be seen on labium.

**hare lip** *See* CLEFT LIP.

**harlequin fetus** rare genetic skin condition, congenital ICHTHYOSIS; excess keratin layer results in large, diamond-shaped, reddish skin scales limiting movement, easily become fatally infected; eyes, ears, penis and appendages may be abnormally contracted; diagnosed *in utero* by fetal skin biopsy, amniocentesis, 3D ultrasound.

**Hartmann's solution** sodium chloride, sodium lactate, calcium and potassium phosphate solution used intravenously as systemic alkalizer and to replace fluids and electrolytes.

**Hashimoto's disease** postpartum transient autoimmune thyroiditis; occurs in 10% of mothers within 12 months of birth; mild hyperthyroidism followed by hypothyroidism; causes fatigue, painless goitre; may mimic postnatal depression. Recovery usually spontaneous, may recur in next pregnancy or lead to permanent hypothyroidism.

**hashish** hemp plant extract: *Cannabis sativa*; smoked or chewed for euphoric effect; marijuana. Not recommended in pregnancy, as long-term use adversely affects mother or fetus.

**head, fetal** *See* FETAL SKULL.

**headache** pain in head; physiological in first trimester as progesterone dilates cerebral blood vessels; after 20 weeks' gestation may be due to fulminating pre-eclampsia, impending ECLAMPSIA. **Spinal h.** complication of epidural anaesthesia; inadvertent puncture of dura mater causes cerebrospinal fluid loss; persists for several days.

**headbox** Perspex box placed over baby's head into which additional oxygen can be administered.

**head circumference** measurement of suboccipitobregmatic diameter (33 cm) or occipitofrontal diameter (35 cm) of baby's head.

**head fitting** manual attempt to fit non-engaged fetal head into maternal pelvic brim at term or in labour to exclude CEPHALOPELVIC DISPROPORTION; ultrasound provides more accurate, detailed information to assess if vaginal delivery possible.

**Heaf test** form of tuberculin testing.

**healing** restoration of structure and function of injured or diseased tissues, including blood clotting, inflammation and repair.

**health** state of complete physical, mental and social well-being, not merely absence of disease or infirmity.

**health centre** strategically placed community building providing full range of primary healthcare, commonly focused around general practitioner services and facilities for minor surgery.

**Health and Safety at Work Act** legislation dealing with welfare, health and safety of employers and employees; defines structure and authority for regulation and enforcement of workplace health, safety and welfare within United Kingdom.

**health promotion** information and education of individuals, families and communities to prevent disease, improve health and well-being.

**health technology** technological methods for diagnosis and treatment, e.g. medical devices, diagnostic techniques, surgical procedures and other therapeutic interventions.

**health visitor** registered nurse with social and preventive medicine training responsible for health promotion, disease prevention in mothers and children under 5; midwife liaises with HV when care of mother and baby is transferred after tenth postnatal day.

**hearing test** screening test within National Newborn Hearing Screening Programme for early diagnosis and treatment of hearing loss, including OTOACOUSTIC EMISSIONS TEST and AUTOMATED AUDITORY BRAINSTEM RESPONSE TEST (AABR).

**heart** organ that pumps blood into arteries for transfer to every part of body; cardiac output increased in pregnancy due to increased blood volume, body weight, metabolism, size of uterus. **H. disease in pregnancy** pre-existing heart disease may worsen in pregnancy due to extra pressure exerted on heart and circulation; seen more frequently in pregnancy than previously due to delayed motherhood, morbid obesity, immigrant populations, survival to adulthood of girls with **congenital h. disease**; commonest indirect cause of maternal death. Antenatal care shared between obstetrician and cardiologist. **H. defects** include TETRALOGY of Fallot, PATENT DUCTUS ARTERIOSUS. **H. failure** inability of heart to pump sufficient blood to assure normal flow through circulation. *H. murmur* sound in heart region other than normal heart sounds.

**heartburn** burning sensation in chest due to regurgitation of stomach contents into lower oesophagus. In pregnancy, due to relaxation of cardiac sphincter of stomach; may be worse at night, relieved by sleeping propped up on pillows; antacid medications give transient relief.

**heat shield** Perspex shield placed over low-birthweight and/or sick baby in incubator to prevent radiant and convective heat loss.

**Hegar dilators** series of graduated dilators to dilate cervix uteri.

**Hegar's sign** (also known as Goodell's sign) pregnancy sign. Bimanual examination at 6–8 weeks gestation identifies firm cervix and softened isthmus.

**Hellin's law** UK formula to calculate incidence of multiple pregnancy: twins, 1:89 pregnancies; triplets, $1:89^2$; quadruplets, $1:89^3$; less indicative of true incidence, as ASSISTED REPRODUCTION increases chance of multiple pregnancy.

**HELLP syndrome** *H*aemolysis, *E*levated *L*iver proteins, *L*ow *P*latelets, severe coagulation; complication of pregnancy-induced hypertension, occurs from 32–34 weeks' gestation or within 48 hours of birth. Signs, symptoms: malaise, nausea, vomiting, upper abdominal pain, tenderness, non-specific viral-like symptoms; minimal or absent hypertension, proteinuria. Diagnosis: full blood and platelet count, coagulation studies, liver function tests. Positive D-DIMER TEST in pre-eclampsia predictive of those at risk of HELLP. Complications: PLACENTAL ABRUPTION, DISSEMINATED INTRAVASCULAR COAGULATION, renal failure, pulmonary oedema, liver haematoma or rare, usually fatal, hepatic rupture; intrauterine growth retardation, birth asphyxia, fetal/neonatal death. Treatment: intensive/high-dependency care to stabilize condition, expedite birth, prevent complications; corticosteroids to correct abnormal biochemistry, aid fetal maturity. Blood product transfusions to correct coagulopathies; liver transplant if severe hepatic problems.

**HELPERR** mnemonic to aid memory of shoulder dystocia management: *H*elp; *E*pisiotomy; *L*egs (MCROBERTS MANOUVRE); supra*p*ubic *P*ressure; *E*nter vagina (internal rotation); *R*emove posterior arm; *R*oll mother over, try again. *See* APPENDIX 4.

**hemiplegia** paralysis of one side of body.

**hemisphere** half-sphere; one of two halves of cerebrum.

**heparin** anticoagulant formed in liver, circulates in blood. Used to treat thrombosis, subcutaneous or intravenous: prevents conversion of prothrombin to thrombin; rapidly excreted. Does not cross placenta, not excreted in breast milk. Side effects: bleeding, bruising, allergic reactions; heparin-induced thrombocytopenia (rare, potentially life threatening). Long-term use may cause osteoporosis. Protamine sulphate counteracts overdose, but in excess may be anticoagulant. Women on anticoagulants must avoid all herbal remedies that may potentiate anticoagulation.

**hepatic** pertaining to liver.

**hepatitis** inflammation of liver, usually caused by blood-borne viral infection, notifiable disease in UK. *H. A* worldwide endemic acute infection, spread primarily through ingestion of contaminated water; mother-to-baby transmission at birth is rare. Vaccination available. Strict hygiene measures reduce cross-infection risks. *H. B* serious infection; some people are carriers, later developing chronic active hepatitis or fatal hepatic failure unless liver transplant available. If transmitted from mother to baby, immunization given; if baby develops infection, increased risk of later chronic liver disease, cirrhosis, cancer. Spread sexually, via blood transfusion, sharing contaminated needles. *H. C* spread via blood, blood products, sharing intravenous needles, etc.; screening offered to high-risk drug users, hepatitis B/HIV-positive mothers. Most infected people have no symptoms or transient nausea, jaundice. Long-term effects: B-cell lymphoma, chronic liver disease; no vaccination available; optimal delivery route and safety of breastfeeding not yet confirmed.

**hepatomegaly** enlargement of liver.

**hepatosplenomegaly** enlargement of liver and spleen.

**herbal medicine** therapeutic use of plants. All herbal remedies act pharmacologically; many contraindicated in pregnancy, labour, breastfeeding; most interact with medication, many have anticoagulant effects. Avoid routine use in pregnancy; discontinue 2 weeks before elective surgery. Midwives must be adequately trained to advise on herbal remedies. *See also* RASPBERRY LEAF, GINGER.

**hereditary** transmissible or transmitted from parent to offspring; genetically determined.

**heredity** inheritance from parents and ancestors by offspring of physical and mental characteristics, transmitted in genes.

**hermaphrodite** having characteristics of both sexes; partial development of both male and female sex organs; true hermaphrodites rare, but PSEUDO-HERMAPHRODITISM relatively more common.

**hernia** protrusion of peritoneum, abdominal structures through cavity wall defect. *Diaphragmatic h.* protrusion into thorax of abdominal contents due to serious congenital malformation; emergency surgery needed. *Femoral h.* protrusion of bowel loop through femoral canal. *Hiatus h.* protrusion of part of stomach through diaphragm into thorax, may cause severe heartburn in pregnancy. *Inguinal h.* protrusion of bowel through inguinal canal into groin or scrotum; commoner in males, may be present at birth. *Umbilical h.* protrusion of bowel through gap in recti at umbilicus; usually heals spontaneously.

**heroin** morphine-based narcotic used therapeutically as analgesic; also abused illicitly for euphoric effects; can lead to dependence.

**herpes** inflammatory skin eruption; small vesicles. *H. gestationis* pemphigoid autoimmune skin eruption of erythematous blisters in second or third trimester, causing severe irritation; unknown origin, unrelated to herpes virus *H. simplex* or *labialis* 'cold' sore on face or lip. *Genital h.* lesions on cervix, vulva, surrounding skin in women, on penis in men, usually due to type 2 virus. Caesarean section recommended to prevent neonatal herpes if clinical genital tract herpes present within 2 weeks of birth. ***Congenital h. simplex*** serious neonatal generalized vesicular rash, causing encephalitis and death. ***H. zoster*** shingles; painful condition caused by chickenpox virus; eruption follows course of cutaneous nerves.

**heterogeneous** dissimilar, made up of different characteristics.

**heterosexual** 1. pertaining to, characteristics of, or directed towards opposite sex. 2. person sexually attracted to opposite sex.

**heterozygous** carrying dissimilar genes, e.g. man whose blood is rhesus positive, but who may transmit either rhesus-positive or rhesus-negative genes to his children. *cf.* HOMOZYGOUS.

**hiatus** space or gap. ***H. hernia*** See HERNIA.

**Hibitane** See CHLORHEXIDINE.

**high-frequency oscillation ventilation** respiratory ventilation method for extreme prematurity, may be with NITROUS OXIDE; pressure used to reach optimum lung expansion; oscillation (bounce) added to aid gas distribution.

**high-performance liquid chromatography** chromatographic technique that separates compound mixtures to identify, quantify and purify individual components of mixture; used in diagnosis of PHENYLKETONURIA.

**higher education institution** university providing degree and diploma programmes, e.g. midwifery training.

**highly active antiretroviral therapy** See ANTIRETROVIRAL THERAPY.

**hilot** See TRADITIONAL BIRTH ATTENDANT.

**hindwaters** amniotic fluid surrounding fetus, separated from forewaters below presenting part.

**hip examination** neonatal examination to detect developmental hip dysplasia, either by ORTOLANI'S TEST or BARLOW TEST. *See also* CONGENITAL HIP DISLOCATION.

**Hirschsprung's disease** congenital absence of parasympathetic nerve ganglia in anorectum or proximal rectum, leading to absence of peristalsis, enlargement of colon, constipation and obstruction; requires surgical correction. Also called *aganglionic megacolon* or *congenital megacolon*.

**hirsute** hairy. May be seen in POLYCYSTIC OVARY SYNDROME.

**histamine** chemical substance produced in tissue injury; dilatation and increased permeability of capillaries; counteracted by antihistamine drugs; may be factor in anaphylactic shock.

**histogram** graph in which values found in statistical study are represented by lines or symbols placed horizontally or vertically to indicate frequency of distribution.

**histology** visualization of minute structure, composition and function of tissues and organs.

**history taking** detailed record of woman's medical, surgical, obstetric and family history, current pregnancy and lifestyle, taken at first antenatal appointment; forms basis for planning pregnancy, birth and postnatal care. *See also* BOOKING.

**Hodge pessary** devise to correct retroversion of uterus.

**holism** philosophy viewing individual as a functioning whole rather than composite of several systems; mind–body–spirit approach.

**holistic** pertaining to holism; women's physical, emotional, psychological, social, spiritual needs considered interdependent; woman treated as complete person, not merely for presenting condition.

**Homans' sign** pain in calf when foot is dorsiflexed and leg extended; sign of deep vein thrombosis.

**home birth** *Planned h. b.* woman's choice to give birth at home, with community midwife, or INDEPENDENT MIDWIFE; midwife is legally obliged to provide care even when not medically advised. *Unplanned h. b.* baby born unexpectedly or prematurely at home, or when pregnancy is concealed. *See also* UNASSISTED BIRTH.

**home help service** social services department providing domestic and housekeeping assistance to those in need, short term or long term; payment is according to means.

**homeopathy** complementary, energy-based medicine; does not act pharmacologically; unlike HERBAL MEDICINE, will not interact with drugs. Midwives must be appropriately trained to advise on/treat women with homeopathy. *See also* ARNICA.

**homeostasis** ability of body systems to maintain stability, continually adjusting to optimal condition e.g. temperature maintenance.

**homo-** prefix pertaining to similarity, same.

**homogeneous** having same nature, of same composition throughout.

**homologous** having same structure or pattern.

**homosexual** 1. pertaining to same sex. 2. person sexually attracted to someone of same sex.

**homozygous** having a pair of genes that are the same; e.g. homozygous rhesus-positive man can only transmit rhesus-positive genes, and all his children will be rhesus positive even if mother is rhesus negative. *cf.* HETEROZYGOUS.

**hookworm** parasitic roundworm; enters body through skin, usually of feet, migrates to intestines, attaches to intestinal wall, sucks blood, causing blood loss, anaemia; common in insanitary tropical, sub-tropical conditions.

**horizon** specific anatomical stage of embryonic development, of which 23 have been defined, beginning with unicellular fertilized egg and ending 7–9 weeks later with beginning of fetal stage.

**hormone** chemical substance secreted into bloodstream by endocrine gland and exerting effect on some other part of body.

**hourglass constriction** uterine CONSTRICTION RING in third-stage labour; rare cause of placental retention; treatment: anaesthesia.

**Hughes syndrome** *See* ANTIPHOSPHOLIPID SYNDROME.

**human chorionic gonadotrophin** pregnancy hormone produced by embryo, later by TROPHOBLAST; prevents corpus luteum from disintegrating, maintains progesterone to sustain pregnancy; may influence immune tolerance of pregnancy. Present in maternal blood, urine; basis of early pregnancy testing. Levels raised in multiple pregnancy, chorion carcinoma, Down syndrome.

**Human Fertilisation and Embryology Act 2008** law regulating human embryos outside body; sex selection of offspring for non-medical reasons banned; same-sex couples recognized as legal parents of children conceived with donated sperm, eggs, embryos; restricts use of HFEA data to enable infertility treatment research.

**Human Fertilisation and Embryology Authority** statutory regulatory body overseeing use of gametes and embryos in fertility treatment and research; licenses UK centres performing ASSISTED CONCEPTION techniques and undertaking human embryo research.

**human immunodeficiency virus (HIV)** blood-borne retrovirus, pandemic in developing world; transmitted via sexual contact, blood transfusion, sharing contaminated needles, vertical transmission from mother to baby; primarily destroys immune cells, adversely affecting immune system, leads to ACQUIRED IMMUNE DEFICIENCY SYNDROME; prophylactic measures: antiretroviral drugs, avoid vaginal birth, breastfeeding unless viral load very low to reduce incidence of vertical transmission. Care of HIV-positive mothers shared between obstetrician and genitourinary physician.

**human milk banking** service to collect, screen and dispense human milk donated by breastfeeding mothers; milk can be given to babies whose mothers are unable to produce sufficient milk, especially preterm and sick neonates.

**human papillomavirus** virus causing genital warts, cancer of vagina, vulva, cervix, anus in women and penis and anus in men; transmitted through skin-to-skin contact; most common sexually transmitted infection. Infection usually temporary but if persistent, high risk of developing precancerous cervical lesions, leading to invasive cervical cancer; cancer of throat or tongue may result from oral sex. HPV infection can reduce fertility. Vaccination offered to all girls aged 12–13 in UK.

**human placental lactogen** placental hormone that aids growth and development of breast, thought to resemble growth hormone and affect carbohydrate metabolism.

**humerus** bone of upper arm.

**humid** moist.

**humidity** degree of moisture in atmosphere.

**Huntington's disease** chorea; rare hereditary disease; appears in adulthood from 30–45 years of age; mental deterioration, speech disturbance; degenerative changes in cerebral cortex, basal ganglia cause quick involuntary movements; total incapacitation, death.

**Hutchinson's teeth** typical notching of borders of upper incisor teeth occurring in congenital syphilis.

**hyaline** resembling glass. *H. membrane* protein material in alveoli of babies with respiratory distress syndrome; baby has increasing difficulty breathing, with expiratory grunting and rib and sternal recession; preterm babies and those of diabetic mothers particularly at risk; caused by lack of SURFACTANT in lungs, demonstrated at post-mortem examination.

**hyaluronidase** enzyme that hastens absorption of drugs into body tissues. Found in testes, present in semen; increases permeability of connective tissue; disperses cells of corona radiata around newly released ovum, facilitating entry of spermatozoon to ovum.

**hydatidiform mole** vesicular mole; benign TROPHOBLAST neoplasm, precursor of CHORIOCARCINOMA, appears as collection of hydropic vesicles. Incidence: 1 in 2000 pregnancies. Early pregnancy nausea and vomiting often severe but no embryonic development occurs. Treatment: uterus evacuated surgically; regular tests to ensure no regrowth of vesicles which could progress to choriocarcinoma; advise to refrain from conceiving for 2 years.

**hydraemia** 'watering down' of blood, excess plasma in relation to proportion of red blood cells; occurs physiologically in pregnancy.

**hydralazine** antihypertensive vasodilator drug administered intravenously by slow bolus injection or by infusion; safe in pregnancy and breastfeeding; contraindicated in women with tachycardia.

**hydramnios** excessive accumulation of amniotic fluid. *See* POLYHYDRAMNIOS *and* OLIGOHYDRAMNIOS.

**hydro-** prefix signifying water or hydrogen.

**hydrocele** swelling due to fluid accumulation, especially in tunica vaginalis surrounding testicles; common in newborn, usually disappears spontaneously.

**hydrocephalus** congenital malformation; increased cerebrospinal fluid distends ventricles of brain. Often incompatible with life; if mild, baby can be treated by surgery to divert cerebrospinal fluid from ventricles into bloodstream. Suspected antenatally if head fails to engage or persistent breech presentation or through observation of very large fetal head; usually detected on ULTRASOUND SCAN.

**hydrochloric acid** strong acid secreted into gastric juice; chemical symbol, HCl. Very acidic gastric juice (pH $\leq 2.0$) aspirated into lungs; main cause of bronchospasm in MENDELSON SYNDROME.

**hydrocortisone** hormone secreted by adrenal cortex. Synthetic preparations may be used for skin disorders.

**hydrogen** gas that combines with OXYGEN to form water ($H_2O$); symbol H.

**hydrogen ion concentration** proportion of HYDROGEN ions in blood; determines blood pH.

**hydrogen ions** HYDROGEN atoms carrying positive electrical charge; cations.

**hydromeningocele** protrusion of meninges-containing fluid through defect in skull or vertebral column.

**hydromyelomeningocele** defect of spine marked by protrusion of the membranes and tissue of spinal cord, forming fluid-filled sac.

**hydronephrosis** collection of urine in pelves of kidney, causing kidney atrophy due to constant pressure of fluid until whole organ becomes one large cyst; may be congenital, due to malformation of kidney or ureter, or acquired, resulting from obstruction of ureter by tumour or stone, or back pressure from stricture of urethra.

**hydropic vesicles** fluid-filled sacs, or blisters.

**hydrops fetalis** severe oedema of fetus caused by blood incompatibility, usually resulting in either STILLBIRTH or neonatal death.

**hydrosalpinx** distension of fallopian tube by aqueous fluid.

**hydrotherapy** therapeutic use of water to relieve discomfort and promote well-being; e.g. labouring in birthing pool.

**hygiene** health science. *Communal h.* maintenance of community health by provision of pure water supply, efficient sanitation, good housing, etc.

**hygroscopic** readily absorbing moisture.

**hymen** fold of skin, partly occluding vaginal introitus in virgin; ruptured during sexual intercourse, leaving small tags of skin called *carunculae myrtiformes*. *Imperforate h.* membrane that completely occludes vaginal orifice.

**hyoscine (scopolamine)** antisalivary and amnesic drug.

**hyper-** prefix meaning 'excessive' or 'above normal'.

**hyperbilirubinaemia** excess of bilirubin in circulating blood.

**hypercalcaemia** abnormally high concentration of calcium in blood. *Idiopathic h.* neonatal condition; vitamin D intoxication, elevated serum calcium levels, increased skeletal density, mental deterioration and nephrocalcinosis.

**hypercapnia** abnormal increase in carbon dioxide in blood.

**hyperdactyly** presence of supernumerary digits on hand or foot.

**hyperemesis** excessive vomiting. *H. gravidarum* serious complication of pregnancy, severe, persistent vomiting, weight loss of more than 3 kg or 5% on booking weight; cause not fully understood.

**hyperglycaemia** excess of glucose in blood (normal adult value is 3.3–5.3 mmol/L; 60–95 mg/100 mL). Persistent hyperglycaemia is sign of DIABETES MELLITUS.

**hyperkalaemia** abnormally high blood concentration of potassium.

**hypernatraemia** abnormally high serum sodium concentration; plasma sodium above 150 mmol/L; usually due to water depletion and extracellular fluid loss, or excess salt intake e.g. if excessive salt added to artificial milk feeds or baby dehydrated; convulsions occur, can lead to brain damage. Prevention, if baby has diarrhoea: low-sodium feeds, 25%–50% normal strength.

**hyperphenylalaninaemia** excess serum phenylalanine, PHENYLKETONURIA.

**hyperplasia** multiplication of cells, occurs in uterus in pregnancy.

**hyperprolactinaemia** increased prolactin in blood; associated with infertility, may lead to galactorrhoea (excessive or spontaneous milk flow); may cause impotence in men.

**hyperpyrexia** excessive body temperature, over 40°C (104°F).

**hypersalivation** abnormally increased secretion of saliva, PTYALISM.

**hypertension** abnormally high blood pressure, occurring in several diseases, e.g. acute or chronic nephritis, coarctation of aorta. *Essential h.* raised blood pressure, unknown cause, in person otherwise healthy; common in adult population; if untreated or uncontrolled, may lead to damage of blood vessels in heart, brain and kidneys. In pregnancy, blood pressure of 140/90 mm Hg or rise of more than 15–20 mm Hg above first-trimester level is regarded as upper limit of normal. *Pregnancy-induced h.* hypertension in pregnancy, with or without proteinuria, may lead to eclampsia.

**hyperthyroidism** thyrotoxicosis; excessive thyroid gland activity resulting in raised basal metabolic rate and exophthalmos.

**hypertonic** 1. relating to hypertonia, excess tone or tension, as in blood vessel or muscle. *H. action of uterus* abnormal excess uterine muscle tone; very painful contractions, brief respite with inadequate relaxation, prolonged labour; mother becomes exhausted; fetus hypoxic. Mother may benefit from EPIDURAL ANALGESIA, intravenous oxytocin; Caesarean section needed if no progress. 2. applied to solutions stronger than physiological saline, e.g. hypertonic saline.

**hypertrophy** growth, increase in cell size. *See also* HYPERPLASIA.

**hyperventilation** over-breathing; excess carbon dioxide removed from blood; transient respiratory alkalosis common; may occur in labour. Symptoms: faintness, palpitations, pounding heart, muscular spasm of hands, feet. Reassurance to encourage return to normal breathing usually rectifies situation.

**hyperviscosity** excessive viscosity of blood, e.g. in polycythaemia when number of red blood cells is increased; venesection to remove excess red cells may be necessary.

**hypervolaemia** abnormal increase in circulating plasma volume.

**'hypno-birthing'** deep visualisation and relaxation to prepare women for birth. Midwives must be adequately trained to use 'hypno-birthing'. *See also* HYPNOSIS.

**hypnosis, hypnotherapy** deep relaxation, trance-like state; person acts under influence of some external suggestion. *Clinical h.* applied use of hypnotherapeutic suggestions for specific clinical reasons, e.g. birth preparation, needle phobia. Midwives must be adequately trained to use hypnosis.

**hypnotic** agent that produces sleep.

**hypo-** prefix meaning 'lacking in' or 'below normal'.

**hypocalcaemia** low blood calcium. *Neonatal h.* can occur within 48 hours of birth or from fifth to eighth days of life; convulsions occur, especially if baby fed on unmodified cows' milk high in phosphorus; very rare complication of EXCHANGE TRANSFUSION.

**hypocapnia** diminished CARBON DIOXIDE level in blood.

**hypochondria** morbid preoccupation or anxiety with one's health.

**hypochondrium** region of ABDOMEN.

**hypochromic** deficient in pigmentation or colouring, as with red blood cells deficient in iron.

**hypodactyly** less than usual number of digits on hand or foot.

**hypodermic** beneath skin, e.g. injection into subcutaneous tissue. *H. syringe* plastic or glass syringe for hypodermic injections.

**hypofibrinogenaemia** deficiency of fibrinogen in blood; rare, serious cause of postpartum haemorrhage, often associated with disseminated intravascular coagulation, severe placental abruption, amniotic fluid embolism, intrauterine death.

**hypogastric arteries** branches of internal iliac arteries; in fetus pass out into umbilical cord to carry deoxygenated blood to placenta.

**hypogastrium** *See* ABDOMEN.

**hypoglycaemia** abnormally low blood sugar; may develop in diabetic woman if insufficient carbohydrate ingested. *Neonatal h.* blood glucose level below 1.7 mmol/L in term baby, below 1.2 mmol/L if low birthweight; may occur soon after birth in baby of diabetic mother if too much insulin produced for extrauterine needs, or within 24–48 hours of birth in SMALL FOR GESTATIONAL AGE BABY, or in any baby after severe asphyxia, due to lack of glycogen in liver. Fits, APNOEA may occur, lead to brain damage. Prevention in babies at risk: early feeding, hourly screening during first few days of life.

**hypomagnesaemia** abnormally low magnesium content of blood, manifested chiefly by neuromuscular hyperirritability.

**hypomenorrhoea** infrequent menstruation.

**hyponatraemia** deficiency of blood sodium; salt depletion; sodium concentration less than 135 mmol/L. Symptoms: muscular weakness and twitching, progressing to convulsions if unrelieved.

**hypopituitarism** SHEEHAN SYNDROME; anterior pituitary gland deficiency; may occur after severe postpartum haemorrhage; failure of lactation, subsequent amenorrhoea, sterility.

**hypoplasia** under-development of part or organ. *Adj* hypoplastic.

**hypoprothrombinaemia** lack of prothrombin in blood causing bleeding. *See* HAEMORRHAGIC DISEASE OF NEWBORN.

**hypospadias** urinary meatus opens on undersurface of penis.

**hypostatic** pertaining to decreased movement. *H. pneumonia* may develop if mother with eclampsia, lies supine for long periods.

**hypotension** blood pressure below normal. *Postural h.* temporary fall in blood pressure on standing, causes dizziness, fainting; common in pregnancy. *Supine h.* occurs if woman lies flat on back; weight of pregnant uterus compresses inferior vena cava returning blood to heart; causes maternal dizziness, fainting, fetal heart changes.

**hypotensive** pertaining to low blood pressure. *H. drugs* drugs that lower blood pressure, e.g. HYDRALAZINE, BUPIVACAINE HYDROCHLORIDE.

**hypothalamus** part of brain near third ventricle; controls pituitary gland activity, sympathetic and parasympathetic nervous systems, food intake and temperature regulation.

**hypothermia** subnormal body temperature. *Neonatal h.* baby may lose heat rapidly due to body's large surface area, especially if not dried well at birth; worse in preterm infants who lack brown fat to help maintain temperature. Extreme chilling causes baby to use up energy and oxygen; if temperature falls below 35°C, neonatal cold injury develops, which may lead to death.

**hypothesis** theory presented as basis for argument or discussion.

**hypothyroidism** condition resulting from deficiency of thyroid secretion: cretinism in babies, myxoedema in adults.

**hypotonia** deficient muscle tone.

**hypotonic** lacking tone. *H. uterine action* weak, ineffective contractions; leads to prolonged labour unless intravenous oxytocin used. *H. solution* solution more dilute than physiological saline.

**hypovolaemia** abnormally low circulating blood volume.

**hypovolaemic** pertaining to hypovolaemia. *H. shock* haemorrhagic shock; occurs after antepartum or postpartum haemorrhage. Emergency treatment required to maintain airway, administer OXYGEN, replace fluids intravenously; volume of fluid required estimated via central venous pressure line. Midwife should assist with emergency treatment, maintain contemporaneous records, keep woman calm and avoid her overheating.

**hypoxaemia** low OXYGEN tension in arterial blood; low PCO$_2$.

**hypoxia** diminished OXYGEN tension in body tissues. *See* ANOXIA.

**hysterectomy** removal of uterus. *Abdominal h.* removal via abdominal incision. *Subtotal h.* removal of body of uterus only. *Total h.* removal of body of uterus and cervix. *Vaginal h.* removal *per vaginam*. *Wertheim h.* in addition to uterus, fallopian tubes and ovaries, parametrium, upper vagina and all local lymphatic glands are excised: successful method of treatment of cervical cancer.

**hysteria** psychoneurosis; varied symptoms but no organic disease.

**hystero-** pertaining to uterus. *H-oophorectomy* excision of uterus and one or both ovaries. *H-salpingectomy* excision of uterus and one or both uterine tubes. *H-salpingography* radiography of uterus and uterine tubes after instillation of contrast medium. *H-scope* instrument used to gain access to uterus *per vaginam*.

**hysterotomy** operation performed between 12 and 24 weeks' gestation; incision into abdominal wall and uterus to remove ovum or evacuate contents of uterus.

**iatrogenic** caused by treatment.

**ibuprofen** non-steroidal anti-inflammatory and analgesic drug; avoid in first two trimesters of pregnancy but suitable for use postnatally.

**ichthyosis** rare congenital skin abnormality characterized by scaliness and desquamation of skin of whole body.

**icterus** jaundice; yellow staining of skin and mucous membranes due to excess bile pigments in blood and tissues. *I. neonatorum* jaundice of newborn. *I. gravis neonatorum* severe jaundice of newborn, usually caused by rhesus ISOIMMUNIZATION.

**ICSI** *See* INTRACYTOPLASMIC SPERM INJECTION.

**identical** exactly alike. *I. twins* twins of same sex developed from single fertilized ovum; MONOZYGOTIC TWINS.

**identification of baby** babies born in hospital or birth centre should have two labels attached to their wrists, which state name, sex, date and time of birth, in order to avoid errors which could mean baby being given to wrong mother. Information should match case notes and are repeated on cot card. Name bands should remain on baby until transfer home from hospital. If information on wristbands becomes illegible or one band is lost, two new name bands should be prepared, verified by mother and put onto baby's wrists in mother's presence, and replacement documented in notes.

**idiopathic** of unknown cause.

**idoxuridine** analogue that prevents replication of DNA viruses; used topically in herpes simplex keratitis.

**ileocaecal valve** valve at junction of the ileum and the caecum.

**iliococcygeus muscle** deep muscle in pelvic floor, originating from fascial covering of obturator internus muscle and directed posteriorly and medially; converges with pubococcygeus where it inserts into coccyx and lower sacrum.

**ileum** last part of small intestine, terminating at caecum.

**ileus** paralysis of wall of gut; functional obstruction preventing peristaltic action; complication of Caesarean section and other abdominal operations. *Meconium i. See* CYSTIC FIBROSIS.

**iliac** pertaining to ilium. *I. crest* crest of hip bone. *I. fossa* large shallow depression forming much of inner surface of ilium above pelvic brim.

**iliopectineal** pertaining to ilium and pubes. *I. line* ridge crossing innominate bone from sacroiliac joint to *I. eminence*, small protrusion marking fusion of ilium and os pubis.

**ilium** upper broad part of innominate bone.

**imaging** production of diagnostic images, e.g. radiography, ultrasonography, scintigraphy.

**imipramine** tricyclic antidepressant drug used in treatment of perinatal psychiatric disorders, considered safe

http://dx.doi.org/10.1016/B978-0-7020-6906-2.00009-7

in pregnancy. Withdrawal effects may occur in babies of mothers who take it during pregnancy; therefore gradual withdrawal before delivery is usually advocated to reduce effects on baby.

**immature** not mature, insufficiently developed.

**immune** protected against infectious diseases, foreign tissue, foreign non-toxic substances and other ANTIGENS. *I.-reactive trypsin test* blood test to diagnose cystic fibrosis.

**immunity** resistance of body to infectious diseases, foreign tissues, foreign non-toxic substances, other antigens. *Humoral i.* occurs in body fluids; concerned with antibody and complement activities; dependent on B lymphocytes maturing into plasma cells responsible for forming antibodies. *Cell-mediated* or *cellular i.* involves activities that destroy alien, harmful cells; dependent on T lymphocytes concerned with delayed immune responses, e.g. rejection of transplanted organs, defence against some bacterial diseases, allergic reactions, certain autoimmune diseases. *Acquired i.* immunity in response to ANTIGEN; involves change in behaviour of cells, production of antibody as primary response, then sensitization; secondary response produced more quickly, is more marked. *Active i.* natural, i.e. from infectious diseases, or artificial, i.e. from injection of living or dead organisms or products as toxins and toxoids. *Passive i.* natural, e.g. maternal immunoglobulin G (IgG) via placenta protects infant from various infectious diseases for a few months, or acquired, e.g. temporary immunity following injection of antibodies of human

GAMMA GLOBULIN or of animal origin. *Natural* or *innate i.* non-specific; provided by intact cellular epithelial barriers, humoral substances, e.g. COMPLEMENT and LYSOZYME; affected by genetic factors, age, race and hormone levels.

**immunization** rendering immune. *See* VACCINATION.

**immunoglobulin** Ig antibody; chemical compound in GAMMA GLOBULIN; major component of humoral immune response system, synthesized by lymphocytes and plasma cells, found in serum, other body fluids, tissues. IgA, two types with antiviral properties, secretory IgA present in non-vascular fluids, e.g. colostrum, breast milk; IgD, found in trace quantities in serum; IgE, reaginic antibody, increased with allergy; IgG, most abundant, major antibody in secondary humoral response of immunity, crosses placenta; IgM, principally concerned with primary antibody response.

**immunological pregnancy test** diagnostic method for pregnancy: increased serum or urinary HUMAN CHORIONIC GONADOTROPHIN (HCG) detected with immunological techniques, e.g. latex particle agglutination or anti-hCG antibody 'sandwich' assay.

**immunology** science of structure and function of immune system, innate and acquired immunity and laboratory techniques involving interaction of antigens with specific antibodies.

**impacted** driven into, wedged, lodged in narrow strait, e.g. impacted shoulder presentation.

**impaired fasting glucose** metabolic state between normal glucose homeostasis and true diabetic state. Fasting

**Immunization Schedule for Children from Birth to Age 18 Years**

| AGE DUE | IMMUNIZATION |
| --- | --- |
| 3 days | BCG (if tuberculosis in family in previous 6 months); hepatitis B vaccine if mother HBsAg positive |
| 2 months | Diphtheria, tetanus, pertussis (whooping cough), polio and *Haemophilus influenzae* type b (Hib)<br>Pneumococcal infection (PCV)<br>Rotavirus<br>Meningitis B |
| 3 months | Diphtheria, tetanus, pertussis (whooping cough), polio and *Haemophilus influenzae* type b (Hib), second dose<br>Meningitis C<br>Rotavirus, second dose |
| 4 months | Diphtheria, tetanus, pertussis (whooping cough), polio and *Haemophilus influenzae* type b (Hib), third dose<br>Meningitis B, second dose<br>Pneumococcal infection (PCV), second dose |
| 12–13 months | *Haemophilus influenzae* type b (Hib) with meningitis C<br>Meningitis B, second dose<br>Mumps, measles, rubella (MMR)<br>Pneumococcal infection (PCV), third dose |
| 2, 3 and 4 years plus school years 1 and 2 | Children's influenza vaccine annually (nasal spray) |
| From 3 years 4 months to 5 years | Diphtheria, tetanus, pertussis (whooping cough), polio<br>Measles, mumps and rubella (MMR) |
| Girls, 12–13 years | Human papillomavirus (HPV) |
| 13–18 years | Diphtheria, tetanus, polio (booster)<br>Meningitis ACWY |

glucose concentration is lower than those required to diagnose diabetes mellitus, but higher than normal reference range.

**impaired glucose tolerance** metabolic state between normal glucose homeostasis and true diabetic state. Carbohydrate metabolism slightly raises post-prandial blood glucose levels of $\geq 7.8$ mmol/L.

**imperforate** having no opening. *I. anus* congenital malformation in which anal sphincter is closed; requires surgery. May occasionally be masked by leaking of meconium through fistular connection to vagina, bladder or urethra.

**impetigo** skin blisters, raw patches on trunk and buttocks of baby, usually due to STAPHYLOCOCCI or STREPTOCOCCI; severe form, PEMPHIGUS NEONATORUM, is highly contagious.

**Implanon** long-active progestogen contraceptive implant.

**implant** introduction into body tissues of drugs or tissue.

**implantation** act of planting or setting in, e.g. of fertilized ovum in endometrium. *I. bleeding* nidation or decidual bleeding; vaginal bleeding at time and from site of embedding of blastocyst; coincides closely with first missed menstrual period and may cause erroneous calculation of estimated date of delivery.

**implementation** third stage of midwifery care process; preceded by ASSESSMENT and planning, followed by EVALUATION.

**impotence** absence of sexual power; man is unable to achieve or maintain penile erection of sufficient rigidity to perform sexual intercourse successfully. *Adj* impotent.

**impregnate** 1. to saturate or instill. 2. to render pregnant.

**imprinting** species specific, rapid learning in critical period of early life in which social attachment and identification are established.

**inborn errors of metabolism** rare inherited disorders, occurs in 1:5000 births, mainly due to enzyme deficiencies, usually autosomal recessive; includes PHENYLKETONURIA and GALACTOSAEMIA.

**incarcerated** imprisoned, held fast. *Retroverted i. gravid uterus* retroverted pregnant uterus that does not antevert spontaneously; by 14 weeks' gestation it becomes trapped under sacral promontory and cannot rise out of pelvis; may lead to acute retention of urine, abortion or, very rarely, SACCULATION OF UTERUS.

**incest** sexual activity between persons closely related; marriage is legally or culturally prohibited. *Adj* incestuous.

**incidence** number of particular events occurring in population in given period, e.g. number of stillbirths per 1000 live births per annum.

**incident** event. *Pl* incidents. *Critical i.* any event occurring within maternity services (or other healthcare setting) that has stressful impact sufficient to overwhelm coping skills of individual or group, typically sudden, powerful events outside range of ordinary clinical experience. Any midwife involved in critical incident should have opportunity to debrief and reflect on event with named supervisor of midwives; managerial evaluation may include all staff involved considering how similar event may be avoided.

**incidental haemorrhage** uncommon vaginal bleeding due to extraplacental causes, e.g. cervical polyps, erosion, acute vaginitis, cervical carcinoma; diagnosed on speculum examination, rarely leads to dangerous haemorrhage; treatment is that of cause.

**inclusion criteria** characteristics that prospective research subjects must have to be included in the study.

**incompatible** mutually repellent, unsuitable for combination; possible cause of miscarriage due to mismatch between ovum and sperm.

**incompatibility** state of being incompatible, applied to blood or chemicals, etc.

**incomplete miscarriage** See MISCARRIAGE.

**incontinence** inability to control excretory functions. *I. of urine* enuresis. *Stress i.* involuntary escape of urine resulting from strain on orifice of bladder, as in coughing, sneezing or laughing. *Faecal i.* may occur after delivery if mother sustains third-degree tear involving anal sphincter.

**incoordinate** lacking in harmony. *I. uterine action* failure of POLARITY, resulting in weak, ineffectual contractions with delay in first stage of labour and poor, irregular cervical dilatation; oxytocic drugs are used to coordinate rather than accelerate uterine action.

**incubate** to place in optimal situation with suitable temperature, humidity, oxygen concentration for development of living matter.

**incubation period** time elapsing between invasion of body by pathogenic micro-organisms and clinical manifestation of disease, e.g. chickenpox, 14–15 days; diphtheria, 2–4 days; measles, 10–14 days; mumps, 14–28 days; rubella, 17–18 days; scarlet fever, 2–4 days; smallpox, 10–14 days; whooping cough, 7–14 days.

**incubator** 1. apparatus providing suitable environment for low-birthweight or sick babies. 2. heated apparatus used to culture micro-organisms in laboratory.

**independent midwife** self-employed midwife; contracts directly with pregnant women; practice must be contemporary, research based and of highest standard; midwife is personally accountable for practice, must notify intention to practise in each area of work.

**independent prescribers** midwives who have successfully completed approved course to make diagnoses, prescribe medication appropriate to field of expertise and competence, including all prescription-only medicines, some controlled drugs.

**index notation** small raised number used to indicate number of times a quantity must be multiplied by 10, e.g. $100 = 10 \times 10 = $ index $10^2$. Fractions of unit – index have minus sign representing number of times quantity should be divided by 10, e.g. $0.1 = 1/10 = $ index $10^{-1}$; $0.01 = 1/100 = $ index $10^{-2}$.

**indigenous** occurring naturally in certain locality.

**indirect antiglobulin test (IAT)** used in matching of blood products before blood transfusion. *See* COOMBS' TEST.

**indomethacin** anti-inflammatory, analgesic, antipyretic agent, used in arthritic disorders and degenerative bone disease; prostaglandin inhibitor, reducing uterine activity; may also be used in neonates to treat PATENT DUCTUS ARTERIOSUS.

**induction** causing to occur. *I. of labour* artificially starting labour with prostaglandin pessaries, amniotomy or intravenous oxytocin, performed when fetal or maternal health is endangered, e.g. poor fetal growth or well-being, maternal diabetes, hypertension, cardiac or renal disease, poor obstetric history, antepartum haemorrhage, breech presentation, postmaturity. *See also* BISHOP SCORE.

**inertia** sluggishness. *Uterine i.* hypotonic uterine action; inefficient contraction of myometrium; may cause prolonged labour.

**inevitable** that which cannot be avoided. *I. abortion* See ABORTION. *I. haemorrhage* See PLACENTA PRAEVIA.

**infant** baby from birth to 1 year of age. *I. feeding* breast and artificial feeding. *Preterm i.* baby born before 37 weeks' gestation.

**infant mortality rate** number of registered INFANT deaths for every 1000 registered live births in any given year.

**infanticide** murder of INFANT.

**infantile paralysis** POLIOMYELITIS.

**infarct** area of necrosis in organ caused by local ischaemia. *Placental i.* necrosis due to obstruction of local circulation caused by fibrin deposits in INTERVILLOUS spaces, so that any VILLI in area die from ischaemia; initially deep red, subsequently changing through brown and yellow to white after about a week. Infarcts occur in PLACENTAL ABRUPTION and hypertensive conditions, e.g. pre-eclampsia; large areas of infarct may cause fetus to die or be SMALL FOR GESTATIONAL AGE.

**infarction** formation of an infarct. *Pulmonary i.* necrosis of lung tissue, caused by embolus.

**infection** invasion of tissues by pathogenic micro-organisms, entering body through nose, mouth, vagina, open wounds or contact with FOMITES. Body forms ANTIBODIES, INFLAMMATION occurs. *Aerobic i.* infection caused by aerobe. *Airborne i.* infection by inhalation of organisms in water droplets or dust particles. *Anaerobic i.* infection caused by ANAEROBE. *Cross i.* infection transmitted between patients. *Droplet i.* due to inhalation of respiratory pathogens in liquid particles exhaled by infected person. *Endogenous i.* 1. infection due to reactivation of organisms in dormant focus, e.g. tuberculosis; 2. caused by organisms present in or on body. *Exogenous i.* caused by organisms not normally present in body but which gain entrance from others' body or from environment. *Nosocomial i.* hospital-acquired infection. *Opportunistic i.* caused by micro-organism not normally causing disease but which may do so when person's resistance lowered, e.g. after severe postpartum haemorrhage. *Secondary i.* infection occurring during or after treatment of existing infection. *Sexually transmitted i.* infection transmitted by intimate, oral or rectal contact.

**inferior longitudinal sinus** venous sinus within tentorium cerebelli; drains blood away from head; joins with great vein of Galen and straight sinus at *confluens sinuum*, which tears if excess or rapid fetal skull moulding occurs, leading to tentorial tears and intracranial haemorrhage. See FETAL SKULL.

**infertility** complete inability to conceive; may be primary or secondary. *See also* SUBFERTILITY.

**infestation** animal parasites on or within body.

**infibulation** process of fastening, e.g. joining wound edges with clasps during surgery; performed in FEMALE GENITAL MUTILATION when labia are joined together to reduce vestibular introitus.

**infiltration** entrance and diffusion of liquid. *I. analgesia* injection of lidocaine (lignocaine) into tissues.

**inflammation** series of tissue changes as reaction to mechanical, chemical or bacterial trauma; heat, swelling, pain, redness, loss of function occurs. *Acute i.* of sudden onset, marked, progressive signs. *Chronic i.* inflammation, slow progress, formation of new connective tissue.

**influenza** acute, epidemic, viral respiratory tract infection, with fever, generalized aching, limb pain and minor respiratory symptoms; in severe cases, pneumonia may follow due to secondary bacterial infection.

**informed consent** providing sufficient information to enable mother to make decision based on knowledge and understanding of positive and negative aspects of situation.

**infra-** prefix meaning 'below'.

**infundibulum** funnel shaped; fimbriated end of fallopian tube.

**infusion** 1. process of extracting soluble principles of substances (especially drugs) by soaking in water. 2. treatment by introducing fluid into body, e.g. dextrose or saline.

**ingestion** introduction of food and drugs by mouth.

**inguinal** relating to groin. *I. canal* channel through abdominal wall, above POUPART'S LIGAMENT, through which spermatic cord and vessels pass to testicle in male; contains round ligament of uterus in female. *I. hernia* See HERNIA.

**inhalational analgesia** nitrous oxide and oxygen inhaled from specially-designed machines, used as pain relief in labour. See ENTONOX.

**inheritance** passing on of certain genetic characteristics from parents to child *Autosomal dominant i.* abnormal gene from one parent can cause disease, even though matching gene from other parent is normal, i.e. abnormal gene dominates. *Autosomal recessive i.* both genes in pair abnormal i.e. both parents carry defective gene. *Mendelian i.* means by which genes and traits are passed from parents to children. *X-linked inheritance*. mode of inheritance in which one pair of genes carries a particular characteristic, one gene being dominant over the other; 50% chance of baby being affected.

**inhibin** hormone secreted by gonads in both men and women, inhibit production of FOLLICLE-STIMULATING HORMONE. Control production of gametes and embryonic and fetal development. *Inhibin A.* biochemical MARKER used in second-trimester Down syndrome screening: affected pregnancies have increased levels, but levels may also be influenced by smoking. Inhibin A results are added to results of TRIPLE TEST to calculate risk of Down syndrome, i.e. QUADRUPLE TEST.

**inhibition** arresting or restraining.

**inhibitor** agent that interferes with or inhibits reaction.

**iniencephaly** rare congenital neural tube defect that combines extreme retroflexion of head with severe defects of spine.

**injection** introduction of liquid into body via syringe or other instrument. *Epidural i.* into epidural space. *Intradermal i.* into skin. *Intramuscular i.* into muscles. *Intrathecal i.*

into theca of spinal cord. *Intravenous i.* into vein. *Subcutaneous i.* below skin.

**inlet (pelvic)**   brim, or entrance to true pelvis. See PELVIS.

**innate**   inborn; present in individual at birth.

**inner cell mass**   group of cells in blastocyst cavity from which amniotic membrane and fetus develops.

**innervation**   nerve distribution to organ or part of body.

**innominate**   without a name. *I. artery* branch of aortic arch. *I. bone* hip bone of fused ilium, ischium, os pubis. See PELVIS.

**inoculation**   introduction into body of protective substance, e.g. antitoxin or vaccine.

**inquest**   legal or judicial inquiry into some matter of fact. *Coroner's i.* held in cases of sudden, unexplained death to determine cause.

**insemination**   introduction of semen into vagina or cervix. *Artificial i.* insemination by other means than sexual intercourse.

**insertion**   attachment point, e.g. of muscle to bone, cord to placenta.

**insidious**   applied to disease, condition developing imperceptibly.

**insomnia**   inability to sleep.

**inspection**   looking. Initial part of antenatal abdominal examination: midwife observes mother's abdomen for size, shape, scars, STRIAE GRAVIDARUM, presence of LINEA NIGRA and fetal movements.

**inspiration**   drawing in breath.

**instillation**   pouring liquid into cavity drop by drop, e.g. into eye.

**instrumental delivery**   vaginal birth of baby with instruments, e.g. FORCEPS, VACUUM EXTRACTOR, SYMPHYSIOTOMY.

**insufficiency**   inadequate function. *Placental i.* failure of placenta to fulfill its function adequately, often associated with pre-eclampsia, essential hypertension, chronic nephritis, postmaturity, heavy smoking; fetus is SMALL FOR GESTATIONAL AGE or dies *in utero.*

**insufflation**   blowing of gas, fluid or powder into cavity. *I. of the fallopian tubes* blowing of CARBON DIOXIDE or methylene blue dye via uterus into fallopian tubes to test patency.

**insulin**   hormone produced in islets of Langerhans in pancreas that regulates carbohydrate metabolism; deficiency causes DIABETES MELLITUS; overdosage of insulin preparations leads to HYPOGLYCAEMIA. *I.-like growth factor* hormones that stimulate protein synthesis; involved in uterine, placental and early embryonic growth. *I. resistance* lowered response to insulin, causes body to produce larger quantities of insulin to maintain blood glucose. May lead to metabolic dysfunctions of diabetes, metabolic syndrome (X), OBESITY and POLYCYSTIC OVARY SYNDROME.

**integrated test**   two-stage Down syndrome screening test: maternal blood is assessed for PREGNANCY-ASSOCIATED PLASMA PROTEIN-A (PAPP-A) and NUCHAL TRANSLUCENCY ultrasound scan is performed; later, TRIPLE or QUADRUPLE TEST is performed. Results of both stages are combined with maternal age-related Down syndrome risk for overall result; test is controversial, as parents are not informed of results until second stage is complete.

**intention to practise**   statutory requirement of UK-registered midwives intending to practise; completed annually and at any time when midwife intends to provide midwifery care in health authority other than usual one.

**inter-** prefix signifying 'between'.

**interaction** quality, state or process of (two or more things) acting on each other. *Drug i.* action of one drug on effectiveness or toxicity of another.

**intercellular** between cells, i.e. the tissue spaces.

**intercostal** between ribs. *I. muscles* those of chest wall.

**intermittent** having intervals or pauses, not continuous, e.g. intermittent uterine contractions to allow fetal oxygenation.

**intermittent mandatory ventilation** method of weaning baby from ventilator by gradually reducing ventilator pressure and respiratory rate settings.

**intermittent positive pressure ventilation** respiratory therapy using VENTILATOR to treat patients with inadequate breathing, e.g. babies who are preterm or suffering from respiratory difficulties. *See also* VENTILATION, RESPIRATORY DISTRESS SYNDROME.

**internal** pertaining to the inside *I. bimanual compression* emergency management of severe postpartum haemorrhage; right fist inserted in vagina towards anterior vaginal fornix, left hand applies abdominal pressure behind uterus, pulls it forwards towards symphysis pubis. Hands are pushed together, compressing uterus and placental site, pressure maintained until uterus contracts, remains retracted. *See also* APPENDIX 2, POSTPARTUM HAEMORRHAGE *I. conjugate See* DIAGONAL CONJUGATE. *I. os* cervical opening into body of uterus.

**International Baby Food Action Network** organizational network aiming to reduce infant, child mortality, promote breastfeeding.

**intersex** abnormality of sex chromosomes, gonads, sex hormones or genitalia. *See* KLINEFELTER SYNDROME *and* TURNER SYNDROME.

**interspinous** between the (ischial) spines. *See* PELVIS.

**interstitial** between body tissues.

**intertrigo** erythematous skin eruption on apposed surfaces, e.g. groin or armpit, caused by moisture, warmth, friction, sweat retention and infection; usually treated with good hygiene measures and application of zinc oxide talcum powder.

**intervillous** between (chorionic) villi; intervillous spaces allow maternal arterial blood to cascade around terminal placental villi where gaseous exchange and transport of amino acids, glucose, minerals and vitamins take place.

**intestine** part of alimentary canal between stomach and anus. *Small i.* first 7 m (20 ft) from pylorus to caecum, consisting of duodenum, jejunum and *ileum. Large i.* 2 m in length; consists of caecum, vermiform appendix, ascending, transverse, descending and pelvic colon, rectum; completes digestive process; eliminates waste.

**intra-** prefix signifying 'within'.

**intracellular** within cell. *I. organisms* those that invade cells, e.g. gonococci. *I. fluid* fluid within cells of body.

**intracranial** within cranium. *I. membranes* meninges covering brain; vertical fold in midline between cerebral hemispheres forms falx cerebri, joining posteriorly horizontal fold of tentorium cerebelli, which separates cerebellum and cerebrum. Membranes contain blood vessels (sinuses); undue pressure or trauma during delivery may cause tearing of membranes and sinuses leading to cerebral haemorrhage. *I. pressure* pressure exerted by cerebrospinal fluid within subarachnoid space and ventricles of brain, measured by monitoring pressure within cerebral ventricles.

**intracytoplasmic sperm injection** *in vitro* fertilization procedure, usually for male infertility, or when sperm donor is used; single sperm injected directly into oocyte.

**intraepithelial** within the epithelium.

**intragastric** within stomach. *I. tube feeding* artificial feeding, e.g. by nasogastric tube.

**intrahepatic cholestasis of pregnancy** idiopathic condition, occurs in 7 per 1000 pregnancies. Usually third trimester; resolves spontaneously after delivery, often recurs in next pregnancy; possibly due to bile metabolism changes, inherited oestrogen hypersensitivity, geographical, environmental factors; bile accumulation in maternal blood, nocturnal pruritus without rash, in extremities or more generally, fatigue, insomnia; later mild jaundice persists until delivery, dark urine, pale stools, abdominal pain, nausea, vomiting. Increased serum bile acid affects placental blood flow, fetal steroid metabolism. Risks: preterm labour, fetal compromise, meconium staining, stillbirth. Investigations: blood tests for bile acids, alkaline phosphatase, bilirubin, transaminases, hepatic viral studies, hepatobiliary tract ultrasound scan, autoantibody screen. Treatment:

local antihistamines, vitamin K to prevent hypoprothrombinaemia, elective delivery after 35 weeks' gestation.

**intramuscular** within or into muscle.

**intrapartum** within or during parturition or labour.

**intraperitoneal** within peritoneal cavity. *I. transfusion* introduction of rhesus-negative red blood cells to replace haemolyzed rhesus-positive cells in rhesus isoimmunization, to prolong life of fetus.

**intrathecal administration** method of administering drugs via spinal canal, as in spinal anaesthesia.

**intrauterine** within uterus. *I. contraceptive device* contraceptive device inserted in uterine cavity increases tubal motility, renders endometrium less favourable for implantation, may increase prostaglandin production, increasing likelihood of expulsion of conceptus. *I. death* death of fetus in utero. *I. growth restriction* fetal growth less than normal. Causes: hypertension, pre-eclampsia, diabetes mellitus, smoking, alcohol misuse, major medical conditions, drugs, young or elderly mothers, malnourished, underweight women; multiple pregnancy, chromosomal and genetic disorders, intrauterine infection; placental abruption, placenta praevia, abnormal cord insertion, single umbilical artery, chorioamnionitis. Fetal growth may be asymmetrical (acute): fetal weight out of proportion with length and head circumference, or symmetrical (chronic): all measurements in proportion. Symmetric growth in genetically small babies treated in accordance with gestational age.

*See also* SMALL FOR GESTATIONAL AGE baby. *I. transfer* transfer of pregnant woman to maternity unit with facilities for neonatal intensive care, e.g. very preterm labour. *I. transfusion* antenatal procedure to treat severe fetal anaemia of HAEMOLYSIS from maternal rhesus ALLOIMMUNIZATION or due to PARVOVIRUS B19 infection; performed in specialist fetal medicine centre to avoid risk of miscarriage, preterm labour, fetal death. CORDOCENTESIS determines fetal haemoglobin levels, facilitates accurate calculation of transfusion requirements. May be repeated every 2–3 weeks until birth of baby safer than continuing pregnancy.

**intravascular** within blood vessel. *I. coagulation* blood clotting in circulation. *See* DISSEMINATED INTRAVASCULAR COAGULATION.

**intravenous** within vein.

**intraventricular haemorrhage** serious cerebral haemorrhage occurring in preterm infants below 34 weeks' gestation causing APNOEA and death; most common lethal condition in very-low-birthweight infants; diagnosed by COMPUTED TOMOGRAPHY or REAL-TIME SCANNER (ultrasound).

**intrinsic** relating to quality of structure or substance, which is inherent within itself.

**introitus** entrance to cavity of body, e.g. entrance to vagina.

**intubation** introduction of tube. *Endotracheal i.* introduction of catheter into trachea; e.g. in asphyxiated infant, under direct vision laryngoscopy, then controlled pressure oxygen or air insufflation.

**intussusception** prolapse of one part of intestine into lumen of immediately adjacent part, causing intestinal obstruction; may occur during first year of life.

**inversion** in genetics, rearrangement of part of chromosome.

**inversion of uterus** turning inside out of uterus, rare, serious labour complication, usually due to mismanaged third-stage labour; occasionally spontaneous. Sudden profound maternal shock, severe abdominal pain, with bleeding if there is placental separation. On palpation, concave-shaped fundus felt, or no uterus felt at all if inversion complete, uterus in cervix or vagina, felt on vaginal examination or visible at vulva. Raise foot of bed to reduce tension and shock; summon doctor to replace uterus. If replacement of totally inverted uterus impossible, place it inside vagina to reduce traction on fallopian tubes and ovaries. Severe shock treated by replacing fluids, blood, narcotic analgesia; general anaesthetic to replace uterus manually or hydrostatic method used. In rare cases, hysterectomy required. *Acute i.* spontaneous in third-stage labour, or due to forceful fundal pressure or umbilical cord traction applied when uterus relaxed and placenta incompletely separated; causes extreme shock; uterus must be replaced immediately.

**in vitro** within glass, observable in test tube, in artificial environment. *I. v. fertilization* artificial fertilization of ovum harvested from woman, combined with spermatozoa under laboratory conditions; fertilized ovum is replaced in woman's uterus.

**in vivo** within living body.

**involution** returning to normal size after enlargement, e.g. uterus after labour by process of ischaemia and AUTOLYSIS. Soluble end product removed by bloodstream; thrombosed uterine blood vessels are self-digested, new vessels form; placental site contracts and disappears below pubic bone by sixth or seventh week. *See also* SUBINVOLUTION.

**iodide** compound of iodine.

**iodine** non-metallic element with distinctive odour, obtained from seaweed. *Tincture of i.* preparation most commonly used. Radioactive iodine is used to evaluate thyroid activity. *See also* ISOTOPE.

**ion** electrically charged atom(s) formed when electrolyte dissolves in water. HYDROGEN ions carry positive charge; hydroxyl ions negative charge. HYDROGEN ion concentration of fluid determines its acidity, expressed as its pH.

**iron** metallic element, constituent of haemoglobin. Iron compounds ingested in food are converted for use by action of stomach hydrochloric acid, which separates iron from food and combines with it in form readily assimilated by body; vitamin C enhances and administration of alkali hampers iron absorption. Adult requires 15 mg iron daily. Iron deficiency anaemia common in pregnancy due to increased demands on mother's blood; iron-rich foods advised, supplements may be prescribed. *I. deficiency anaemia See* ANAEMIA.

**ischaemia** local insufficiency of blood supply.

**ischaemic** pertaining to ischaemia. In ischaemia kidneys secrete RENIN to act on serum plasma protein, produce ANGIOTENSIN I, converted to angiotensin II by lung enzyme, causes vasoconstriction, increases peripheral resistance,

blood pressure. Angiotensin II influences sodium, water retention, increases aldosterone secretion, raising blood pressure. *I. heart disease* coronary artery disease in which narrowed or blocked arteries lead to hypertension, angina, myocardial infarction. Incidence in pregnancy is increasing due to pregnancies later in life and to morbid obesity.

**ischial** pertaining to ischium.

**ischiocavernosus muscle** muscle extending from ischium of pelvis to clitoris or penis, aiding in their erection.

**ischiococcygeus muscle** muscle extending from pelvic ischium to coccyx; posterior portion of levator ani muscle.

**ischium** lower posterior part of innominate bone of pelvic girdle.

**isoimmunization** immunization within species, as in rhesus-negative woman if rhesus-positive. *See also* RHESUS INCOMPATIBILITY.

**isolation** separation of infected person from those not infected.

**isometric** maintaining, or pertaining to, same length; of equal dimensions.

**isoniazid** antibacterial compound used for treating tuberculosis.

**isotonic** of same strength or tension. *I. solution* of same osmotic pressure as fluid with which it is compared, e.g. normal saline is isotonic with blood plasma.

**isotope** form of element having same atomic number, i.e. number of protons in nucleus, as another element, but different number of NEUTRONS; leads to instability, often with emission of radioactivity, making even minute quantities identifiable with Geiger counter.

**isoxsuprine hydrochloride** beta-adrenergic stimulant used as vasodilator in peripheral vascular disease and cerebrovascular insufficiency; used intravenously to arrest preterm labour by relaxing myometrium.

**isphaghula** oral laxative that works by increasing faecal mass.

**isthmus** *See* UTERUS.

**itching in pregnancy** pruritus; abdominal skin itching common; women with generalized itching or itching starting on palms should be referred to obstetrician as may be due to INTRAHEPATIC CHOLESTASIS OF PREGNANCY, hepatic or thyroid disease, lymphoma or scabies.

**Jacquemier's sign** blueness of vaginal lining due to increased blood supply in early pregnancy.

**Jarisch-Herxheimer reaction** reaction to endotoxin-like products released by death of micro-organisms within body during antibiotic treatment. Causes acute febrile illness, chills, myalgia, headache, hypotension, tachycardia.

**jaundice** icterus; yellow staining of skin, sclera, mucous membranes from excess bile pigments in blood, tissues. *Haemolytic j.* bile pigment from haemoglobin of haemolyzed erythrocytes. *Obstructive j.* bile pigment present as constituent of bile. Pregnancy jaundice rare but serious consequence of HYPER-EMESIS GRAVIDARUM, ECLAMPSIA, INTRAHE-PATIC CHOLESTASIS OF PREGNANCY, acute liver atrophy, hepatitis or drugs. *Breast milk j.* raised unconjugated bilirubin may occur in breastfed baby; milk steroid inhibits glucuronyl transferase-conjugating activity. *Infectious j.* may be due to infectious hepatitis or leptospirosis. *Physiological j.* due to haemolysis of excess fetal erythrocytes no longer required; red blood cells break down to fat-soluble bilirubin, conjugate into water-soluble bilirubin, liver enzyme, glucuronyl transferase, aids excretion. Baby's immature liver causes bilirubin to accumulate in blood, leak into tissues, skin and sclerae to become yellow. Phototherapy needed if serum bilirubin very high to avoid kernicterus. *See also* SERUM BILIRUBIN.

**jejunum** small intestine from duodenum to ileum.

**jelly** soft, resilient substance, usually colloidal semi-solid mass. *Contraceptive j.* non-greasy jelly inserted in vagina to prevent conception.

**jitteriness** neonatal tremulous twitching, occasional colic contractions. Differentiate from seizures: when pressure is applied to tremulous limb, movement stops with jitteriness, continues if it is a seizure.

**Johnson manoeuvre** technique to replace uterus manually in acute INVERSION; steady pressure applied to fundus with palm of hand, towards vaginal posterior fornix, then towards umbilicus.

**joint** articulating bone junction, enabling motion and flexibility.

**joule (J)** international (SI) unit, measures food energy.

**jugular** concerning neck. *J. veins* carry blood away from head.

**justominor pelvis** small gynaecoid pelvis, diameters reduced proportionately.

**juxtaposition** apposition; side by side or close together.

http://dx.doi.org/10.1016/B978-0-7020-6906-2.00010-3

**kalaemia** potassium in blood.

**kalium** potassium; symbol K.

**Kallman syndrome** delayed or absent puberty, impaired sense of smell, form of hypogonadotropic hypogonadism that affects production of hormones responsible for sexual development.

**kanamycin** broad-spectrum antibiotic effective against many gram-negative bacteria, some gram-positive and acid-fast bacteria.

**kangaroo care** system aimed at promoting closeness between mother and preterm or ill baby by positioning baby between mother's breasts, encouraging skin-to-skin contact.

**Kaposi's sarcoma** multifocal, metastasizing, malignant reticulosis with angiosarcoma features, major feature of AIDS.

**karyo-** prefix, 'nucleus'.

**karyotype** number and structure of chromosomes in cell nucleus, normally 46 chromosomes: 22 autosomal pairs (AUTOSOMAL INHERITANCE), 1 pair of sex chromosomes (XX female, XY male). Karyotyping identifies chromosome size, aids diagnosis of disorders, e.g. DOWN SYNDROME.

**Kell blood system** group of antigens on erythrocyte surface, important determinants of blood type; targets for autoimmune or alloimmune diseases that destroy red blood cells.

**keloid** overgrowth of fibrous tissue in scar.

**keratin** tough protein that forms base of horny tissues.

**keratitis** inflammation of cornea.

**kernicterus** bilirubin toxicity; yellow staining of kernel cells in brain's basal ganglia; occurs in severe neonatal jaundice, in rhesus ISOIMMUNIZATION; unconjugated serum bilirubin above 350 μmol/L (20 mg/100 mL) (lower in preterm or seriously ill baby). Signs: irritability, fits, athetoid arm movements; mental or neurological disability, death. Treatment: replacement blood transfusions or phototherapy.

**Kernig's sign** person unable to straighten leg at knee joint when thigh supported at right angle to trunk; sign of meningitis.

**ketoacidosis** electrolyte imbalance; ketosis and lowered blood pH.

**ketones** acetone, acetoacetic acid, β-hydroxybutyric acid; normal metabolic products of lipids and pyruvate in liver, oxidized by muscles; acetone also arises spontaneously from acetoacetic acid; excess ketones are excreted in urine, as in diabetes mellitus.

**ketonuria** ketones in urine.

**ketosis** excess ketones, with sweet breath odour, e.g. in uncontrolled DIABETES MELLITUS, from raised fatty acid metabolism, impaired carbohydrate metabolism. Eating carbohydrate reverses it.

**kick chart** *See* FETAL MOVEMENT CHART.

**kidneys** two bean-shaped organs near lower thoracic, upper lumbar vertebrae, behind peritoneum. Cortex

http://dx.doi.org/10.1016/B978-0-7020-6906-2.00011-5

and medulla with 1 million nephrons. Functions: maintain water balance, solute content, osmotic pressure, plasma pH; regulate blood pressure; waste product excretion, especially nitrogen. *See also* ISCHAEMIA.

**Kiellands forceps** obstetric forceps with sliding lock with no pelvic curve; enable rotation of fetal head to occipitoanterior position.

**kilo-** prefix indicating 'one thousand', e.g. kilogram (kg), 1000 grams; kilocalorie (kcal), 1000 calories.

**kilocalorie** unit of energy, 1000 calories; measures body heat and food energy. Pregnant or breastfeeding women need 2500 kcal/day; term baby needs 110 kcal/kg body weight/day.

**Kiwi** commercially produced suction cup for ventouse birth; allows greater control than other types.

*Klebsiella* genus of gram-negative bacteria.

**Klebs–Löffler bacillus** diphtheria bacillus.

**Kleihauer test** blood test to confirm presence of fetal cells in maternal circulation after ANTEPARTUM HAEMORRHAGE, placental ABRUPTION etc.; false-negative results occur with haemolysis of fetal cells in maternal circulation, e.g. after rhesus sensitization.

**Klinefelter syndrome (XXY syndrome)** additional X chromosome in males; incidence about 1:500–1:1000 male births; detected antenatally from CHORIONIC VILLUS SAMPLING, AMNIOCENTESIS; in child from language or developmental delay; in adult from sterility or gynaecomastia; treatment involves testosterone administration.

**Klumpke paralysis, Klumpke palsy** lower arm and hand paralysis, wrist drop; due to eighth cervical,

first dorsal nerve injury in lower BRACHIAL PLEXUS; may occur in birth of extended arms in breech birth, or from excess anterior shoulder traction in cephalic birth.

**knee–chest position** maternal position encouraged in event of cord prolapse, prevents fetal pressure on cord: raising pelvis and buttocks causes fetus to gravitate towards maternal diaphragm.

**knee presentation** knee below buttocks in breech presentation.

**Kocher forceps** artery forceps; used to clamp umbilical cord; artificial membrane rupture.

**Konakion** *See* PHYTOMENADIONE.

**Koplik spots** small, irregular, red buccal and lingual mucosa spots with tiny bluish white centre; may occur in early stage of measles.

**Korotkoff sounds** sounds heard in artery while pressure in inflated cuff reduced, enabling blood pressure measurement. *Korotkoff 1* clear rhythmical tapping as cuff is deflated, represents systolic pressure. *Korotkoff 2* murmur, swishing sound. *Korotkoff 3* crisp, intense tapping. *Korotkoff 4* muffled, low-pitched sound, easier to record in pregnancy than *Korotkoff 5* no sound; represents diastolic pressure. In pregnancy, muffled tapping may be heard to 0 when cuff fully deflated.

**kraurosis vulvae** dryness, atrophy of vulva.

**kwashiorkor** severe protein deficiency; symptoms in babies and children include oedema, impaired growth and development, abdominal distension, pathological liver changes, pigmentation changes of skin and hair.

**kyphosis** posterior curvature of spine.

# I

**labetalol hydrochloride** oral or intravenous alpha- and beta-adrenergic receptor blocker used in hypertension.

**labia** lips. *L. majora* large fold of flesh surrounding vulva. *L. minora* lesser fold within. *Sing* labium.

**labial** pertaining to labia.

**labile** unstable, liable to variation. *L. hypertension* blood pressure that varies between normal and higher level.

**labour** parturition, childbirth. *Augmentation of l.* artificial acceleration of labour by membrane rupture or oxytocin infusion in prolonged labour. *Induction of l.* medical means of starting labour by artificial membrane rupture, vaginal or intravenous hormone administration; may be performed for POST-DATES PREGNANCY, or when maternal or fetal condition compromised by continuation of pregnancy. *Normal l.* spontaneous onset after 37 weeks' gestation, vertex presentation, single fetus; completed within 24 hours, no maternal or fetal trauma; physiology depends on interaction between uterus, maternal pelvis and fetus. First stage: cervical effacement, dilatation; FUNDAL DOMINANCE facilitates uterine POLARITY: contraction and RETRACTION in upper segment, contraction and relaxation in lower segment. Second stage: from full cervical dilatation until baby's birth. Third stage: separation and expulsion of placenta and membranes, haemorrhage control. *Obstructed l.* fetus unable to negotiate pelvic canal, presenting part does not descend despite good contractions. Causes: contracted bony pelvis, soft pelvic mass; malpresentation, malposition, fetal abnormality. Dangers: uterine rupture, fetal death. Diagnosis: severe maternal pain, tachycardia, pyrexia, oliguria, ketonuria; abdominally, uterus is 'moulded' around fetus, constant hypertonia, fetal parts not felt. Treatment: relieve pain, dehydration, shock, Caesarean section, manipulative or destructive delivery of baby to save mother's life. *Precipitate l.* completed in less than 2 hours; risks: haemorrhage, uterine inversion, birth injury due to rapid head moulding and birth. *Preterm l.* occurs after 24, before 37 weeks' gestation. *Spurious l.* contractions but no cervical dilatation; false labour.

**laceration** tear. *Perineal l. See* PERINEAL.

**lacrimal** pertaining to tears. *L. ducts* minute openings at inner end of eyelid convey lacrimal fluid into nose to mix with nose secretions. *L. glands* organs at upper, outer surface of eyeball; provide fluid to keep conjunctiva moist, free from infection by action of LYSOZYME, except in neonate.

**lactalbumin** main protein in human milk, easily digested by baby.

http://dx.doi.org/10.1016/B978-0-7020-6906-2.00012-7

**lactase** enzyme produced by cells in small intestine; splits LACTOSE into MONO-SACCHARIDES, GLUCOSE, and GALACTOSE.

**lactation** secretion of milk by breasts.

**lactational** pertaining to lactation.

**lacteals** lymphatics of intestine that absorb split fats.

**lactic acid** acid produced in hypoxia, e.g. in blood of asphyxiated baby, causes ACIDAEMIA; also produced in gut by lactose fermentation through action of bacilli.

**lactiferous** conveying milk, e.g. lactiferous ducts, tubules.

***Lactobacillus acidophilus*** Döderlein bacillus; gram-positive bacillus, normal vaginal inhabitant in reproductive years; converts glycogen to lactic acid, inhibits growth of other organisms; predominates in stools of breastfed babies.

**lactoferrin** iron-binding protein in human milk; bacteriostatic on ESCHERICHIA COLI.

**lactogen** substance enhancing lactation. ***Human placental l.*** placental hormone with lactogenic, luteotrophic and growth-promoting activity; inhibits maternal insulin in pregnancy; disappears from blood immediately after birth.

**lactoglobulin** globulin in milk.

**lactotroph** anterior pituitary gland prolactin cell.

**lactose** milk sugar, DISACCHARIDE. ***L. intolerance*** inability to tolerate lactose due to insufficient LACTASE; causes diarrhoea; treatment: lactose-free milk; avoid confusion with GALACTOSAEMIA.

**lactosuria** lactose in urine; not glycosuria; often occurs in lactation period and towards term; not clinically significant.

**lactulose** oral laxative; takes up to 48 hours to take effect.

**laked** blood in which haemoglobin separated from red blood cells.

**LAM** contraception: Lactation, Amenorrhoea, 6-month time period.

**Lamaze method** birth preparation training mind and body to modify pain perception in labour.

**lambda** posterior fetal skull fontanelle, from the Greek letter lambda (λ).

**lambdoidal suture** suture between occipital bone, two parietal bones.

**lamivudine** antiretroviral drug to treat HIV/AIDS and hepatitis B.

**lamotrigine** anticonvulsant drug to treat epilepsy and bipolar disorder.

**Lancefield's classification** classification of haemolytic streptococci into groups on basis of serological action.

**Landsteiner system** blood group classification; O, A, B, AB, depends on presence/absence of agglutinogens A and B in erythrocytes.

**Langerhans islets** pancreatic cells, produce insulin to control carbohydrate metabolism; disease causes DIABETES MELLITUS.

**Langhans cell layer** cytotrophoblast; inner layer of TROPHOBLAST.

**lanugo** fine hair, covers fetus, disappears by term or just after birth.

**laparoscope** instrument for examining peritoneal cavity.

**laparoscopy** examination of interior of abdomen with laparoscope.

**laparotomy** exploratory opening of abdominal cavity.

**large for gestational age baby** baby weighing above 90th centile.

**laryngeal** pertaining to larynx. ***L. oedema*** oedema of larynx, may occur in severe pre-eclampsia, pregnancy-induced hypertension. ***L. stridor***

noise made by baby on inspiration, exacerbated by crying; usually due to LARYNGOMALACIA.

**laryngomalacia**  laxity of larynx in baby, may be due to delayed development of supporting tissues; associated with respiratory, neuromuscular, gastroenterological problems. Symptoms: stridor, feeding difficulty, ear, nose, throat problems; if severe, low oxygen disrupts normal growth; may take 2 years to resolve.

**laryngoscope**  endoscopic instrument to inspect larynx and vocal cords, aid insertion of endotracheal tube.

**larynx**  upper tracheal organ; muscular, cartilaginous frame, lined with mucous membrane; vocal cords are spread across it, with glottis in space between cords.

**laser**  surgical and diagnostic device; transfers electromagnetic radiation into intense, nearly non-divergent beam of monochromatic radiation; immense heat and power at close range.

**last menstrual period**  date of last normal menstrual period aids estimated date of delivery; *implantation bleeding* may be misinterpreted as normal menstruation; check if vaginal bleeding was of normal duration, at time expected for last period.

**latent**  hidden, not manifest. *L. phase* apparently inactive period in early first-stage labour.

**lateral**  relating to side. *L. sinuses* sinuses in FETAL SKULL; from confluence sinuum along outer edge of TENTORIUM CEREBELLI; carry blood to internal jugular veins; FALX CEREBRI attached to tentorium, with risk of tearing, bleeding from great cerebral vein.

**'laughing gas'**  *See* NITROUS OXIDE.

**lavage**  washing out cavity.

**lavender oil**  aromatherapy oil; relaxing, hypotensive, analgesic; may aid uterine action. Use with caution in early pregnancy; avoid with oxytocin or epidural anaesthesia, anti-hypertensive drugs. Midwives must be appropriately trained to use AROMATHERAPY.

**laxative**  medicine to loosen bowel contents; encourages evacuation. Mild laxative safe in pregnancy; strong laxative is purgative, may stimulate uterine activity and trigger bleeding.

**lead professional**  midwife, obstetrician or general practitioner who takes primary responsibility for mother's care.

**learning difficulty**  disability affecting babies with cerebral palsy, chromosomal disorders e.g. Down syndrome.

**Lea's shield**  reusable vaginal barrier contraceptive; cup-shaped device inserted into vagina to prevent sperm from entering cervix.

**Leboyer method**  birth system in which baby is born gently in calm, tranquil environment, thought to reduce shock of birth process.

**lecithin**  complex molecule of protein and fatty acid in lining of lung; e.g. SURFACTANT that helps keep lungs open. Produced in fetal lung, flows into amniotic fluid; measured to determine fetal maturity. *L–sphingomyelin ratio* lecithin, but not sphingomyelin, increases as pregnancy progresses; L/S ratio increases with fetal lung maturity; if 2 or more, little risk of respiratory distress in neonate.

**Lee–Frankenhauser plexus**  nerve network, third and fourth sacral, hypogastric and ovarian nerves, relating to cervical area of uterus.

**left lateral position** birth position; mother lies on left side, upper right leg supported by assistant. May aid uterine contractions, fetal rotation; enables midwife to view perineum clearly.

**left occiput anterior position** fetal position with occiput pointing to left iliopectineal eminence of maternal pelvis; sagittal suture in right oblique diameter of pelvis; most common fetal position.

**leg cramps** common late pregnancy symptom, due to increasing weight, uterine pressure on leg veins, reduced muscle tone; exacerbated by calcium or magnesium deficiency, prolonged sitting, inadequate fluid intake, high-heeled shoes.

**leiomyoma** smooth muscle tumour (fibroid), commonly in uterus.

**Leopold manoeuvres** in abdominal examination, techniques to determine fetal presentation, position. *See also* PAWLIK GRIP.

**leptin** hormone that regulates energy balance, suppresses hunger.

**leptospirosis** *See* WEIL'S DISEASE.

**lesion** injury, wound, morbid structural change in organ.

**'let down' reflex** neurogenic process stimulating release of milk from breasts, e.g. when mother hears her baby crying.

**leucine** amino acid vital for infant growth, adult nitrogen equilibrium.

**leucocyte** white blood corpuscle.

**leucocytosis** increased blood leucocytes, usually due to infection.

**leucopenia** decreased leucocytes in blood.

**leucorrhoea** white, mucoid, non-irritating vaginal discharge from cervical

glands, moistens vaginal membranes; increases at ovulation, premenstrually, in pregnancy, stimulated by sexual excitement; normally white, inoffensive, non-irritating unless infection present.

**leukaemia** malignant blood disease, abnormal leucocytosis, reduced erythrocytes, blood platelets; causes anaemia, increased infection risk, haemorrhage.

**levallorphan** antagonist to analgesic narcotics.

**levator** muscle that raises part. *L. ani* broad pelvic floor muscle.

**levetiracetam** anti-epilepsy medication.

**levonorgestrel** progestogen used in some oral contraceptives.

**lignocaine hydrochloride** local anaesthetic used for perineal infiltration before episiotomy and perineal repair.

**lie, fetal** relation of long axis of fetus to long axis of mother's uterus, normally parallel with longitudinal lie; in abnormal lie fetus lies across uterus, i.e. transverse or oblique lie, obstructs labour.

**ligament** tough fibrous tissue band, connects bones or supporting internal organs. *Broad l.* not a true ligament: peritoneal fold, adjacent to uterus, covers fallopian tubes. *Round l.* extend from uterine cornua to labia majora. *Uterine l.* transverse cervical (cardinal), pubocervical, uterosacral.

**ligamentum arteriosum** vestiges of ductus arteriosus.

**ligamentum teres** vestiges of umbilical vein.

**ligamentum venosum** vestiges of ductus venosus.

**ligation** process of applying ligature.

**ligature** thread, usually of nylon or wire, to tie blood vessels. *Living l.* rearrangement of uterine muscle fibres in pregnancy produces 'criss-cross' arrangement; in third stage of labour, after placental separation and expulsion, muscle fibres clamp the open sinuses at placental site to prevent excessive haemorrhage.

**lightening** physical relief from reduced pressure under diaphragm when fetal head descends into pelvic brim (ENGAGEMENT); consequent lowering of fundal height; usually occurs around 36 weeks' gestation in nullipara, but not until onset of labour in multipara.

**light for dates** *See* SMALL FOR GESTATIONAL AGE BABY.

**linea** line. *L. alba* tendinous central area of abdominal wall into which transversalis and oblique muscles are inserted. *L. nigra* in pregnancy, temporarily pigmented linea alba between umbilicus and pubis, due to raised melanocytic hormone from pituitary gland.

**linezolid** antibiotic drug, active against gram-positive bacteria resistant to other antibiotics.

**lipase** ENZYME in breast milk and pancreatic juice; splits fat into fatty acids; pancreatic lipase not present in large amounts; baby who is not breastfed is less able to digest fats.

**lipid** fatty substance insoluble in water, soluble in alcohol; important part of diet, normally present in body tissues.

**liquor amnii** *See* AMNIOTIC FLUID.

**liquor volume** amount of amniotic fluid in amniotic sac, peaks at 28 weeks' gestation. *See* OLIGOHYDRAMNIOS, POLYHYDRAMNIOS *and* AMNIOTIC FLUID INDEX.

*Listeria monocytogenes* gram-positive bacteria causing listeriosis.

**listeriosis** infection caused by *Listeria monocytogenes*; upper respiratory disease, septicaemia, meningitis, encephalitis. May cause miscarriage, stillbirth, preterm labour, congenital infection. Transmission: eating infected unpasteurized dairy produce, direct contact with infected animals or contaminated soil. In pregnancy, avoid mould-ripened cheese, e.g. Brie, unpasteurized meat, fish or vegetable pâtés; cook chilled foods, poultry well.

**lithium carbonate** mood-stabilizing drug for bipolar disorder; pregnancy use increases risk of cardiac conditions, EBSTEIN ANOMALY, fetal hypothyroidism, diabetes insipidus, macrosomia, FLOPPY BABY SYNDROME.

**lithopaedion** very rare condition; fetus develops outside uterus, dies and becomes petrified due to lime salt deposition.

**lithotomy position** mother lies on back with thighs and legs flexed, abducted, held in place with lithotomy poles; used for forceps, breech birth, perineal suturing. Lift legs into/out of stirrups simultaneously to avoid hip dislocation due to joint laxity.

**litigation** legal action taken if suspected negligence or malpractice.

**litmus paper** blotting paper impregnated with litmus, pigment used to identify fluid reactions; blue litmus is turned red by acids; red litmus is turned blue by alkalis.

**liver** large wedge-shaped gland in right hypochondrium and epigastrium. Essential for bile formation; plasma protein production, except GAMMA GLOBULINS; glycogen, iron, vitamins A, D, E, K storage; fat, protein, carbohydrate metabolism; detoxication of drugs, other substances; ERYTHROCYTE formation; PROTHROMBIN, FIBRINOGEN production; heat production; bacterial phagocytosis.

**liver function tests**   tests to assess liver function: albumin; liver enzymes; aminotransferases, e.g. aspartate aminotransferase, alanine aminotransferase; alkaline phosphatase; prothrombin clotting time; bilirubin.

**livid**   cyanotic; blueness of venous congestion, inadequate OXYGEN.

**lobe**   section of organ, separated from other parts by fissures.

**lobule**   small segment or lobe, one of smaller divisions making up lobe. *Adj* lobular.

**local anaesthetic**   pain-relieving drugs e.g. epidural anaesthesia.

**Local Supervising Authority**   local organization monitoring quality of midwifery practice.

**lochia**   vaginal discharges continue for 2–6 weeks after labour or miscarriage; contain placental site blood, decidual shreds, vaginal epithelial cells, uterine debris, e.g. amniotic fluid, vernix caseosa, meconium. *L. alba* (white) contains white blood cells, mucus; *L. rubra* (red) fresh, then stale blood; *L. serosa* (pink) contains fewer red, more white cells. Red, profuse lochia or sudden cessation may indicate subinvolution, infection, retained products, imminent haemorrhage. *Sing* lochium.

**locked twins**   rare cause of obstructed labour; bodies and heads of twins are caught together; precludes normal vaginal birth.

**locus**   place, site. In genetics, specific site of gene on chromosome.

**lofepramine**   tricyclic antidepressant drug.

**long-acting reversible contraception**   contraceptive methods, more effective than daily or weekly contraceptives; injectable progestogens, intrauterine devices or hormones, subdermal implants.

**longitudinal study**   investigation involving observations of same group at sequential time intervals; valuable for studying human individual or organizational development or change.

**lordosis**   exaggerated lumbar curve; in pregnancy due to musculoskeletal laxity from relaxin and progesterone; worsened by poor posture. Weight of uterus pulls body forward; mother leans backward to compensate, puts extra strain on sacroiliac joints, causes backache. Posture, exercise, ergonomics advice may help.

**Løvset's manoeuvre**   technique to deliver fetal shoulders in breech presentation, when arms extended; fetus rotated through half-circle, keeping back uppermost, posterior arm brought into anterior position below symphysis pubis to be born; fetus then rotated half-circle in reverse direction and other arm is similarly born.

**low-birthweight baby**   baby weighing 2.5 kg or less at birth; may be preterm, small for gestational age or both; may be well or ill. *See also* SMALL FOR GESTATIONAL AGE BABY *and* PRETERM.

**low cavity forceps delivery**   method of delivery when fetal head at pelvic floor and visible at vulva, using Wrigley's forceps or similar.

**lower uterine segment**   part of uterus between vesicouterine peritoneal fold superiorly and junction of uterus and cervix inferiorly.

**lumbar** pertaining to lumbar vertebrae in lower back. *L. puncture* introduction of hollow needle into subarachnoid space, usually between fourth and fifth lumbar vertebrae, to withdraw cerebrospinal fluid for diagnostic purposes, relieve pressure or introduce drugs.

**lumbopelvic cylinder** pelvic area comprising transabdominus muscles, diaphragm, multifidus, pelvic floor muscles.

**lumbosacral** relating to lumbar and sacral vertebrae or regions.

**lumen** space inside tube.

**lumpectomy** surgical excision of local lesion (benign or malignant).

**lungs** two conical respiratory organs; air tubes (bronchi, bronchioles) terminating in air spaces (alveoli), occupy most of thoracic cavity. During respiration lungs supply blood with oxygen inhaled from outside air and dispose of waste carbon dioxide in exhaled air.

**lupus** chronic skin disease, many different manifestations. *L. anticoagulant* antiphospholipid antibodies, present particularly if history of repeated miscarriages. *See* SYSTEMIC LUPUS ERYTHEMATOSUS.

**luteal** pertaining to CORPUS LUTEUM. *L. phase* second part of menstrual cycle, from day after ovulation, to onset of next menstrual period; usually 14 days.

**lutein** yellow pigment in corpus luteum.

**luteinizing hormone** anterior pituitary hormone; with follicle-stimulating hormone causes ovulation of mature follicles and secretion of oestrogen by ovary; aids corpus luteum formation. Stimulates development of testicular interstitial cells, testosterone secretion in men.

**luteotropin** prolactin.

**lymph** body fluid derived from interstitial fluid, carried in lymphatic vessels back to bloodstream; lymph nodes occur at intervals throughout lymphatic vessels, acting as filters.

**lymphatic** pertaining to lymph *L. vessels* vessels carrying lymph.

**lymphocytes** white blood cells, formed mainly from lymphoid tissue in bone marrow and thymus.

**lymphoedema** condition in which intercellular spaces contain abnormal amounts of lymph due to obstruction of lymph drainage.

**lyse** to cause disintegration of cell or substance.

**lysin** cell-dissolving substance present in blood serum.

**lysis** breaking down, as of red blood cells in haemolysis.

**lysozyme** antibacterial (gram-positive) agent present in all tissues and secretions, particularly tears and breast milk.

**maceration** softening, breaking down of skin from prolonged exposure to moisture; discoloration, tissue softening, peeling, disintegration of skin e.g. dead fetus retained in uterus for over 24 hours; may cause DISSEMINATED INTRAVASCULAR COAGULATION.

**Mackenrodt ligaments** transverse, cardinal ligaments supporting uterus in pelvic cavity.

**macro-** prefix meaning 'large'.

**macrocyte** abnormally large red blood corpuscles found in megaloblastic anaemia of pregnancy resulting from folic acid deficiency.

**macronutrient** essential nutrient; e.g. calcium, phosphorus, magnesium, potassium; daily requirement >100 mg.

**macrophage** large, mononuclear, phagocytic cells (PHAGOCYTES) in reticuloendothelial system, derived from monocytes; occur in blood vessel walls, loose connective tissue; mobile when stimulated by inflammation; interact with lymphocytes to facilitate antibody production.

**macroscopic** discernible with naked eye.

**macrosomia** large baby, birthweight above 97th centile for gestation or over 4–4.5 kg at term.

**magnesium** metal, symbol Mg; in intra- and extracellular fluids; excreted in urine, faeces; minute quantities essential for enzyme activity. Normal serum level approximately 1 mmol/L; deficiency causes nervous system irritability, tetany, vasodilatation, convulsions, tremors, depression, psychotic behaviour.

**magnesium sulphate** intravenous or intramuscular saline to control eclampsia via reversing cerebral vasospasm, increasing cerebral blood flow. Side effects: flushing, nausea, vomiting, palpitations, headaches. Toxicity (above 5 mmol/L) causes poor patellar reflexes, muscle paralysis, slurred speech, pulmonary oedema, respiratory, cardiac arrest. Antidote: intravenous calcium gluconate.

**magnetic resonance imaging** technique using magnetic and radio waves passed through body, signals converted to computer image. Enables fetal brain, spinal cord examination in utero, although fetal movements may adversely affect image quality.

**maintenance order** court order requiring regular payments for child care by spouse in case of separation or divorce.

**mal-** prefix meaning 'impaired' or 'ill'. *Grand m.* generalized convulsive seizure, loss of consciousness. *Petit m.* momentary loss of consciousness without convulsive movements. *See* EPILEPSY.

**malabsorption** impaired intestinal nutrient absorption. *M. syndrome* subnormal intestinal absorption of dietary constituents, with excessive nutrient loss in stools.

**malacia** tissue softening. *Osteomalacia* softening of bone tissue, may cause deformity of pelvic bones.

http://dx.doi.org/10.1016/B978-0-7020-6906-2.00013-9

**malaise** feeling of general discomfort and illness.

**malar** pertaining to malar bone of face or adjacent area.

**malaria** notifiable tropical infection from mosquito bites, with protozoan parasites in erythrocytes; causes periodic fever, sweating, chills, rigors, even years later. Prophylaxis essential before, during, after travel to malaria areas; proguanil and chloroquine are safe in pregnancy; avoid Maloprim in first trimester.

**male reproductive system** two sperm-producing testes in scrotum; sperm are collected by fine tubular epididymis, conveyed by vas deferens to seminal vesicles for storage. At ejaculation prostate gland adds fluid to sperm, which pass into urethra inside erect penis; during sex, sperm are deposited in posterior vaginal fornix.

**malformation** congenital or acquired anatomical abnormality.

**malignant** becoming progressively invasive, resulting in death, as in cancer, with metastasis. *M. disease in pregnancy* about 1:1000–1500 pregnancies complicated by cancer; incidence increases in older mothers; pregnancy may adversely affect course of disease; abnormal cells may metastasize to placenta and fetus. Diagnosis in pregnancy: need to consider effects of disease and treatment on continuation of pregnancy and fetomaternal condition.

**Mallory-Weiss syndrome** bleeding from mucosal laceration at junction of stomach and oesophagus; may occur in HYPEREMESIS GRAVIDARUM.

**malnutrition** poor nutritional quantity or quality, causing deficiency syndromes.

**Malpighian body** glomerulus and Bowman capsule of kidney.

**malposition** misplaced siting of organ or part in relationship to neighbouring structures. *Fetal m.* cephalic presentation other than normal, well-flexed anterior position, e.g. occipitoposterior.

**malpractice** professional misconduct or negligence, unreasonable lack of skill or fidelity in professional duties, illegal or immoral conduct, by omission or inclusion. In midwifery, malpractice results in injury, unnecessary suffering or death of mother or baby.

**malpresentation** fetal presentation other than vertex; breech, face, brow or shoulder presentation; failure to diagnose can lead to obstructed labour, uterine rupture, fetal or maternal death.

**malrotation** neonatal developmental abnormality; incomplete rotation of small bowel leads to obstruction, vomiting, abdominal distension; surgical correction usually necessary.

**Malström vacuum extractor** See VACUUM EXTRACTOR.

**maltase** sugar-splitting enzyme, converts maltose to glucose, present in pancreatic and intestinal juice.

**maltose** sugar (disaccharide) formed when starch is hydrolyzed by amylase.

**mamma** breast.

**mammary** pertaining to breasts.

**mammilla** nipple.

**mammography** breast radiography; routine screening procedure to diagnose cancer and other breast disorders.

**Managing Obstetric Emergencies and Trauma** course in practical skills and procedures needed for life-threatening situations.

**mandelic acid**  urinary antiseptic for nephritis, pyelitis, cystitis.

**mandible**  bone forming lower jaw.

**mania**  psychiatric disorder; acceleration of mental processes, associated with BIPOLAR DISORDER; may follow childbirth.

**manipulation**  using hands, e.g. to change position of fetus.

**mannitol**  osmotic diuretic used for forced diuresis and in cerebral oedema; not recommended in pregnancy but may be used for ACUTE TUBULAR NECROSIS after postpartum haemorrhage. Not to be added to whole blood.

**manoeuvre**  manual procedure to facilitate birth of baby, delivery of placenta. *See* EXTERNAL CEPHALIC VERSION, LØVSET'S MANOEUVRE *and* MAURICEAU–SMELLIE–VEIT MANOEUVRE.

**manometer**  instrument to measure pressure or tension of liquids or gases. *See* SPHYGMOMANOMETER.

**Mantoux test**  intradermal injection of old tuberculin to determine susceptibility to tuberculosis; positive reaction, weal developing within hours, signifies previous infection has conferred immunity.

**manual**  with hand. *M. removal of placenta* emergency procedure to remove retained placenta when no medical aid available; antiseptic cream applied to gloved hand, inserted in vagina; umbilical cord followed up to uterus, placenta; other hand supports uterus abdominally. From separated placental edge, remainder peeled off uterine wall, withdrawn; may need BIMANUAL COMPRESSION to control bleeding; risk of shock greater when no anaesthetic used.

**Manual removal of the placent**

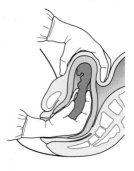

**maple syrup urine disease**  autosomal-recessive genetic disorder; deficiency of enzyme needed for metabolism of branched-chain amino acids; clinical manifestation: physical and learning disabilities, feeding difficulties, characteristic odour of urine.

**marasmus**  severe malnutrition and weight loss in babies; associated with protein–calorie deficiency, usually with normal appetite and mental alertness; related to KWASHIORKOR.

**Marcaine**  *See* BUPIVACAINE HYDROCHLORIDE.

**Marfan syndrome**  autosomal-dominant genetic disorder of connective tissue (chromosome 15); causes abnormally long fingers, toes, myopia, retinal detachment, glaucoma, scoliosis; major heart problems, aortic aneurysm. Pregnancy puts extra pressure on heart; 50% risk of child inheriting condition. Monitor carefully; antihypertensives may reduce blood pressure and aortic dilatation.

**marijuana, marihuana**  *Cannabis sativa*; hemp, hashish. Contains

137

pharmacologically active principles; used therapeutically or recreationally for euphoric properties; more potent when smoked and inhaled than ingested. Increased risk of miscarriage, birth defects.

**marker** indicator of increased risk of disease or disorder; several markers are often combined to provide more detailed clinical picture or to increase SENSITIVITY and SPECIFICITY of screening test.

**marrow** soft, organic, sponge-like material in bone cavity; aids erythrocyte, leucocyte, platelet production; destruction by chemical agents or excessive x-ray exposure may cause aplastic anaemia, leukaemia, pernicious anaemia, myeloma, metastatic tumours.

**mask of pregnancy** See CHLOASMA.

**massage** systematic therapeutic stroking or kneading to aid relaxation, circulation, excretion, lower blood pressure; in labour, may ease pain as touch impulses reach brain before pain impulses. *Cardiac m.* intermittent heart compression applied over sternum or directly to heart through opening in chest wall. *Infant m.* promotes maternal–infant bonding; aids growth, physical, psychological development, especially in preterm babies.

**mast cells** connective tissue cells in heart, liver, lungs; release heparin, serotonin, histamine in response to inflammation, allergy.

**mastitis** breast inflammation. *Puerperal m.* infection due to staphylococci or streptococci, enters through cracked nipples; wedge-shaped area of breast tender, red, warm; responds quickly to antibiotics but delay in treatment may lead to breast abscess.

**MAT B1 certificate** form signed by midwife or doctor confirming estimated due date; needed to claim maternity benefits.

**maternal** pertaining to mother. *M. mortality* death due to pregnancy or childbearing. *M. mortality rate* number of maternal deaths per 1000 registered live births and stillbirths.

**maternity** pertaining to childbearing. *M. benefits* in UK, women entitled to maternity allowance; paid time off work for antenatal appointments; free dental care and prescriptions in pregnancy and for 1 year after delivery; if employed, women are entitled to statutory maternity pay and right to return to work. *M. support worker* healthcare practitioner specifically trained to assist midwives and support mothers.

**maternity services liaison committee** local committees to serve interests of maternity service consumers; two-way communication between obstetric, paediatric, anaesthetic and midwifery representatives, prospective and retrospective service users.

**matrix** intercellular substance of tissue, e.g. bone matrix, or tissue from which structure develops, e.g. hair or nail matrix.

**Matthews Duncan expulsion** placental expulsion in which maternal side appears first at end of third stage of labour, often due to low-lying placenta; bleeding heavier than with SCHULTZE EXPULSION.

**maturation** process of ripening or developing, as in cell division when number of chromosomes in germ cell is reduced to half.

**Mauriceau–Smellie–Veit manoeuvre** method to aid birth of aftercoming

**Mauriceau–Smellie–Veit manoeuvre**

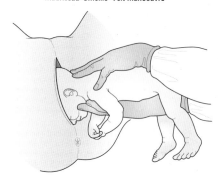

head in breech birth; flexion increased, jaw and shoulder traction applied; allows better control over birth of head than BURNS–MARSHALL MANOEUVRE.

**Maxolon** *See* METOCLOPRAMIDE.

**MBRRACE-UK** Mothers and Babies: Reducing Risk through Audits and Confidential Enquiries in the UK.

**McRoberts manoeuvre** technique of anterior rotation of symphysis pubis; mother brings knees up to chest in order to release impacted fetal shoulders in SHOULDER DYSTOCIA. *See also* APPENDIX 4.

**mean** average; numerical value intermediate between two extremes. *M. corpuscular haemoglobin* indicates average amount of haemoglobin in red blood cells; low levels indicate reduced oxygen-carrying capacity of blood; MCH concentration of <25 pg may indicate ALPHA THALASSAEMIA trait. *M. corpuscular volume* measures red blood cell size, decreased in iron deficiency anaemia,

increased in vitamin $B_{12}$ deficiency anaemia.

**measles** infectious notifiable viral disease. *See* IMMUNIZATION.

**meatus** opening, passage. *Auditory m.* opening leading into auditory canal. *Urinary m.* where urethra opens to exterior.

**mechanism of labour** sequence of movements made by fetus during labour to facilitate passage through maternal pelvis.

**meconium** greenish-black fetal intestinal substance, passed per rectum in first few days of life; contains bile pigments, salts, mucus, intestinal epithelial cells, amniotic fluid. *M. aspiration syndrome* inhalation of meconium-containing fluid, as in babies who were hypoxic in utero; causes severe respiratory distress. *M. ileus* gross bowel distension with congealed meconium, as in CYSTIC FIBROSIS.

**median** situated in median plane, midline of body. *M. nerve* nerve originating in brachial plexus, innervates muscles of wrist and hand. *M. plane* imaginary plane passing longitudinally through body from front to back, dividing it into right and left halves.

**mediastinum** 1. median septum or partition. 2. mass of tissues and organs separating sternum in front and vertebral column behind; contains heart, large vessels, trachea, oesophagus, thymus, lymph nodes, other structures and tissues.

**medical** pertaining to medicine.

**medicine** 1. drug or remedy. 2. art and science, diagnosis and treatment of disease, maintenance of health. 3. non-surgical treatment of disease, as opposed to surgery.

**Medicines Act 1968 and amendments** law relating to prescribing, supply, administration of medicines; prescription-only medicines, including controlled drugs, pharmacy medicines, general sale list. Midwives exempt from some restrictions, able to supply and administer antiseptics, aperients, sedatives, analgesics, local anaesthetics, oxytocics, agents for maternal and neonatal resuscitation.

**Medicines and Healthcare Products Regulatory Authority (MHRA)** Department of Health agency to safeguard public health by ensuring that medicines and medical devices are effective and safe.

**medium** 1. agent by which something is accomplished or impulse is transmitted. 2. substance providing correct nutritional environment for growth of micro-organisms; culture medium.

**medium-chain acyl-coenzyme A dehydrogenase deficiency** inherited autosomal-recessive metabolic disorder; occurs in 1:6000 UK births; 25% cot death rate. Lack of medium-chain acyl-coenzyme A dehydrogenase to metabolize stored fat into energy so fats not completely broken down; causes hypoglycaemia, toxin accumulation; poor feeding, drowsiness, lethargy, seizures, unconsciousness, brain damage, infection, apparent sudden infant death. Screening is via NEWBORN BLOOD-SPOT SCREENING PROGRAMME test.

**medroxyprogesterone acetate (Depo-Provera)** single-dose intramuscular contraceptive, effective for 12 weeks, useful after rubella vaccination, partner's vasectomy or if unable to manage other methods; risk of heavy bleeding if used before fifth postnatal week.

**medulla** central or inner portion of organ. *M. oblongata* lowest part of brainstem between pons varolii and spinal cord, seat of vital centres, i.e. cardiac, respiratory, vasomotor centres.

**mega-** word element meaning 'large'; units of measurement designating $10^6$ (one million) times.

**megaloblastic anaemia** large, nucleated, immature red cells in bone marrow (megaloblasts) circulate in blood; anaemia due to folic acid deficiency; epileptic women on long-term PHENYTOIN SODIUM more prone.

**meiosis** cell division; germinal epithelium in either ovary or testis gives rise to gamete containing only one CHROMOSOME from each pair, i.e. haploid number (23); normally diploid (46).

**melaena** dark, altered blood in stools; occurs in haemorrhagic disease of newborn; may be accompanied by HAEMATEMESIS.

**melanin** dark pigment in hair, choroid coat, etc., sometimes in malignant tumours. Increased pigmentation occurs in pregnancy due to raised melanocytic hormone; causes LINEA NIGRA, darkening of areolae of nipples, facial CHLOASMA.

**melanocyte-stimulating hormone** anterior pituitary gland peptide; influences formation or deposition of melanin in body.

**melasma** *See* CHLOASMA.

**membrane** thin tissue covering surface of some organs and body cavity linings. *M. sweep* procedure *per vaginam*; examining fingers 'sweep' round cervical os to loosen membranes, initiate labour; may be performed around 41 weeks' gestation to reduce need for labour induction. *Mucous m.* contains secreting cells, lines all cavities connected directly or indirectly with skin. *Fetal m.* CHORION and AMNION.

**menaquinone** vitamin K$_2$.

**menarche** onset of menstruation at puberty.

**Mendel's laws** pattern, first shown by Gregor Mendel; transmission of inherited characteristics, some dominant, others recessive.

**Mendelson syndrome** marked bronchial, alveolar irritation; causes dyspnoea, cyanosis, tachycardia, severe bronchospasm, pulmonary oedema, hypotension, death; occurs when acidic gastric juice inhaled during general anaesthesia; anaesthetist may request midwife to apply prophylactive CRICOID pressure during intubation.

**meninges** membranes covering brain and spinal cord: dura mater, arachnoid and pia mater.

**meningitis** meninges inflammation; viral form develops after common childhood illness, e.g. chickenpox, measles; bacterial form more serious with 5% mortality rate, 25% risk of long-term deafness, epilepsy, permanent brain damage. Symptoms: initially flu-like, making diagnosis difficult; constant headache, confusion, drowsiness, pyrexia with cold extremities, abdominal pain, vomiting, diarrhoea, rapid respirations, joint or muscle pain. Three cardinal signs and symptoms: neck stiffness, sensitivity to light and red/purplish spots, which do not blanch on pressure. Babies may present with fever, vomiting, muscle dystonia, high-pitched moan or whimpering cry, irritability when handled, refusal to feed, neck retraction, arching of back, lethargy, convulsions, tense, bulging fontanelle. Urgent treatment: hospital admission, antibiotics (for bacterial form); prognosis better with prompt treatment. *See also* IMMUNIZATION, NOTIFIABLE DISEASES.

**meningocele** congenital deformity; protrusion of meninges through skull or spinal column; cerebrospinal fluid-filled cyst. *See also* SPINA BIFIDA.

**meningoencephalocele** hernial protrusion of meninges and brain substance through defect in skull.

**meningomyelocele** hernial protrusion of meninges and spinal cord through defect in vertebral column.

**meniscocyte** sickle cell.

**menopause** cessation of menstruation. *Induced m.* cessation induced by operation or irradiation.

**menorrhagia** excessive menstrual discharge.

**menses** menstruation.

**menstrual** pertaining to menstruation. *M. cycle* cyclical event, normally every 28 days. Bleeding begins on day

1 due to fall in progesterone, lasts 4–5 days; endometrium is shed to basal layer. In secretory phase, rising oestrogen from pituitary gland triggers ovary to mature one Graafian follicle; endometrium thickens in anticipation of pregnancy. Follicle ripens 14 days *before* next cycle, ovulation releases ovum to traverse fallopian tube towards uterus. Progesterone rises; sustained in event of pregnancy assist embryonic embedding and development; if no conception occurs, ovum passes to uterus, hormone fall causes thickened endometrium to be shed with ovum and blood. Ruptured uterine follicle degenerates due to falling hormones (corpus luteum).

**menstruation** discharge of blood from uterus, at approximately 4-week intervals; commences at puberty, lasts until menopause.

**mental** 1. pertaining to mind. 2. pertaining to chin.

**mentoanterior** fetal position with chin directed anteriorly in pelvis; similarly, mentolateral and mentoposterior.

**mentum** chin; denominator in face presentation.

**meperidine** pethidine (USA).

**meptazinol (Meptid)** opioid analgesic causing less respiratory depression than pethidine; relatively quick onset but short action, 2–4 hours; side effects include nausea, vomiting.

**mercury** element; symbol Hg. Liquid heavy metal in clinical thermometer (expands with heat); in SPHYGMOMANOMETER (heavier than water, so short tube can record wide variation in pressure).

**mesentery** membranous fold attaching various organs to body wall, especially peritoneal fold attaching small intestine to dorsal body wall. *Adj* mesenteric.

**mesoderm** cells between ectoderm and endoderm cell layers in embryo, from which bone, muscle, heart, blood, blood vessels, gonads, kidneys and connective tissues develop.

**mesosalpinx** peritoneum covering fallopian tubes.

**mesovarium** peritoneal fold connecting ovary to broad ligament.

**mestranol** synthetic steroidal oestrogen.

**meta-analysis** analysis and evaluation of results of all accessible research trials on given subject.

**metabolic** pertaining to metabolism.

**metabolism** process of life; tissue cells break down by combustion (catabolism), new protein builds up from end products of digestion (anabolism). *Basal m.* See BASAL METABOLIC RATE. *Inborn errors of m.* genetically determined biochemical disorders; specific enzyme defects produce metabolic block with pathological effects at birth, as in phenylketonuria, or in later life. *Adj* metabolic.

**metanephrine** metabolite of epinephrine, indicator of PHAEOCHROMOCYTOMA.

**metastasis** transfer of disease from one organ to another not directly connected with it. *Pl* metastases; growth of malignant cells or pathogenic micro-organisms distant from primary site.

**metatarsum** part of foot between ankle and toes; five bones (metatarsals) extending from tarsus to phalanges.

**metformin** anti-diabetic drug occasionally used in infertility treatment, polycystic ovary syndrome; not generally used for diabetic control in pregnancy although is not thought to cross placenta.

**methadone hydrochloride** synthetic compound similar to morphine and heroin; may be given to drug addicts as maintenance drug.

**methicillin-resistant *Staphylococcus aureus*** strain of *S. aureus* resistant to 'methicillin-like' antibiotics; carried in nose or on skin without symptoms; spread by direct contact; cause of severe, contagious, hospital-acquired infection.

**methohexitone sodium** intravenous anaesthetic.

**methotrexate** folic acid antagonist, anti-neoplastic agent.

**methyldopa** hypotensive drug for essential hypertension; crosses placenta but does not affect fetus. May cause maternal lethargy, drowsiness, depression; effects are dose dependent. Not suitable for acute hypertension; sudden withdrawal can cause anxiety, insomnia, rebound hypertension; safe when breastfeeding.

**metoclopramide** drug for nausea, vomiting, heartburn.

**metopic suture** frontal suture.

**metritis** inflammation of uterus.

**metro-, metra-** word element meaning 'uterus'.

**metronidazole (Flagyl)** antimicrobial drug effective against anaerobic infections, e.g. *Trichomonas vaginalis*.

**metropathia haemorrhagica** painless excessive menstrual and intermenstrual bleeding, failure of ovulation.

**metrorrhagia** bleeding from uterus independent of menstruation.

**metrostaxis** persistent slight haemorrhage from uterus.

**Michel clips** small metal clips for closing skin wounds.

**miconazole** drug active against fungi, parasites, some bacteria.

**micro-** 1. prefix meaning 'small', microscopic. 2. prefix indicating 'one-millionth', e.g. microgram (μg), one-millionth of gram.

**microbe** micro-organism, pathogenic bacterium. *Adj* microbial.

**microcephaly** abnormally small head with ossified skull bones; baby will have learning difficulties. *See also* ZIKA VIRUS.

**microcytic** having unusually small cells. *See* ANAEMIA.

**micrognathia** unusually small mandible or lower jaw, with receding chin. *See* PIERRE–ROBIN SYNDROME.

**micro-organism** minute living organism e.g. virus, bacterium, visible under microscope.

**microphage** small phagocyte; actively mobile neutrophilic leucocyte capable of phagocytosis.

**micturition** act of passing urine.

**mid-cavity forceps delivery** instrumental delivery with Neville Barnes or Simpson forceps, when fetal head is engaged and presenting part is below ischial spines.

**middle cerebral artery flow** ultrasound measurement of blood flow in middle cerebral artery; if rapid, indicates fetal anaemia. Aids diagnosis of haemolytic disease from maternal ALLOIMMUNIZATION: may indicate INTRAUTERINE TRANSFUSION required.

**midwife** Latin word, means '*with woman*'; female or male midwifery practitioner, defined by International Confederation of Midwives 1972, International Federation of Gynaecologists and Obstetricians 1973. Qualified midwife legally licensed to supervise, care for, advise pregnant, labouring, newly birthed women, conduct births on own responsibility, care for newborn and infant; use preventative measures, detect abnormalities, obtain medical aid, deal with emergencies; provide health, antenatal education, aspects of gynaecology, family planning, preconception, child care.

**midwifery** art and science of caring for women undergoing *normal* pregnancies, labours and puerperia.

**midwifery-led care** woman-centred, non-interventionist, individualized care provided by midwife, with continuity of care and carer.

**mifepristone** progesterone receptor antagonist; abortifacient used in first 8 weeks of pregnancy, and as emergency contraceptive.

**milia** white, hard spots on neonate's nose, chin and forehead, formed from oil glands; disappear spontaneously.

**miliaria** skin condition; prickly heat rash; retention of sweat.

**military attitude** attitude of fetus, neither flexed nor extended.

**milk** secretion of mammary gland. *Human breast m.* contains lipids, 98% as triglycerides, which provide more than 50% of calorific requirements; carbohydrates, mainly lactose, giving 40% of calorific needs; whey-dominant protein, vitamins, minerals, trace elements, anti-infective factors e.g. leucocytes, immunoglobulins, lysozyme, lactoferrin, bifidus factor, hormones, growth factor. *Pasteurized m.* milk heated at 73°C for 15 seconds or 63–66°C for 30 minutes, cooled and bottled. *Sterilized m.* milk heated to 100°C for 15 minutes to render free from bacteria.

**milk flow mechanism, milk ejection reflex** oxytocin released from posterior pituitary gland in response to nerve stimulation contracts MYOEPITHELIAL CELLS; milk forced out of ALVEOLI into ducts and lacteal sinuses, pushed towards nipple; occurs 30–40 seconds after baby takes AREOLA in mouth.

**milli-** prefix, 'one-thousandth', e.g. milligram (mg), one-thousandth of gram; millilitre (mL), one-thousandth of litre; millimetre (mm), one-thousandth of metre.

**mineral** naturally occurring non-organic homogeneous solid substance; 19 occur in body, at least 13 essential to health; obtained from mixed and varied diet of animal and vegetable products.

**Mirena coil** hormonal contraceptive device inserted in uterus for long-term use; releases progestin to thicken cervical mucus to prevent sperm fertilizing ovum.

**miscarriage** fetal expulsion before 24 weeks gestation, i.e. before fetus legally viable. *Complete m.* entire products of conception expelled, no retained products. *Incomplete m.* some products of conception retained in uterus; risk of haemorrhage, requires CURETTAGE. *Habitual m.* three or more miscarriages. *Inevitable m.* irreversible vaginal bleeding. *Missed (silent) m.* non-viable pregnancy; products of conception remain in utero; evidence of fetus but no fetal heartbeat; ultrasound shows ANEMBRYONIC PREGNANCY; expulsion may occur weeks after fetal death. *Spontaneous m.* may be due to blighted ovum, e.g. HYDATIDIFORM, CARNEOUS MOLE. *Threatened m.* vaginal bleeding, abdominal pain before 24 weeks' gestation; may resolve or become inevitable miscarriage.

**misoprostol** oral uterotonic, prostaglandin E1 analogue, for cervical ripening, postpartum haemorrhage, usually given *per vaginam*.

**Misuse of Drugs Act 1971** law on drugs liable to misuse, including controlled drugs; schedules detail safe custody, documentation, record keeping, procedures for destruction.

**Misuse of Drugs Regulations 1973 and amendments** permit midwives to carry and administer controlled drugs; prescription-only medicines; orders specify drugs which can be supplied to midwives for administration without doctor's prescription.

**mitochondria** structures responsible for energy production in cells, located in cytoplasm outside nucleus of cell; each contains chromosome composed of deoxyribonucleic acid (mitochondrial DNA) always transmitted by mother; many genetic conditions are related to changes, in particular mitochondrial genes. *Sing* mitochondrium.

**mitosis** normal process of cell multiplication; nuclear division occurs with each chromosome dividing in two; two identical cells formed. *cf.* MEIOSIS.

**mitral** shaped like mitre. *M. incompetence* defective mitral valve, usually due to scar tissue after endocarditis. *M. regurgitation* result of mild endocarditis, valve closes imperfectly. *M. stenosis* more serious; fibrous tissue causes narrowed orifice, commonest cardiac lesion in childbearing women. *M. valve* bicuspid valve between left atrium and left ventricle of heart. *M. valvotomy* cutting into and widening of narrowed mitral valve to relieve mitral stenosis.

**mittelschmerz** abdominal or pelvic pain occurring between menstrual periods, related to ovulation.

**MMR vaccination** combined live attenuated viruses for immunization against mumps, measles, rubella; offered at one year of age and preschool; risks include neurological, learning disorders e.g. autism.

**mobile epidural** low-dose bupivacaine, sometimes with opiate, administered into epidural space by patient-controlled epidural analgesic system pump; enables mobility in labour; pain relief not as complete as with conventional epidural; normal labour observations monitoring of mother's respiratory rate.

**moclobemide** reversible monoamine oxidase inhibitor drug for depression and anxiety.

**molar** pertaining to mole.

**mole** dead, degenerate ovum. *Carneous m.* uterine mass occurring after fetal death, usually contains blood, fetal, placental tissue. *Vesicular m. See* HYDATIDIFORM MOLE.

**molecule** smallest substance particle, varying number of atoms.

**Mongolian blue spot** grey-blue sacral naevus with excess melanocytes; may be seen at birth in babies of African or Asian parents, occasionally in those of Mediterranean origin; usually disappears in childhood.

**mongolism** *See* DOWN SYNDROME.

**monilia, moniliasis** *See* CANDIDA ALBICANS, THRUSH.

**monoamine** amine with only one amino group. *M. oxidase inhibitors* substances inhibiting monoamine oxidase activity, increase catecholamine and serotonin levels in brain; antidepressants, antihypertensives. Potentiate action of pethidine.

**monoamniotic twins** twins which develop in same amniotic sac.

**monochorionic twins** monozygotic twins developing with single chorion, may be monoamniotic or diamniotic.

**monoclonal** derived from single cell. *M. antibodies* derived from single clone of cells, all with identical molecules and reacting with same antigenic site.

**monosaccharide** simplest form of sugar, e.g. dextrose, glucose.

**monosomy** genetic condition in which one chromosome of a pair is missing the diploid organism.

**monozygotic** derived from single zygote (fertilized ovum). *M. twins* uniovular twins develop from division of one ovum, one spermatozoon: same sex, one placenta, one chorion but two amniotic sacs; developmental abnormalities more common in monozygotic twins than DIZYGOTIC. *See also* MULTIPLE PREGNANCY. *Adj* monozygous.

**mons pubis, mons veneris** area over female pubes.

**Montgomery glands, tubercles** sebaceous glands around nipple, which enlarge during pregnancy.

**mood** state or quality of feeling *M. stabilizers* principle drugs for bipolar disorder: lithium, valproate, carbamazepine; antipsychotics usually discontinued in pregnancy to avoid fetal anomaly risk; anticonvulsants safer. *M. swings* hormonal mood changes in pregnancy, puerperium e.g. depression, anxiety, fear, mania, etc.

**morbid** diseased, relating to diseased parts. *Noun* morbidity.

**moribund** dying.

**morning sickness** colloquial phrase for gestational sickness, as symptoms commonly worse on waking due to hypoglycaemia. *See* NAUSEA *and* VOMITING.

**Moro (startle) reflex** baby's response to sudden movement or noise nearby: quick arm extension then bringing them together; 'embrace' or 'startle' reflex; may be absent in sick or pre-term babies.

**morphine sulphate** principal alkaloid obtained from opium; analgesic for severe pain, may cause respiratory depression.

**mortality** death. *M. rate* death rate of given population, e.g. maternal, neonatal or infant mortality rates.

**morula** fertilized ovum about 4 days after fertilization, resembling small mulberry. *Pl* morulae.

**mosaicism** person with several different types of cell, e.g. in some types of DOWN SYNDROME, not all cells have 47 chromosomes.

**motilin** polypeptide hormone secreted by intestinal cells; increases gut motility, pepsin secreted in presence of duodenal acid and fat.

**motor nerves** nerves conveying motion impulses from nerve centre to muscle.

**mould** fungus, e.g. *Penicillium*.

**moulding** overriding of fetal cranial bones at sutures and fontanelles during birth; head is squeezed, changes shape and length. *Normal m.* in vertex presentation fetal head well flexed; suboccipitobregmatic and biparietal diameters decrease as bones overlap; mentovertical diameter lengthens. *Abnormal m.* excessive or extremely rapid changes in diameters from abnormal position in cephalic presentation; causes tearing of falx cerebri and tentorium cerebelli, leading to intracranial haemorrhage, death.

**movements (fetal)** *See* 'QUICKENING'.

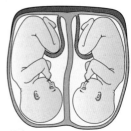

## Placentation of twins

### Monozygotic or dizygotic

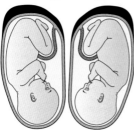

(A) Separate placentae
2 chorions
2 amnions

### Monozygotic

(B) Single placenta
1 chorion
2 amnions

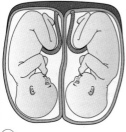

(C) Fused placentae
2 chorions
2 amnions

(D) Single placenta
1 chorion
1 amnion

**A**, Separate placentae. Two chorions. Two amnions. **B**, Single placents.
One chorion. Two amnions. **C**, Fused placentae. Two chorions. Two amnions.
**D**, Single placenta. One chorion. One amnion.

**Moulding**

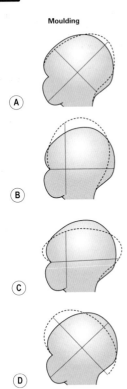

The unmoulded head is indicated by the heavy line **A**, moulding in the occipitoanterior position; **B**, moulding in the persistent occipitoposterior position; **C**, face moulding; **D**, brow moulding.

**moxibustion** Chinese technique to turn breech presentation to cephalic; contraindications as for EXTERNAL CEPHALIC VERSION, plus hypertension. Midwives must be trained to use/advise on moxibustion.

**mucoid** resembling mucus.

**mucopolysaccharidosis** gargoylism; inborn error of metabolism in which mucopolysaccharide builds up in body; distorted features, large spleen, joint movement problems, learning difficulties.

**mucopurulent** containing mucus and pus.

**mucosa** mucous membrane.

**mucous** pertaining to or secreting mucus.

**mucoviscidosis** See CYSTIC FIBROSIS.

**mucus** viscid mucous membrane secretion.

**Müllerian ducts** two embryonic ducts develop into vagina, uterus, fallopian tubes in female; largely obliterated in male.

**multidisciplinary** involving two or more professional disciplines.

**multifactorial** 1. of, pertaining to, or arising through action of many factors. 2. in genetics, arising from interaction of several genes.

**multi-fetal pregnancy reduction** reduction of apparently healthy higher-order multiple pregnancy down to two or even one embryo to improve survival chances; usually performed at 10–12 weeks' gestation by inserting needle under ultrasound guidance, via vagina or abdominal wall into fetal thorax, injecting potassium chloride or saline; all embryos remain in uterus until delivery. See also SELECTIVE FETICIDE.

**multigravida** pregnant woman with at least one previous pregnancy.

*Grande m.* pregnant woman with four or more previous pregnancies. *See also* MULTIPARA. *Adj* multigravid. *Pl* multigravidae.

**multipara** woman who has given birth to more than one VIABLE infant. *Adj* multiparous. *Pl* multiparae.

**multiple of the median** measurement used in biochemistry reports, with 1 indicating median or middle range of scores; more accurate than the mean as less likely to be skewed by extreme results; 0.5 indicates half median and 2 indicates twice median amount.

**multiple pregnancy** pregnancy with more than one fetus. Twins occur naturally in about 1 in 80 pregnancies, more with assisted conception; triplets occur in 1 in 802 pregnancies (1 in 6400); quadruplet pregnancies in 1 in 803 pregnancies (1 in 512,000). Pregnancy complications: POLYHYDRAMNIOS, HYPERTENSION, GESTATIONAL DIABETES, TWIN-TO-TWIN TRANSFUSION SYNDROME. Labour complications: malpresentations, premature membrane rupture, prolonged labour, cord prolapse, premature placental expulsion, postpartum haemorrhage.

**multiple sclerosis** chronic, progressive disease; damage to nerve cell sheaths in brain and spinal cord; symptoms: numbness, speech impairment, uncoordinated muscles, blurred vision, fatigue.

**multivariate analysis** analysis of data collected on several different variables but all having relevance to study; data analysis indicates effects of each variable and their interactions.

**mumps** notifiable viral disease; attacks parotid, submaxillary glands; may cause male infertility. *See also* MMR VACCINATION.

**murmur** periodic auscultatory sound of short duration, cardiac or vascular origin, often associated with disease or abnormality.

**muscle** bundle of long, slender cells, or fibres; relax and contract, producing movement. Uterine muscle, myometrium, also retracts in labour: muscle fibres retain some shortening occurring with contractions; assists in progressive passage of fetus down birth canal.

**muscular dystrophy** genetic, painless, degenerative myopathy; gradual muscle weakening, atrophy. *Duchenne m. d.* sex-linked recessive disease carried by women; sons have 50% chance of inheriting disease.

**musculoskeletal system** in pregnancy, progesterone, relaxin cause joint laxity, increased lumbar lordosis, causing backache, abdominal muscle stretching, separation of symphysis pubis and sacroiliac joints, tilting of pelvic angle; fluid retention around median nerve can cause CARPAL TUNNEL SYNDROME. Neonatal musculoskeletal anomalies include POLYDACTYLY, SYNDACTYLY, limb reduction, TALIPES, hip dysplasia, ACHONDROPLASIA, OSTEOGENESIS IMPERFECTA.

**mutation** change in form or other characteristic; in genetics, change in gene from parent to offspring.

**mutagenicity** property of being able to induce genetic mutation.

**myasthenia** muscular debility or weakness. *M. gravis* autoimmune disease with mild to life-threatening muscle weakness, fatigue and exhaustion, aggravated by activity, relieved by rest; affects ocular and other cranial muscles, tends to fluctuate in severity, responds to cholinergic drugs.

**mycobacterium** gram-positive bacterium (see GRAM STAIN) distinguished by acid-fast staining, e.g. *Mycobacterium tuberculosis*.

**myelomeningocele** spinal cord deformity, most serious form of SPINA BIFIDA.

**myocardium** thick, middle cardiac wall, composed of cardiac muscle. *Adj* myocardial.

**myoclonic seizures** fits involving single or multiple jerks of upper or lower extremities.

**myoepithelial cells** branched contractile epithelial cells surrounding each ALVEOLUS in breast tissue.

*See also* MILK FLOW MECHANISM, BREAST *and* LACTATION.

**myoma** benign tumour of muscle tissue.

**myomectomy** removal of myoma, e.g. uterine fibroids.

**myometrium** uterine muscle.

**myxoedema** hypothyroidism; underactive thyroid gland; facial, limb, hand oedema; dry rough skin; hair loss; slow pulse; low temperature; slow metabolism; mental dullness; treated with preparations of thyroid gland. Congenital hypothyroidism causes CRETINISM.

**Naboth (Nabothian) cyst** mucus-filled cyst on ovarian surface.

**Naegele pelvis** rare asymmetrical pelvis due to congenital failure of one sacral ala to develop fully.

**Naegele rule** method to estimate date of delivery: subtract 3 months from first day of last normal menstrual period, add 7 days; adjusted if menstrual cycle is more than or less than 28 days.

**naevus** birthmark; dilated superficial blood vessels. *Pl* naevi.

**naloxone hydrochloride (Narcan)** antidote to narcotics, e.g. pethidine; 0.01 mg/kg of estimated body weight is administered to baby if APGAR SCORE low and mother had narcotic in labour; observe baby for respiratory difficulties for first 24 hours.

**nano-** prefix indicating 'one-thousand-millionth', e.g. nanogram (ng), one-thousand-millionth of gram.

**napkin/nappy rash** skin rash on baby's buttocks, commonly ammoniacal dermatitis; erythema, vesicles, thrush, psoriasis, perianal erythema.

**Narcan** *See* NALOXONE.

**narco-** prefix denoting 'stupor'.

**narcosis** unconsciousness produced by narcotic drug.

**narcotic** habit-forming drugs; produce narcosis, insensibility, stupor, only available on prescription; e.g. morphine, heroin, pethidine.

**nares** nostrils.

**nasal** pertaining to nose. *N. flaring* neonatal opening of nares on inspira-

tion, to minimize airway resistance effect by maximizing diameter of upper airways. *N. obstruction* occlusion of nostrils in neonates causes cyanosis, unsuccessful attempts to breathe through mouth; sign of CHOANAL ATRESIA.

**nasogastric tube** soft rubber or plastic tube inserted via nostril into stomach to enable instilling of liquid food or other substances, or for withdrawing gastric contents.

**nasojejunal feeding** method of feeding baby on a ventilator or one receiving continuous inflating pressure (cip) by mask or nasal tube; catheter is passed via nose to jejunum; used to avoid aspiration dangers of nasogastric tube feeding.

**nasopharynx** part of pharynx above soft palate.

**National Childbirth Trust (NCT)** charitable organization providing antenatal classes, breastfeeding counselling, postnatal support.

**National Health Service (NHS)** established 1948 to provide free accessible healthcare to all in UK.

**National Institute for Health and Clinical Excellence (also known as NICE)** authority that assesses clinical and cost effectiveness of new and existing health technologies, providing guidance to NHS on their adoption.

**National Screening Committee** Department of Health advisory body; assesses, implements, monitors UK

http://dx.doi.org/10.1016/B978-0-7020-6906-2.00014-0

screening programmes e.g. antenatal, newborn and child health screening.

**National Service Frameworks** NHS policies defining care standards for major medical issues e.g. maternity, children's care.

**natural childbirth, active birth** approach to birth advocating avoidance of intrapartum intervention, technology, analgesia; encourages parents to participate in childbirth experience.

**natural family planning** fertility awareness, rhythm method of contraception in which intercourse is avoided at stage of menstrual cycle when woman is most fertile, or using a barrier method.

**natural induction of labour** complementary therapies and remedies to encourage onset of labour, e.g. ACUPUNCTURE, ACUPRESSURE, REFLEXOLOGY, AROMATHERAPY. Midwives must be trained to advise on/use complementary therapies; women should be cautioned on risks. *See also* CASTOR OIL, CLARY SAGE, NIPPLE STIMULATION, PINEAPPLE, RASPBERRY LEAF.

**nausea** sensation, need to vomit, occurs in almost 90% of pregnancies, commonly in first trimester but may persist throughout pregnancy; may be accompanied by heartburn, hypersalivation, constipation, headaches. *See also* VOMITING, HYPEREMESIS GRAVIDARUM.

**navel** umbilicus.

**necro-** prefix meaning 'dead'.

**necrobiosis** degeneration, tissue death e.g. of uterine fibroids in second trimester.

**necropsy** post-mortem examination.

**necrosis** death of tissue.

**necrotizing enterocolitis** inflammatory bowel disease associated with neonatal septicaemia if previous asphyxia, respiratory distress, hypoglycaemia, hypothermia, cardiovascular disease; bacteria proliferate, penetrate bowel wall in areas of ischaemic damage. Oedema, ulceration, bowel wall haemorrhage, peritonitis; treated with parenteral nutrition, antibodies, surgery for perforation.

**negligence** in law, failure to do something that a reasonable person of ordinary prudence would do in certain situations; may provide basis for lawsuit. Midwife has legal duty to provide reasonable care for women.

*Neisseria gonorrhoeae* microorganism causing GONORRHOEA.

**nem** unit of nutrition equivalent to nutritive value of 1 g breast milk.

**neo-** prefix meaning 'new'.

**neomycin** broad-spectrum antibiotic; intestinal antiseptic.

**neonatal** pertaining to first 4 weeks of life. *N. mortality rate* number of deaths of neonates per 1000 live births in a year.

**neonate** newborn up to 4 weeks old.

**neonatology** paediatric medicine specialism dealing with disorders of newborn baby.

**neoplasm** new growth, e.g. tumour; neoplasia.

**nephrectomy** excision of kidney.

**nephritis** kidney inflammation. *Acute n.* kidney lesion, often after streptococcal infection; lumbar pain, pyrexia, oedema, poor renal function, urine contains albumin, blood, renal tubule casts; serum urea rises; may lead to chronic nephritis, permanently impaired renal function, oedema, proteinuria, hypertension, raised blood urea, subfertility. Increased risk of miscarriage, PRE-ECLAMPSIA.

**nephron** functioning kidney unit: glomerulus, Bowman capsule, tubule system; about one million nephrons in each kidney.

**nephropathy** disease of kidneys.

**nephrosis** renal disease.

**nephrotic syndrome** degeneration of renal tubules; may follow acute nephritis; excessive fluid accumulates due to protein loss, decreased serum albumin. Treatment: diuretics, high protein diet, steroids, immunosuppressants.

**nerve** bundle of fibres enclosed in sheath which transmits impulses between part of body and nerve centre. *Motor (efferent) n.* conveys impulses for movement from nerve centre to muscle. *N. fibre* prolongation of nerve cell, conveys impulse to or from part that it controls. *Sensory (afferent) n.* conveys sensations from sense organs to nerve centre. *Vasomotor n.* either dilator or constrictor of blood vessels.

**nerve block** local analgesic blocking impulses passing along nerves, e.g. EPIDURAL ANALGESIA.

**nervous** 1. pertaining to, or composed of, nerves. 2. unduly excitable. *N. system* body system that correlates adjustments and reactions of organism to internal and environmental conditions; central nervous system composed of brain, spinal cord; peripheral nervous system subdivided into voluntary and autonomic systems.

**netilmicin** aminoglycoside antibiotic, may cause ototoxicity; may be used in serious maternal infection where benefits outweigh risks.

**neural tube defect** structural anomaly of brain or spinal cord causing ANENCEPHALY or SPINA BIFIDA.

**neuritis** nerve inflammation.

**neuroblast** embryonic nerve cell.

**neuroblastoma** malignant tumour of immature nerve cells, most often occurs in children.

**neurogenic shock** collapse, acute shock from insult to nervous system, e.g. uterine INVERSION.

**neurohormonal** pertaining to nerves and hormones and coordination. *N. reflex* process in LACTATION physiology; nerves and hormones work in harmony to control 'LET DOWN' REFLEX.

**neurological assessment of newborn** performed shortly after birth with baby awake, alert, not crying; assessed for neck retraction, limb posture and hyperextension or hyperflexion, jittery or abnormal involuntary movements, high-pitched or weak cry; any may indicate antenatally acquired or perinatal neurological disorder.

**neuromuscular** pertaining to nerves and muscles and coordination. *N. harmony* intrapartum relationship between upper and lower uterine segments; upper uterine segment contracts and retracts, lower segment and cervix contract and dilate.

**neuron, neurone** nerve cell; conducting cell of nervous system: cell body, nucleus, surrounding cytoplasm, axon, dendrites.

**neuropeptides** natural substances produced at neural synapses in central nervous system; modulate pain perception; opiate-like; ENDORPHINS, ENKEPHALINS.

**neurosis** functional nervous system disturbance; emotional instability, no obvious structural change in nerve substance.

**neurotensin** neuropeptide implicated in release of luteinizing hormone

153

and prolactin; interacts with dopaminergic system.

**neutral** neither acid nor alkaline.

**neutral thermal environment** environmental temperature range over which heat production, oxygen consumption, nutritional requirements for growth are minimal, provided body temperature normal.

**neurotransmitters** endogenous chemicals which transmit signals from neuron to target cell across synapse.

**neutron** neutral particle found with protons in nucleus of atom.

**Neville Barnes forceps** obstetric forceps for operative vaginal delivery; allow downward traction of high head into pelvis.

**nevirapine** antiviral drug for treatment of HUMAN IMMUNODEFICIENCY SYNDROME (HIV) in pregnancy.

**Newborn and Infant Physical Examination** physical examination of baby offered just after birth, repeated at 6–8 weeks; includes examination of eyes, heart, hips, testes; may be performed by doctor or suitably trained midwife.

**newborn blood-spot screening programme** national screening of babies to diagnose and treat early PHENYLKETONURIA, congenital HYPOTHYROIDISM, SICKLE CELL DISEASE, CYSTIC FIBROSIS and MEDIUM CHAIN ACYL-COENZYME A DEHYDROGENASE DEFICIENCY; blood-spot sample taken on sixth day of life.

**NHS number** ten-digit number, unique identifier for each patient. *NHS Number for Babies* allows midwives to request NHS number for every baby after birth; ensures baby offered NEWBORN BLOOD-SPOT SCREENING PROGRAMME, ensures results made available to health visitor when duty of care is transferred from midwife.

**niacin** water-soluble B complex vitamin in liver, yeast, bran, peanuts, lean meats, fish, poultry; required for enzyme synthesis.

**NICE** *See* NATIONAL INSTITUTE FOR HEALTH AND CARE EXCELLENCE.

**nidation** embedding of fertilized ovum in endometrium of uterus.

**nifedipine** calcium channel blocker, antihypertensive, anti-anginal, sometimes used for preterm labour.

**nipple** small conical projection in centre of breast; gives outlet to milk; tip contains 15–20 small lactiferous ducts. *Accessory n.* rudimentary nipple anywhere in line from breast to groin. *Retracted n.* nipple drawn inwards; may be sign of breast cancer. *N. stimulation* practice towards term to try to accelerate cervical ripening, trigger uterine contractions through natural release of oxytocin; also used to trigger oxytocin release to aid placental separation and control postpartum haemorrhage.

**nitrofurantoin** antibacterial drug for urinary tract infection; may cause neonatal haemolysis if given to mother at term.

**nitrogen** element, symbol N; gas forming nearly 80% of atmospheric air; constituent of all protein foods and substances.

**nitrous oxide** 'laughing gas'; gas and oxygen (50% of each; Entonox), to relieve pain in labour premixed in single blue and white cylinder approved by Nursing and Midwifery Council for use by midwives. Excreted via lungs; may cause giggling, loss of control, nausea. *N. O. ventilation* neonatal ventilation method; N₂O inhaled with each ventilation breath, working directly on pulmonary vessels with minimal effect on systemic circulation; reduces need for EXTRACORPOREAL MEMBRANE OXYGENATION.

**nociceptor** sensory receptor, responds to stimuli e.g. pain by sending nerve signals to spinal cord and brain, causing pain perception.

**nocturia** night-time urination; in pregnancy, usually due to pressure on bladder from uterus, or presenting part (after ENGAGEMENT).

**node** small swelling, knot or protuberance of tissue, normal or pathological. *Adj* nodal.

**nodule** small solid node detected by touch.

**nominal group technique** group process involving problem identification, generating ideas to resolve problem, decision making.

**non-accidental injury** injury caused to baby: bone fractures, intracranial haemorrhage, giving of poisons and dangerous drugs, sexual abuse, starvation, other physical assault; commonly inflicted by parents or adult responsible for child care.

**non-accidental head injury** presence of unexplained fractures in baby's long bones with evidence of subdural haematoma; caused by violent shaking producing whiplash effect, rotation of head, results in vomiting, convulsions, irritability, coma, death. Previously shaken baby syndrome.

**non-anomalous** not deviating from normal, as in genetics.

**non-disjunction** failure of chromosome pair to separate during meiosis, or paired chromatids during mitosis.

**Non-invasive Prenatal Testing** test for DOWN, EDWARD, PATAU SYNDROME without invasive procedures; 99% detection rate; not yet available on NHS.

**non-maleficence** legal duty to avoid harming interests of others.

**non-shivering thermogenesis** baby's use of brown adipose tissue in mediastinum, around nape of neck, between scapulae, around kidneys, adrenal glands, to produce heat in times of cold stress.

**non-specific urethritis** common sexually transmitted disease caused by various organisms, notably *Chlamydia trachomatis*.

**non-steroidal anti-inflammatory drugs** analgesics with no narcotic effects, anti-pyretic, anti-inflammatory; includes: aspirin, ibuprofen, diclofenac, naproxen, indomethacin. Not used in third trimester, may cause premature closure of fetal ductus arteriosus, fetal renal dysfunction, necrotizing enterocolitis, intracerebral haemorrhage, oligohydramnios, preterm labour. Exception: aspirin used with heparin for women with ANTIPHOSPHOLIPID ANTIBODIES. Indomethacin used short-term as tocolytic and to reduce liquor volume in polyhydramnios. Maternal side effects: gastrointestinal bleeding, peptic ulceration, thrombocytopenia, allergy.

**non-stress test** cardiotocography performed when pregnancy is prolonged; expectation of two ACCELERATIONS of $\geq 15$ above BASELINE in 20-minute period, plus fetal reaction, assessed by movement; may be extended to 40 minutes, but if trace is non-reactive, or other irregularities, further assessment of AMNIOTIC FLUID volume, BIOPHYSICAL PROFILE, contraction stress testing.

**noradrenaline (norepinephrine)** catecholamine neurotransmitter of most sympathetic post-ganglionic neurons and certain tracts in nervous system, released from adrenal medulla in response to sympathetic stimulation, primarily hypotension, producing vasoconstriction, increased heart rate, raised blood pressure.

**norethisterone** progestogen used in contraceptive pill, and for premenstrual syndrome and other menstrual disorders.

**normetanephrine** metabolite of norepinephrine, excreted in urine and found in certain tissues; marker for catecholamine-secreting tumours such as PHAEOCHROMOCYTOMA.

**normo-** normality, e.g. normotensive, normal blood pressure.

**normoblasts** immature nucleated red blood cells; normally remain in bone marrow until maturity, released into circulation in certain anaemias.

**notifiable diseases** certain transmittable diseases must be reported to designated government authority to allow monitoring, prediction of possible outbreak or epidemic. Includes: encephalitis, MENINGITIS, poliomyelitis, infectious hepatitis, food poisoning, botulism, group A streptococcal disease, scarlet fever, MALARIA, measles, meningococcal septicaemia, mumps, RUBELLA, TUBERCULOSIS, whooping cough, diphtheria, tetanus, cholera, anthrax, Legionnaire's disease, brucellosis, leprosy, rabies, yellow fever.

**notification** See INTENTION TO PRACTISE; BIRTH, NOTIFICATION OF.

**nucha** nape of neck.

**nuchal** pertaining to back of neck. *N. fold* fat pad at back of fetal neck, measured on ultrasound scan at anomaly scan. Measurement of $\geq 6$ mm increases chance of DOWN SYNDROME, TURNER SYNDROME. *N. translucency* subdermal collection of lymphatic fluid at back of fetal neck, visualized at 14 weeks' gestation; if increased may indicate chromosomal or structural abnormalities, neuromuscular problems. See PREGNANCY-ASSOCIATED PLASMA PROTEIN-A, COMBINED TEST *and* INTEGRATED TEST. *N. displacement* breech labour complication, arm is displaced behind baby's neck.

**nuclear family** parents and their children living together in household, without extended family living with them or nearby.

**nuclear magnetic resonance** magnetic nuclei in magnetic field absorb and re-emit electromagnetic energy, at specific resonance frequency depending on strength of magnetic field. Signals elicited are used for chemical analysis or MAGNETIC RESONANCE IMAGING.

**nuclear factor kappa B protein** complex controlling DNA transcription, cytokine production, cell survival; regulates immune response.

**nucleic acids** complex, long-chain compounds of high molecular weight in cells of all living organisms, forming genetic material of cell and directing synthesis of protein within cell. See DEOXYRIBONUCLEIC ACID (DNA) *and* RIBONUCLEIC ACID (RNA).

**nucleus** essential part of cell containing chromosomes; division is vital for new cell formation. *Basal n.* group of brain nerve cells; may be bilirubin-stained in neonatal jaundice, causing KERNICTERUS.

**nullipara** woman who has never given birth to a VIABLE, child. *Adj* nulliparous.

**nurse** 1. professional qualified in nursing. 2. to provide services to promote, maintain, restore health. 3. to nourish at breast.

**nursery** place set aside for care of children and infants. *Day n.* for children under school age of working mothers provided by local authority social services department and private or voluntary bodies registered and supervised by local authority. *N. school* school for children between 2.5 and 5 years provided by local education authority.

**Nursing and Midwifery Council** statutory UK regulatory organization for nursing, midwifery, health visiting professions in order to protect public; responsible for quality assurance of education programmes; maintains registers of practitioners; professional conduct rules, documents to guide professional practice.

**Nursing and Midwifery Order 2001** statutory instrument established by NURSING AND MIDWIFERY COUNCIL; specifies NMC duties; certain amendments made 2008.

**nutrition** food assimilation process for nourishment; balanced diet contains adequate essential nutritional elements, i.e. proteins, vitamins, minerals, fats, carbohydrates, fluid.

**NuvaRing** prescription combined hormonal contraceptive vaginal ring, releases low-dose progestin, oestrogen over 3 weeks.

**nystagmus** involuntary, rapid, rhythmic movement of eyeball.

**nystatin** antibiotic used to treat superficial fungal infections, e.g. candidiasis, administered orally or as vaginal pessary.

**obesity in pregnancy** excessive body fat; body mass index (BMI) above 30. Complications: menstrual, fertility issues, pregnancy hypertension, gestational diabetes, urinary tract infection, difficulty determining fetal position, large for gestational age baby, Caesarean section, poor wound healing, postpartum haemorrhage, thrombophlebitis; significant risk factor for maternal death. *Morbid o.* women with booking BMI above 40.

**oblique** slanting. *O. lie* long axis of fetus lies between oblique diameters of pelvis; may cause shoulder presentation, obstructed labour, risk of cord or arm prolapse, ruptured uterus, haemorrhage, fetal or maternal death.

**oblongata** *See* MEDULLA OBLONGATA.

**observational study** epidemiological study of events without intervention of investigator.

**obsessive compulsive disorder** psychiatric anxiety disorder: obsessive thoughts, compulsive actions, e.g. cleaning, checking, counting, hoarding; may occur postnatally as hormones fluctuate, or may pre-exist, leading to relapses during and after pregnancy.

**obstetric** pertaining to obstetrics. *O. cholestasis. See* INTRAHEPATIC CHOLESTASIS OF PREGNANCY. *O. conjugate* pelvic diameter from sacral promontory to upper inner border of symphysis pubis, approximately 11 cm. *O. history* detailed information taken at booking of all previous pregnancies, including miscarriages, terminations, labours, puerperia, babies. *O. shock* collapse associated with childbirth due to circulatory failure, most commonly from haemorrhage or trauma as in acute uterine inversion, or septicaemia caused by gram-negative organisms.

**obstetrician** doctor specializing in care of women with abnormal pregnancies, labours and puerperia.

**obstetrics** medical specialism; pregnancy, labour and puerperium.

**obstipation** intractable constipation.

**obstructed labour** no advance of presenting part in labour despite strong uterine contractions; occurs at pelvic brim or outlet. Mother is distressed, anxious, tachycardic, pyrexial, has ketonuria, oliguria, vomiting, persistent abdominal pain; uterus appears 'moulded' around fetus; on palpation abdomen continuously hard, fetal parts not felt, fetal heart sounds absent; fetal death from anoxia occurs. On examination, vagina hot, dry, oedematous; high head, excessive caput succedaneum, thick 'curtain' of cervix hanging round and below. Multipara may suffer uterine rupture, death; primigravida may develop secondary uterine inertia. Treatment: summon doctor urgently; analgesia, intravenous fluids to combat pain, shock, dehydration; take blood for cross-matching. Immediate Caesarean section if possible, even if fetus dead; in isolated areas fetal

http://dx.doi.org/10.1016/B978-0-7020-6906-2.00015-2

destructive operation may be required to save mother's life, although risk of uterine rupture. *See also* BANDL'S RING.

**obturator** anything that closes an opening. *O. foramen* opening in antero-lateral aspect of innominate bone, closed by fascia, muscle.

**occipital** relating to occiput.

**occipitoanterior** fetal occiput is directed to front of mother's pelvis.

**occipitolateral, occipitotransverse** fetal occiput is to side of mother's pelvis as it enters brim, either right or left sided; if uterine contractions are efficient, usually turns to occipito-anterior position as occiput reaches resistance of pelvic floor.

**occipitoposterior** fetal occiput directed towards right or left sacroiliac joint of maternal pelvis; fetal attitude often military or deflexed; occurs in about 10% of pregnancies. On examination, abdomen appears flattened below umbilicus, high deflexed fetal head and limbs felt over large area on both sides of midline; fetal heart sounds heard in middle and over flank. Vaginal examination: high head, bregma anterior or central. Fetal head may flex at pelvic floor: long rotation to occipito-anterior position, normal birth. Risks: prolonged labour, difficult birth, cord prolapse, infection, fetal hypoxia, intracranial haemorrhage. DEEP TRANSVERSE ARREST requires forceps delivery, or head is born FACE-TO-PUBES.

**occiput** back of head, from lambdoidal suture to nape of neck.

**occlusive cap** rubber contraceptive cap to cover cervix; obstructs entrance of spermatozoa, used with spermicidal gel or cream.

**occult** obscure or hidden from view. *O. blood test* microscopic or chemical examination of faeces, urine, gastric juice, etc., to determine presence of blood not otherwise detectable. *O. cord prolapse* hidden umbilical cord prolapse when cord lies alongside, rather than in front of presenting part.

**ocular** pertaining to eye.

**odds of being affected given positive result** term to describe chances of positive screening test result being correct, i.e. proportion of people with positive screening result who have condition; positive predictive value.

**oedema** excess fluid, due either to excess formation or to failure of absorption, often first recognized by excess weight gain (occult oedema), then by pitting on pressure. Approximately 50% of pregnant women develop mild physiological ankle oedema towards term, normal unless accompanied by other signs and symptoms, e.g. hypertension. In puerperium, ankle oedema often worsens temporarily, as kidneys are unable to cope immediately with excretion of excess fluid resulting from autolytic process of INVOLUTION. Pathological oedema occurs with chronic renal disease, PRE-ECLAMPSIA, ECLAMPSIA, severe heart disease, severe anaemia and malnutrition. *Pitting o.* severe oedema in which pressure leaves persistent depression in tissues.

**oesophageal** pertaining to oesophagus. *O. atresia* absence of oesophageal opening; maternal POLYHYDRAMNIOS may occur as fetus is unable to swallow saliva; in neonate, saliva comes out of mouth continuously as clear mucus; stiff tube should be passed via mouth immediately after birth to ensure oesophageal patency; often accompanied by TRACHEO-OESOPHAGEAL FISTULA.

**oesophagus** canal from pharynx to stomach; 22.5 cm long in adult.

**oestradiol** ovarian hormone; potent naturally occurring OESTROGEN.

**oestriol** ovarian hormone; relatively weak human oestrogen.

**oestrogens** hormones, oestradiol, oestriol, oestrone; produced by ovary, adrenal gland, testis, fetoplacental unit; facilitates development of female secondary sexual characteristics, acts on genitalia to produce environment suitable for fertilization, implantation, nutrition of embryo. In pregnancy, stimulate growth of uterus, duct system in breasts. Influence water and electrolyte retention to suppress ovulation, inhibit lactation in pregnancy. *Adj* oestrogenic.

**oestrone** OESTROGEN isolated from urine in pregnancy and from human placenta; also prepared synthetically.

**ofloxacin fluoroquinolone** antibiotic sometimes used for gonorrhoea.

**olanzapine** antipsychotic drug for bipolar disorder and schizophrenia, usually discontinued in pregnancy.

**olfaction** sense of smell.

**oligo-** prefix denoting insufficiency.

**oligaemia** deficiency in volume of blood.

**oligohydramnios** reduced amniotic fluid, associated with fetal renal agenesis, limb deformities, intrauterine growth retardation.

**oligomenorrhoea** scanty menstruation.

**oligospermia** deficiency of spermatozoa in semen.

**oliguria** diminished urine secretion; may occur with impaired renal function after severe placental abruption, haemorrhage, pre-eclampsia, eclampsia.

**ombudsman** person appointed to receive and investigate complaints about unfair administration and failures in health services; does not pass judgement on clinical matters.

**omentum** peritoneal fold from stomach to nearby abdominal organs.

**Omnopon** *See* PAPAVERETUM.

**omphalitis** umbilical cord stump infection; superficial cellulitis spreading to involve entire abdominal wall; may progress to necrotizing fasciitis or systemic disease.

**omphalocele** umbilical hernia. *See* EXOMPHALOS.

**omphalus** umbilicus.

**onco-** word element meaning 'tumour', 'swelling', 'mass'.

**oncology** study of tumours.

**onych(o)-** word element meaning 'nails'.

**onychia** inflammation of nail bed.

**ooblast** primitive cell from which ovum ultimately develops.

**oocyte** immature ovum.

**oophor(o)-** word element meaning 'ovary'.

**oophorectomy** removal of ovary.

**oophoritis** inflammation of ovary.

**oophorosalpingectomy** surgical removal of ovary and fallopian tube.

**operative delivery** instrumental birth by forceps, ventouse, vacuum extraction or Caesarean section.

**operculum** mucus plug in cervical canal in pregnancy; shed at start of labour. *See* 'SHOW'.

**ophthalmia neonatorum** purulent discharge from eyes of newborn; most commonly caused by CHLAMYDIA TRACHOMATIS.

**ophthalmic** pertaining to eye.

**ophthalmoscope** instrument for inspecting interior of eye.

**opiate, opioid** powerful habit-forming analgesic, narcotic drugs; e.g. opium, morphine, codeine; heroin; methadone, pethidine, phenazocine; also narcotic antagonists. Long-term use may cause neonatal withdrawal. Naloxone, antidote to PETHIDINE, is opiate antagonist but has no narcotic properties.

**opportunistic** micro-organism not normally causing disease but capable of doing so in some circumstances; disease or infection caused by such organism.

**opsonin** substance that coats bacteria, making them more easily phagocytosed, e.g. antibody.

**optic** pertaining to vision.

**oral** pertaining to mouth. *O. contraceptive pill* combined oral contraceptive pill contains both oestrogen and progesterone; also progestogen-only pill, often prescribed for breast-feeding women and when combined pill is contraindicated.

**orbit** bony cavity containing eyeball.

**orbital ridge** bony rim of orbit.

**orchi(d)(o)-** word element meaning 'testis'.

**orchidopexy** operation, releases undescended testis, places them in scrotum.

**orchitis** inflammation of testis.

**organ** part of body with particular function.

**organic** pertaining to structure of organ.

**organism** individual animal or plant.

**organogenesis** origin or development of organs.

**orgasm** apex and culmination of sexual excitement.

**orifice** opening in body, e.g. mouth, vagina.

**oropharynx** part of pharynx between soft palate and upper edge of epiglottis.

**-orrhaphy** suffix meaning 'repair' or 'suturing', e.g. perineorrhaphy.

**orthostatic** standing erect. *O. albuminuria* albuminuria occurring when individual is upright but not after rest in bed.

**Ortolani's test** diagnosis of CONGENITAL HIP DISLOCATION; 'click' or popping sensation felt on reversing movements of abduction and rotation of hip with baby's knees flexed. *See also* BARLOW TEST.

**os** 1. bone. 2. opening. *External o.* opening of cervix into vagina. *Internal o.* junction of cervical canal with uterine cavity. *O. uteri* opening of uterus into vagina, dilates progressively in labour.

**Osiander sign** uterine artery pulsation through lateral fornices, felt on vaginal examination in early pregnancy.

**osmolality** concentration of solution in terms of osmoles of solutes per kilogram of solvent. *Serum o.* number of dissolved particles per unit of water in serum, used to assess status of hydration. *Urine o.* number of dissolved particles per unit of water in urine.

**osmosis** passage of solvent through semi-permeable membrane into more concentrated solution; clinically important in maintaining adequate body fluids and for proper balance between volumes of extracellular and intracellular fluids.

**osmotic pressure** power of fluid, dependent on its molecular content, to draw another fluid towards it.

**ossification** formation and hardening of bone. *O. centres* seen on radiography at distal end of fetal femoral epiphysis between 35 and 40 weeks' gestation and proximal tibial epiphysis at 37–42 weeks; may help to determine fetal maturity. *See also* ULTRASOUND. Ossification centres on fetal head include frontal bosses, occipital protuberance and parietal eminences.

**osteoblasts** cells that mature and form bone.

**osteogenesis** formation of bone. *O. imperfecta* inherited dominant condition; extremely fragile bones; spontaneous fractures common.

**osteomalacia** adult rickets; painful bone softening, due to severe vitamin D deficiency.

**osteomyelitis** bone inflammation due to pyogenic infection; may cause bone destruction, stiffening of joints if infection spreads, shortening of limbs in children.

**osteopathy** statutorily regulated profession supplementary to medicine in which musculoskeletal manipulation helps to restore structural and functional balance in body; may be effective in treating pregnancy disorders, e.g. backache, carpal tunnel syndrome. *See also* CHIROPRACTIC, CRANIOSACRAL THERAPY.

**osteoporosis** disease, extremely porous bones, subject to fracture, slow healing, occurs especially in women after menopause; may lead to spine curvature from vertebral collapse.

**otitis** ear inflammation. *O. externa* external ear inflammation. *O. media*

infection of middle ear, may occur in neonates. *O. interna* labyrinthitis.

**otoacoustic emissions test** test in Newborn Hearing Screening Programme, based on healthy cochlea producing faint echo when stimulated with sound. Earpiece inserted in baby's ear and clicking sound played; failure to elicit cochlear echo requires further testing. Difficult to interpret if baby unsettled or there is fluid in ear.

**-otomy** suffix meaning 'cutting into', e.g. hysterotomy, incision in uterus.

**outlet** route of exit. *Pelvic o.* inferior opening of pelvis bounded by ischial spines, lower symphysis pubis border, sacrococcygeal joint.

**output** yield, total production. *Cardiac o.* effective volume of blood expelled by ventricle of heart per unit of time (volume per minute), equal to stroke output multiplied by number of beats per time unit used in computation. *Fluid o.* amount of urine passed, usually compared with oral fluid intake.

**outreach clinic** clinic geographically at distance from main maternity department; enables women to access care without inconvenient journeys to hospital.

**ova** plural of ovum.

**ovarian** pertaining to ovary. *O. cyst* tumour of ovary, contains fluid. *O. hyperstimulation syndrome* serious iatrogenic complication of induced multiple ovulation in fertility treatment, potentially life threatening. Risk factors: POLYCYSTIC OVARY SYNDROME, young age, lean physique, human CHORIONIC GONADOTROPHIN administration, multiple pregnancy. *O. pregnancy* fertilized ovum develops in ovary, ECTOPIC pregnancy.

***O. vein syndrome*** obstruction of ureter, commonly right, due to compression by enlarged or varicosed ovarian vein; typically, vein becomes enlarged in pregnancy, symptoms similar to obstruction or infection of upper urinary tract.

**ovariotomy** incision of ovary.

**ovaries** two glandular organs in cavity of female pelvis, attached to posterior fold of broad ligament near fimbriated end of fallopian tube; produce ova, oestrogens, progesterone; aid body changes at puberty and in pregnancy.

**oviduct** passage through which ova leave maternal body or pass to organ communicating with exterior of body.

**oviferous** producing ova.

**ovulation** release of ovum from ovary by rupture of Graafian follicle, normally every 28 days, alternating between two ovaries; occasionally, two or more ova produced; if fertilized, results in multiple pregnancy.

**ovum** egg; reproductive cell of female. *Pl* ova.

**oxidase** enzymes that catalyze reduction of molecular oxygen independently of hydrogen peroxide.

**oxidation** process of combining with oxygen.

**oxprenolol** beta-blocking drug to treat angina, hypertension, cardiac arrhythmias.

**oxygen** element, symbol O; colourless, odourless gas, essential to life. Constitutes 21% of atmosphere; obtained from air, inhaled into lungs. Stored in black and white cylinders for therapeutic use. Lack of oxygen (hypoxia) causes CYANOSIS and ANOXIA leading to neonatal death; oxygen is administered during resuscitation via endotracheal tube. Careful monitoring of oxygen concentration needed in preterm newborns to ensure sufficient oxygen intake to prevent brain damage but not so much as to cause retinopathy leading to blindness.

**oxygenation** addition of oxygen to body, naturally or artificially. Maternal oxygenation may be impaired due to cardiac or respiratory disease, eclampsia, or during general anaesthesia induction if intubation difficult. Fetal oxygenation dependent on maternal oxygenation, adequate placental perfusion and function, fetoplacental circulation, fetal haemoglobin; may be affected by maternal hyper- or hypotension, hypertonic uterine contractions, cord prolapse, rhesus incompatibility, abnormal fetal cardiac function. Poor oxygenation at birth requires resuscitation.

**oxyhaemoglobin** haemoglobin combined with molecular oxygen, form in which oxygen is transported in blood.

**oxytetracycline** broad-spectrum antibiotic of tetracycline group.

**oxytocics** drugs that stimulate uterine contractions, used for induction or acceleration of labour.

**oxytocin** hormone from posterior pituitary gland causing contraction of smooth muscle, e.g. uterine myometrium, myoepithelial cells in breast. Synthetic oxytocin (Syntocinon) may be given intravenously to induce or accelerate labour, or intramuscularly or intravenously to contract uterus after placental delivery, to control haemorrhage. Synthetic oxytocin is combined with

ergometrine to produce Syntometrine. *O. antagonists* TOCOLYTIC drugs
to suppress preterm labour; inhibit
oxytocin and vasopressin; similar

effectiveness but fewer side effects
than other tocolytics.

**oxytocinase** enzyme that metabolizes
oxytocin; produced by placenta.

**pack** large swab or tampon used to control bleeding in wound or abdominal contents during surgery.

**packed cells** fresh blood for transfusion, with some plasma content removed to facilitate cell haemolysis; given when necessary to replace blood cells without overloading circulation with fluid.

**packed cell volume** percentage of blood cells to PLASMA; normal PCV is about 45%.

**PaCO₂** partial pressure of dissolved carbon dioxide which has moved out of cells into bloodstream; reflects alveolar ventilation.

**paediatrician** doctor specializing in paediatrics.

**paediatrics** study of infant and child health and disease.

**paedophilia** abnormal fondness for children; sexual activity of adults with children. *Adj* paedophiliac.

**pain** distress due to stimulation of free nerve endings in small myelinated or unmyelinated nerve fibres in superficial skin layers, some deeper tissues. Impulses transmitted along sensory nerve fibres to spinal cord, then along sensory pathways to thalamus, main sensory relay station of brain. *Abdominal p. in pregnancy* may indicate THREATENED MISCARRIAGE, ECTOPIC PREGNANCY, PLACENTAL ABRUPTION, uterine RETROVERSION or fibroids, urinary tract infection, ovarian cysts, appendicitis, cholecystitis. *Labour p.* increasingly frequent, intense, intermittent abdominal pain from upper uterine segment contractions and dilating cervix. Sacral back pain originates in cervix; if severe, may indicate poor cervical dilatation, prolonged labour. *P. control in labour* woman may require help to ease labour pain, either conventional methods, e.g. INHALATIONAL ANALGESIA, PETHIDINE, MEPTAZINOL or EPIDURAL ANALGESIA, or complementary strategies, e.g. MASSAGE, HYDROTHERAPY, AROMATHERAPY, HYPNOTHERAPY. *See also* AFTERPAINS, GATE CONTROL THEORY, REFERRED PAIN.

**palate** roof of mouth. *Hard p.* bony palate at front. *Soft p.* muscular area behind hard palate. *See also* CLEFT PALATE.

**palliative** agent that relieves but does not cure disease.

**pallor** pale skin, often mottled; in baby, a sign of poor peripheral perfusion; low circulating blood volume or circulatory adaptation and compensation for hypoxaemia; also occurs in anaemia.

**palpation** physical examination by touch; light finger pressure on skin surface to identify condition of parts beneath surface, aiding diagnosis. *See* ABDOMINAL EXAMINATION, VAGINAL EXAMINATION.

**palpitation** sensation of abnormally rapid beating of heart.

**palsy** paralysis. *Bell's p.* facial paralysis, distortion, from facial nerve lesion. *Cerebral p.* persistent qualitative motor disorder occurs before

http://dx.doi.org/10.1016/B978-0-7020-6906-2.00016-4

age 3. **Erb's p.** limp inwardly rotated arm with half-closed hand turned outwards due to brachial plexus damage. **Klumpke p.** hand paralysis and wrist drop from damage to eighth cervical and first thoracic nerve roots.

**Panadol** See PARACETAMOL.

**pancreas** racemose gland about 15 cm long, behind stomach with head in curve of duodenum, tail in contact with spleen; secretes INSULIN from islets of Langerhans and digestive juice.

**pancreatic duct** main excretory duct of pancreas, unites with common bile duct before entering duodenum.

**pandemic** epidemic spreading over wide area.

**panhysterectomy** total removal of uterine body and cervix.

**PaO₂** partial pressure of oxygen in arterial blood; reflects how lung is functioning, but does not measure tissue oxygenation.

**Papanicolaou test** smear test to detect uterine and cervical cancer; spatula passed into cervix, rotated 360 degrees to scrape off surface cells, transferred to glass slide, examined microscopically.

**papaveretum (Omnopon)** analgesic drug, mix of opium alkaloids.

**papilla** small nipple-like eminence. *Pl* papillae.

**papilloma** benign epithelial tumour. *P. virus* sexually transmitted infection, causes anogenital warts (condylomata acuminata), increases cervical carcinoma risk. **Laryngeal p.** rare neonatal condition from infection acquired during vaginal birth.

**papule** small, solid, raised elevation of skin.

**papyraceous** like parchment. *Fetus p.* rare twin pregnancy abnormality; one fetus dies early and is flattened; usually born with placenta.

**para** 1. woman who has produced one or more VIABLE offspring, over 24 weeks' gestation; includes stillbirths: *para 0* NULLIPARA, woman who has not borne a viable baby; *para 1* PRIMIPARA, has given birth to one viable baby; *para 2* or more, MULTIPARA has borne two or more viable babies. GRANDE MULTIPARA woman who has borne five or more viable babies. Miscarriages, terminations not counted; identified by adding $^{+1}$ after number designating viable births, e.g. para $3^{+1}$. *Adj* parous. 2. prefix meaning 'near', e.g. parametrium.

**paracentesis** puncture of cavity wall to draw off fluid. *P. uteri* amniocentesis; abdominal and uterine wall puncture to draw off excess amniotic fluid. See POLYHYDRAMNIOS.

**paracervical block** infiltration of LEE–FRANKENHAUSER PLEXUS with local anaesthetic to relieve cervical dilatation pain in labour. If injected into uterine artery, may cause fetal bradycardia, fetal death.

**paracetamol** oral analgesic, antipyretic; relieves headache, reduces pyrexia; overdose may cause hepatic necrosis. Relatively safe in pregnancy but should be used cautiously.

**paraesthesia** sensation of 'pins and needles' as with CARPAL TUNNEL SYNDROME or in feet after epidural analgesia.

**paralysis** failure of nerve function, especially motor nerve, leading to impairment of voluntary or involuntary

**paralytic** pertaining to paralysis *P. ileus* intestinal blockage without physical obstruction due to intestinal nerve and muscle malfunction; impairs digestive movement; can occur after abdominal surgery e.g. Caesarean section.

**paramedic** emergency medical care professional; ambulance service personnel with specialist training to perform, in emergencies, certain procedures normally undertaken by doctors.

**parametritis** inflammation of PARAMETRIUM; pelvic cellulitis in tissues surrounding uterus; may occur if infection in genital tract.

**parametrium** pelvic connective tissue surrounding lower part of uterus, filling spaces between uterus and related organs.

**paranoia** psychiatric disorder, delusions of persecution, illusions of grandeur focusing on fears for future; often combined with SCHIZOPHRENIA; may occur in POSTNATAL DEPRESSION. *Adj* paranoid.

**paraplegia** central nervous system paralysis of legs and lower body, affecting all muscles within local area. *Adj* paraplegic.

**parasite** plant or animal living in or on another living organism (host) to satisfy all needs. Infections from parasites include TOXOPLASMOSIS, scabies, GIARDIASIS, many tropical diseases.

**parasympathetic nervous system** part of autonomic nervous system; postganglionic nerve fibres, primarily in VAGUS nerves, which serve thoracic and abdominal regions; also in heart, smooth muscles, head and neck glands, pelvic viscera; acetylcholine is secreted from nerve endings, exciting or inhibiting certain activities.

**parathyroid glands** four small endocrine glands associated with thyroid gland; help to maintain plasma calcium levels. *P. g. disorders* rare causes of hypo- or hypercalcaemia in neonates, may be hereditary or deletion of chromosome 22 (DIGEORGE SYNDROME).

**paratyphoid** notifiable infection caused by *Salmonella*.

**parenteral** outside alimentary tract. *P. feeding* introduction of nutritional substances by any route other than alimentary tract.

**parent education** antenatal advice to help parents prepare for labour and parenthood, offered in group setting or on one-to-one basis.

**paresis** partial paralysis affects muscular action but not sensation.

**parietal** related to or attached to wall of cavity. *P. bone* thin, flat bone forming major part of vault of skull. See also FETAL SKULL.

**parity** 1. para; condition of woman having borne viable babies. See PARA. 2. equality; close correspondence or similarity.

**Parlodel** See BROMOCRIPTINE MESYLATE.

**paronychia** common neonatal inflammation of folds of skin surrounding fingernail, usually staphylococcal in origin.

**parotid** near ear. *P. glands* largest of three main pairs of salivary glands, on either side of face, just below and in front of ears.

**parous** having borne one or more viable offspring. See also NULLIPARA and PRIMIPAROUS.

---

muscles supplied by affected nerve. *Facial p.* See BIRTH INJURY. *Infantile p.* POLIOMYELITIS. See also ERB'S PARALYSIS and KLUMPKE PARALYSIS.

**paroxetine (Seroxat)** selective serotonin reuptake inhibitor antidepressant drug for major depression, obsessive-compulsive disorders, post-traumatic stress, panic, anxiety disorders. Contraindicated in pregnancy; may cause miscarriage, fetal cardiac anomalies or, if taken in third trimester, neonatal withdrawal effects.

**paroxysm** 1. sudden recurrence or intensification of symptoms. 2. spasm or seizure. *Adj* paroxysmal.

**partial pressure** *See* PO₂.

**partogram** graphical record of labour progress seen on CARDIOTOCOGRAPH printout; enables assessment of visual patterns of cervical dilatation and descent of presenting part in conjunction with records of maternal and fetal well-being.

**parturient** being in labour; relating to childbirth.

**parturition** labour, childbirth.

**parvovirus B19** droplet-spread viral infection causes 'slapped cheek' syndrome; facial rash, general malaise, fever. Antenatal infection may cause miscarriage, fetal anaemia, fetal death, HYDROPS FETALIS. Diagnosis from maternal serum; INTRAUTERINE TRANSFUSION may correct fetal anaemia; 85% of cases recover.

**pascal** international unit of pressure, corresponding to force of 1 newton per square metre.

**passages** birth canal; bony pelvis and soft tissues of vagina and vulva, through which fetus must pass during birth.

**passenger** fetus, as it traverses PASSAGES.

**passive** not active. **P. immunity** *See* IMMUNITY.

**pasteurization** heating of liquids, e.g. milk to 60°C for 30 minutes; kills pathogenic bacteria and delays other bacterial development.

**Patau syndrome (trisomy 13)** congenital extra chromosome 13; about 1 in 10,000 live births, older mothers more at risk. Affected babies may have weak muscle tone, CLEFT LIP/PALATE, heart defects, skeletal abnormalities, rarely survive infancy. Mosaic Patau syndrome: not all cells have additional chromosome, less severe.

**patella** small, circular, sesamoid bone forming kneecap.

**patent** open. **P. ductus arteriosus** persistence after birth of open lumen in ductus arteriosus between aorta and pulmonary artery; left ventricle of heart over-burdened, diminished aortic blood flow. Indomethacin may close ductus in preterm baby. If severe congenital heart defect in which open ductus arteriosus could be beneficial, prostaglandins given to keep channel open.

**paternity** biological fatherhood; DNA analysis confirms paternity if unsupported mother seeks maintenance from biological father.

**patho-** prefix denoting 'disease'.

**pathogen** micro-organism causing disease. *Adj* pathogenic.

**pathological** pertaining to study of disease.

**pathology** branch of medicine diagnosing and treating essential nature of disease, especially structural and functional changes in tissues and organs in body.

**patient-controlled analgesia** mother may self-administer analgesia, usually intravenously, via mechanical pump, e.g. pethidine. *See also* TRANSCUTANEOUS ELECTRICAL NERVE STIMULATION.

**Patient Group Directions** NHS documents allowing supply of prescription-only medicines to groups of patients, without individual prescriptions; clarified under POMs (Human Use) Amendment Order 2010.

**patulous** distended, open, as in external os of multiparous woman or cervical incompetence.

**Paul–Bunnell test** blood test detects presence of heterophil antibodies to diagnose infectious mononucleosis.

**Pavlik harness** harness to keep hips of infant with congenital hip dysplasia flexed and abducted to 60%.

**Pawlik grip** in abdominal examination, midwife grasps lower pole of uterus between fingers and thumb, spread sufficiently wide apart to accommodate fetal head, to estimate size, flexion, mobility and engagement/non-engagement of fetal head; uncomfortable for mother if not performed gently and slowly.

**pectineal** pertaining to symphysis pubis.

**pectoral** pertaining to chest or breast. *P. muscle pectoralis major* band of muscle separating breast tissue from ribs.

**pedicle** stem of tumour.

**pediculosis** lice infestation of skin or hair.

**pedigree** chart or diagram of individual's ancestors, used in genetics to analyse Mendelian inheritance.

**peduncle** large stalk or pedicle. *Adj* pedunculated.

**peer review** evaluation to ensure quality of midwifery care or professional publications set according to defined criteria set by peers.

**pellagra** niacin deficiency due to poor vitamin B intake or inability to convert tryptophan to niacin; other deficiencies may co-exist.

**pelvic** pertaining to pelvis. *P. bone* hip bone i.e. ilium, ischium, pubis. *P. capacity assessment* abdominal, vaginal or ultrasound assessment of pelvic size and shape related to size, flexion, position of presenting part. *P. cellulitis* See PARAMETRITIS. *P. floor* strong muscle fibre sheets; LEVATOR ANI muscles, support for pelvic organs. *P. floor exercises* muscle-tightening exercises encouraged regularly to reduce risk of urinary or faecal incontinence. *See also* PERINEUM. *P. inflammatory disease* infection of uterine tubes, ovaries, parametrium gut. *See also* PELVIS.

**pelvic girdle** innominate bone and sacrum. *P. g. pain* abnormal ligament and joint mobility, due to relaxin and progesterone, biomechanics, genetics; affects 1 in 300 women. Symptoms: pubic pain, backache, sciatica, abdominal pain; exacerbated by obesity, spinal trauma, multiple pregnancy, grande multiparity. Mother should restrict weight-bearing exercise, avoid abducting hips. Treatment: obstetric girdle, physiotherapy, osteopathy.

**pelvimetry** See PELVIC CAPACITY ASSESSMENT.

**pelvis** bony funnel; anterior and lateral innominate bones, posterior sacrum and coccyx, with muscular floor; contains uterus, fallopian tubes, ovaries, bladder, rectum. Brim: sacral promontory and alae, upper sacroiliac joints, iliopectineal lines, upper borders of pelvic rami, symphysis pubis. Cavity: sacral hollow, sacrospinous ligaments, ischial and pubic bones, symphysis pubis. Anatomical outlet: coccyx, sacrotuberous ligaments, ischial tuberosities, pubic arch. Obstetric outlet: lower aspect of sacrum, ischial spines. *Android p.* masculine-shaped pelvis, triangular or heart-shaped brim, narrow funnel shape, outlet narrower than gynaecoid pelvis. *Anthropoid p.* has long anteroposterior, narrow transverse brim; reverse of gynaecoid pelvis, usually large enough for fetus. *Diagonal conjugate of p.* 12–12.5 cm from apex of pubic arch to sacral promontory. *False p.* bony pelvis above brim: iliac fossae, lumbar spine, abdominal wall, little obstetric significance. *Gynaecoid p.* normal female pelvis, almost round at brim, cavity, outlet, roomy, shallow, ideal shape for childbearing. *High assimilation p.* 5th lumbar vertebra fused to sacrum, angle of inclination of brim increased. *Inclination of p.* brim slopes approximately 55 degrees to horizontal, bony outlet slopes at 15 degrees. *Naegele p.* rare asymmetrical pelvis, only one sacral ala. *Obstetric conjugate of p.* measured from inner upper border of symphysis pubis; 11 cm. *Platypelloid* or *flat p.* oval brim, small anteroposteriorly, wide transversely. *Rachitic p.* flat, kidney-shaped brim. *Robert p.* both sacral alae undeveloped, symphysis pubis sometimes split. *Spondylolisthetic p.* 5th lumbar vertebra slips forwards on sacrum, creates false promontory. *True, anatomical conjugate* measured from sacral promontory to centre of upper symphysis pubis. *True p.* bony pelvis, canal through which fetus passes in vaginal birth. *See also* PELVIC CAPACITY ASSESSMENT, CURVE OF CARUS.

**pemphigus** autoimmune acute or chronic skin disease, with watery blisters. *P. neonatorum* bullous impetigo; extremely infectious, usually due to *Staphylococcus aureus*; needs immediate medical attention, isolation of baby. *Syphilitic p.* occurs rarely in neonate.

**pemphigoid gestationis** See HERPES GESTATIONIS.

**pendulous** hanging down. *P. abdomen* occurs in multigravida, very lax abdominal muscles; uterus falls forwards, abdomen hangs below symphysis pubis; causes discomfort, fetal malpresentation.

**penicillin** antibiotic substance from cultures of mould *Penicillium*.

**penicillinase** enzyme that inactivates penicillin, produced by many bacteria, particularly staphylococci.

**penis** male erectile organ of reproduction and urination; carries urethra, passage for semen and urine. Erectile tissue: corpus cavernosa, either side of urethra and corpus spongiosum, posterior column containing urethra, with tip expanded to form glans penis. Lower two-thirds covered in skin; folded back on itself at tip above glans penis to form prepuce (foreskin), movable double fold which is sometimes excised in CIRCUMCISION.

**pentazocine hydrochloride (Fortral)** synthetic narcotic analgesic.

**pepsin** proteolytic enzyme in gastric juice; catalyst in chemical breakdown of protein to form polypeptides; milk-clotting action similar to RENNIN, facilitating digestion of milk protein.

**peptides** constituent parts of proteins: di-, tri-, tetrapeptides, according to number of amino acids in molecule.

(A) **Classification of the brim of the pelvis.** (B) Pelvic brim

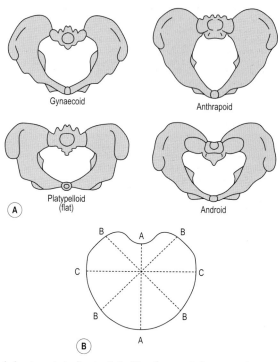

A–A, anteroposterior diameter; **B–B,** oblique diameters; **C–C,** transverse diameter.

**per**  through (Latin), e.g. *per vaginam,* via vagina.

**percentile**  statistical term to show incidence of characteristics; diagrammatic line representing percentage of population with specific characteristic, e.g. babies' weights, lengths: 90th percentile/ centile indicates 90% of population have measurements below that figure; 50th percentile is median or average.

**percussion** tapping surface with fingers to elicit sound to determine condition of underlying organs.

**percutaneous umbilical cord blood sampling** *See* CORDOCENTESIS.

**perforation** hole or break in wall or membranes of organ or structure, occurs when erosion, infection, etc. create weak spot in organ and internal pressure causes rupture.

**performance indicators** 'package' of routine statistics derived nationally; presented visually to highlight relative efficiency of health services comparing one health authority with others.

**peri-** prefix meaning 'around'.

**pericardium** smooth membranous sac around heart; outer fibrous and inner serous coat. *P.6 point* precise ACUPRESSURE point on inner wrists; stimulation of this point may ease sickness.

**Location of Pericardium 6 acupressure point for nausea and vomiting.**

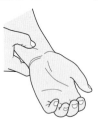

**pericranium** external periosteum of cranial bones.

**perimenopause** time approaching and immediately after complete cessation of menstrual periods (MENOPAUSE); some women experience symptoms, e.g. MENORRHAGIA, hot flushes, mood swings.

**perimetrium** peritoneum of uterus.

**perinatal** around birth. *P. mortality rate* number of stillbirths plus deaths of babies under 1 week old per 1000 total births in any 1 year. *P. period* first week of life.

**perineal** pertaining to perineum. *P. body* muscle and fibrous tissue pyramid from vaginal introitus to anus; pubococcygeus muscles at apex cross at this point. Base: transverse perineal, bulbocavernosus, anal sphincter muscles; downwards movement limited by supporting ligaments. Damage in labour, increased perineal body motility can lead to rectocele, prolapse. *P. infiltration* injection of local anaesthetic into perineum; appropriately trained midwives may perform this prior to episiotomy, perineal repair. *P. laceration* tear in perineum. *First degree:* skin of fourchette only, muscle remains intact. *Second degree:* tear of fourchette skin, superficial perineal muscle, not anal sphincter. *Third degree:* tear of whole perineal body, through anal sphincter into rectum. *Fourth degree:* disrupts anal sphincter muscles, breaches rectal mucosa. *P. repair* suturing of perineal tear or episiotomy; insert tampon to ensure clear visual field, suture vagina, interrupted sutures, from above apex of trauma; suture deep and superficial muscles from centre of incision for good approximation; suture perineal skin; remove tampon, digital rectal examination to ensure no sutures encroach into it.

**Perineal repair (commonly used method)**

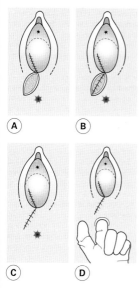

A, vagina sutured with continuous catgut; B, muscle layer sutured with interrupted catgut; C, perineal skin sutured with interrupted catgut or silk; D, rectal examination to exclude rectal involvement.

**perineorrhaphy** repair of perineal body.

**perineum** area from pubic arch to coccyx, with underlying tissues; fibromuscular pyramid between lower third of vagina, anal canal, ischial tuberosities. *See also* PELVIC FLOOR.

**periosteum** connective tissue covering all bones of body; possesses bone-forming potential; point of attachment for certain muscles.

**peripheral** relating to periphery. *P. cyanosis* blueness of extremities, often seen in neonate at birth; APGAR SCORE reduced by one mark, not normally clinically significant, resolves spontaneously.

**periphery** outer surface or circumference.

**peristalsis** wave-like contraction along walls of tubular organ, pressing contents onwards; e.g. in muscle layer of alimentary canal, fallopian tubes; may be visible in PYLORIC STENOSIS.

**peritoneal** pertaining to peritoneum.

**peritoneum** serous membrane. *Parietal p.* lines abdominal cavity. *Pelvic p.* covers pelvic organs, in female forms pouch of Douglas between rectum and uterus and shallow uterovesical pouch between uterus and bladder; peritoneum hanging over fallopian tubes is broad ligament. *Visceral p.* inner layer closely covers organs, including mesenteries. *Adj* peritoneal.

**peritonitis** inflammation of peritoneum due to infection. *General p.* affects whole abdominal cavity. *Pelvic p.* restricted to peritoneum of pelvic cavity; occasional complication of puerperal sepsis.

**periventricular haemorrhage** cerebral bleeding in preterm babies below 34 weeks' gestation. *Grade 1*: bleeding into germinal matrix; *grade 2*: bleeding into lateral ventricles, may cause posthaemorrhagic hydrocephalus; *grade 3*: bleeding into cerebral tissue leads to *grade 4* parenchymal haemorrhage. *P. h. infarction* intraventricular clot in grade 3 bleeding disrupts venous

173

drainage, leads to grade 4 haemorrhage, infarction, cerebral necrosis.

**permeable** able to be penetrated, as in membranes that allow fluids to pass through, e.g. capillary walls (also semipermeable).

**pernicious** highly destructive; fatal. *P. anaemia* anaemia due to failure of gastric secretion of intrinsic factor; treatment: vitamin $B_{12}$. Do not confuse with megaloblastic anaemia.

**peroxide** compound with high quantity of oxygen required to form oxide. *P. of hydrogen* compound of hydrogen and oxygen.

**perphenazine (Fentazin)** oral antiemetic; avoid in first trimester.

**persistent mentoposterior** face presentation: sinciput rotates forwards, chin rotates backwards to sacral hollow; rare cause of obstructed labour, thorax presents at pelvic brim with head.

**persistent occipitoposterior** deflexed vertex presentation: sinciput rotates forwards and occiput rotates backwards to hollow of sacrum; cause of delay in second-stage labour; spontaneous FACE-TO-PUBES delivery possible.

**persistent pulmonary hypertension of newborn** compromised transition from fetal to adult circulation: blood flow mimics fetal circulation, may be due to primary defect in pulmonary vasculature or secondary to factors raising pulmonary vascular resistance, e.g. MECONIUM ASPIRATION SYNDROME. Treatment: nitrous oxide (vasodilator).

**Personal Child Health Record (Red Book)** national health and development record given to parents/carers at baby's birth; also available online (eRedbook).

**Personal Identification Number (PIN)** given to midwife on registration with Nursing and Midwifery Council; enables employers or public to ascertain eligibility to practise as midwife; required when signing Mat B1 certificates.

**perspiration** sweating; excretion of moisture through skin pores; also, salty fluid, largely water, excreted by sweat glands in skin; sodium chloride levels raised in cystic fibrosis.

**pertussis** whooping cough; serious respiratory tract infection due to *Bordetella pertussis*, particularly serious in babies under 3 months, children with asthma. *See* IMMUNIZATION.

**pessary** object inserted into vagina, e.g. contraceptive drug in solvent base, device to maintain anteversion of uterus in early pregnancy. *Prostaglandin p.* pessary inserted into posterior vaginal fornix to aid cervical ripening and labour onset.

**petechiae** small spots caused by minute subcutaneous haemorrhages, seen in purpura, sometimes on face of normal neonate due to venous congestion during birth; feature of congenital RUBELLA, TOXOPLASMOSIS, CYTOMEGALOVIRUS over entire body.

**pethidine hydrochloride** analgesic, antispasmodic opiate drug, relieves labour pain; midwives may carry, administer it intramuscularly. Side effects: nausea, vomiting (antiemetic may be given with it), drowsiness, slowing of labour, neonatal respiratory depression if birth shortly after administration; antidoted by NALOXONE; breastfeeding may be more difficult to establish due to sleepy baby.

**petit mal** mild epileptic attack, momentary loss of consciousness. *See also* GRAND MAL.

**Pfannenstiel incision** transverse abdominal surgical incision just above symphysis pubis.

**pH** denotes alkalinity or acidity of solution; hydrogen ion concentration expressed in moles (mol/L) measured from 0 to 14. Neutral pH 7, acidity pH $\leq$7, alkalinity pH $\geq$7; blood pH 7.4, slightly alkaline. Favourable pH is essential to maintain ACID–BASE BAL-ANCE, enzyme function, other biological systems. Increased acid production of intrapartum hypoxia raises acidity, pH falls; measured on blood sample taken *per vaginam* from fetal scalp.

**phaeochromocytoma** rare, benign catecholamine-secreting adrenal tumour; increased adrenaline causes hypertension with wide diurnal variations, tachycardia, palpitations, sweating. Diagnosis: plasma and urine adrenaline and noradrenaline assays. Vanillylmandelic acid in 24-hour urine sample is greatly increased; surgery usually needed.

**phagocytes** polymorphonuclear leucocytes and monocytes that engulf and digest bacteria and foreign particles.

**phagocytosis** action of PHAGOCYTES. *Adj* phagocytic.

**phalanx** any bone of finger or toe. *Adj* phalangeal.

**phallic** pertaining to penis.

**phantom** 1. image or impression not evoked by actual stimuli. 2. model of body or specific part thereof. *P. pregnancy* pseudocyesis, false pregnancy.

**pharmaceutical** relating to drugs.

**pharmacokinetics** study of drug metabolism and actions, especially absorption, duration of action, distribution in body, excretion.

**pharmacology** science of nature and preparation of drugs. *Adj* pharmacological.

**pharmacopoeia** authoritative publication of standard drug formulae and preparation. *British P.* for use in UK.

**pharmacy** 1. art of preparing, compounding, dispensing medicines. 2. shop or hospital department where medicines dispensed, sold.

**pharynx** back of mouth leading to oesophagus and larynx, communicates with nose through posterior nares and with ears via Eustachian tubes.

**Phenergan** *See* PROMETHAZINE HYDROCHLORIDE.

**phenindione** oral anticoagulant similar to warfarin; avoid in pregnancy, breastfeeding.

**phenobarbital, phenobarbitone** barbiturate drug, depresses cerebral cortex, used for epilepsy, eclampsia, avoid in early pregnancy.

**phenomenology** inductive descriptive approach to research developed from phenomenological philosophy, involving understanding of response of whole human being; focuses on describing experiences as they are lived, e.g. describing a person's pain perception.

**phenothiazines** major tranquillizers, phenothiazine derivatives.

**phenotype** 1. outward, visible expression of hereditary constitution of an organism. 2. individual exhibiting certain phenotype; trait expressed in phenotype.

**phenoxymethylpenicillin** oral antibiotic commonly used for mild streptococcal infections (penicillin V).

**phenylalanine hydroxylase** essential amino acid, normally converted to tyrosine by enzyme from liver.

**phenylketonuria** presence in urine of phenylketones (phenylpyruvates) from incomplete breakdown of PHENYLALANINE to tyrosine; high blood phenylalanine causes learning disabilities, fits, poor muscular coordination; autosomal-RECESSIVE inherited condition, incidence 1:10,000. Diagnosis: NEWBORN BLOOD-SPOT SCREENING PROGRAMME or GUTHRIE TEST performed on day 7 of life. Treatment: low-phenylalanine diet, protein supplements to lower phenylalanine, monitor diet, cognitive development. Those affected often blue-eyed, blond, with defective pigmentation, very sensitive skin, tendency to eczema, musty-smelling urine and sweat due to presence of phenylacetate.

**phenylpyruvic acid** abnormal constituent excreted in urine of those with PHENYLKETONURIA.

**phenytoin sodium (also known as Epanutin)** anticonvulsant drug to control epilepsy; avoid in early pregnancy unless benefits outweigh risks.

**phimosis** constriction of orifice of prepuce so it cannot be drawn back over glans of penis; may require surgery.

**phlebitis** inflammation of deep or superficial vein, usually in leg; may lead to THROMBOSIS or formation of blood clot loosely attached to vein wall, not associated with infection; risk of separation of all or part of clot, leading to EMBOLISM. cf. THROMBOPHLEBITIS.

**phlebothrombosis** deep vein thrombosis.

**phlebotomist** one who performs phlebotomy.

**phlebotomy** venesection, obtaining samples of blood for testing.

**phlegm** sputum; liquid secreted by mucous membranes of respiratory system, expelled by coughing.

**phlegmasia** inflammation. *P. alba dolens* white leg; uncommon puerperal femoral THROMBOPHLEBITIS or PHLEBOTHROMBOSIS due to venous obstruction and/or reflex arterial spasm; leg is swollen, very painful. Treatment: elevate leg without immobilization; antibiotics if due to thrombophlebitis; anticoagulants may also be given.

**phobia** persistent abnormal dread or fear from repressed subconscious inner conflicts; triggers uncontrollable, unreasonable reactions to feared situation, e.g. tocophobia, fear of childbirth.

**phocomelia** congenital absence of proximal portion of limb or limbs; hands or feet attached to trunk by small, irregularly shaped bone.

**phospholipid** lipid containing phosphorus, includes phosphoglycerides, sphingomyelins; major lipids in cell membranes.

**phosphorus** chemical element essential for most metabolic processes; major component of bone mineral phase; found in milk products, meat, fish. Vitamin D, calcium aid absorption. Symbol P.

**photophobia** intolerance of light; symptom of meningitis.

**photosensitivity** abnormal skin sensitivity to sunlight, due in pregnancy to increased melanocytic hormone; also caused by certain drugs, e.g. chlorpromazine.

**phototherapy** fluorescent light treatment to reduce unconjugated bilirubin over 340 µmol/L at term, 210 µmol/L at 34 weeks, 150 µmol/L at 28 weeks in jaundiced neonate; non-toxic photo-degradation products excreted without help of liver enzymes. Side effects: loose green stools, need extra fluid intake; skin rashes, baby's eyes and gonads need covering to prevent problems from light exposure. Prophylactic in bruised preterm babies and in rhesus incompatibility.

**phrenic** pertaining to diaphragm or to mind. *P. nerve* major branch of cervical plexus, carries nerve impulses from inspiratory centre in brain, causing contraction of diaphragm to aid inspiration.

**physiological** pertaining to physiology. *P. anaemia* in pregnancy, low haemoglobin from hydraemia, not clinically significant; haemoglobin fall more than 1–2 gm/dL may indicate pathological ANAEMIA.

**physiological third stage** natural management of third-stage labour; placenta separates from uterine wall; await signs of placental separation: uterus rises in abdomen, feels small, hard, mobile, cord lengthens, small vagina blood loss; placenta and membranes delivered with maternal effort or by CONTROLLED CORD TRACTION. *See also* ACTIVE MANAGEMENT OF FIRST-STAGE LABOUR.

**physiology** science of function of living organisms.

**physiotherapist** practitioner of physiotherapy.

**phytomenadione** vitamin K₁; poorly transferred across placenta, so fetal stores are low, quickly depleted after birth. Synthetic preparation (Konakion) offered orally or intramuscularly after birth to prevent haemorrhagic disease. Oral vitamin K repeated on seventh day of life and, if baby breastfed, again at 1 month and monthly thereafter until solid food and/or milk formula feeding is introduced.

**pia mater** innermost membrane enveloping brain and spinal cord.

**pica** excessive craving to eat unusual foods or inhale aromas of unnatural substances, e.g. petrol, rubber, possibly related to nutritional deficiencies; less common than normal food CRAVINGS.

**pie chart** circular diagram divided into segments showing proportional distribution of observations of particular events.

**Pierre–Robin syndrome** congenital abnormality: MICROGNATHIA, central cleft palate, abnormal attachment of tongue muscles causes respiratory obstruction as tongue occludes pharynx. Treatment: baby nursed prone, tongue pulled forwards to maintain airway; nasal, nasopharyngeal CONTINUOUS POSITIVE AIRWAYS PRESSURE; orthodontic plate to facilitate feeding. Risk of sudden infant death.

**pigment** dye or colouring agent. *Bile p.* BILIRUBIN and biliverdin. *Blood p.* haematin.

**pilonidal** having nest of hairs. *P. cyst* dermoid cyst implanted in natal cleft due to penetration of hairs through skin of natal cleft fold causing sinus and epithelium cell implantation; prone to recurrent infection. *P. depression* non-significant dip in midline near coccyx, seen in newborn baby. *P. sinus* small pericoccygeal sinus, remnant of neural canal; may become infected, necessitating excision.

**pilot study** small-scale version of planned investigation or observation, used to test research design and methodology of larger study.

**Pinard stethoscope** trumpet-shaped fetal stethoscope; placed on mother's abdomen over fetal chest to hear fetal heart sounds.

**pineal** pertaining to pineal body; small conical structure attached to posterior wall of third ventricle of cerebrum, endocrine gland.

**pineapple** bromelain in pineapple thought to contract smooth muscle, eaten by some women to trigger labour contractions. Side effects: diarrhoea, severe allergic reaction, anaphylaxis. Midwives should not advise for natural labour induction.

**pinna** projecting part of ear lying outside head.

**Piriton** See CHLORPHENAMINE (CHLORPHENIRAMINE) MALEATE.

**pituitary gland** major endocrine gland attached to base of brain; controls growth, development, function of other endocrine glands; anterior lobe produces GONADOTROPHIC hormones, GROWTH HORMONE, prolactin, ADRENOCORTICOTROPHIC HORMONE, thyrotrophic hormone; posterior lobe secretes OXYTOCIN, VASOPRESSIN. Pituitary disorders include SHEEHAN SYNDROME, DIABETES INSIPIDUS, hypopituitarism, pituitary tumours. Pituitary insufficiency rare in neonate but investigate prolonged hypoglycaemia and jaundice.

**placebo** substance given to, or procedure performed on, patient or research subject, as in controlled clinical trials of new drugs; effective because person expects it to be, yet it has no intrinsic therapeutic value.

**place of birth** UK women are legally permitted to give birth wherever they choose, irrespective of clinical suitability or service availability; midwives must, by law, attend women wherever they give birth but ensure

mother is able to give informed consent.

**place of safety order** court order permitting removal of child from parental care for safety, or of adults under Mental Health Act, for protection of selves or others.

**placenta** afterbirth; organ sustaining pregnancy, allows transport of nutrients, oxygen, other substances between mother and fetus. Composed of chorionic villi in cotyledons embedded in uterine decidua; villi contain fetal blood vessels, separated by intervillous spaces through which maternal blood circulates. At term, 20 cm diameter, 2.5 cm thick, weight approximately one-sixth of baby's birthweight. Fetal surface: fetal blood vessels radiating from cord insertion, usually central, covered by amnion; chorion continuous with placental edge. Functions: nutrition; glycogen storage; oxygen, carbon dioxide transfer; waste excretion; hormone production; (partial) barrier to protect fetus from some noxious substances. *Battledore p.* cord attached to placental margin. *Bipartite p.* two main lobes. *P. accreta* placenta abnormally attached to myometrium, partial or complete absence of decidua basalis. *P. circumvallata* has dense, raised, white nodular ring of attached membranes doubled back over placental edge. *P. fenestrata* has gap or 'window' in structure. *P. increta* abnormally attached to perimetrium. *P. membranacea* abnormally thin placenta spread over large area of uterus, may occur in PLACENTA PRAEVIA. *P. percreta* chorionic villi abnormally invade perimetrium with total adherence;

hysterectomy needed to control haemorrhage. *Succenturiate p.* separate or accessory lobe joined to main placenta by blood vessels; risk of bleeding if separates from main placenta and retained. *See also* MANUAL REMOVAL OF PLACENTA.

**placenta praevia** placenta inserted in lower uterine segment, causes painless, recurring bleeding as lower uterine segment stretches towards term. *Grade 1 p. p.* edge of placenta encroaches into lower uterine segment; *grade 2 p. p.* whole placenta in lower segment; *grade 3 p. p.* placenta reaches to internal cervical os; *grade 4 p. p.* entire placenta covers cervical os, requires Caesarean section. Fetal malpresentations common; vaginal delivery unsafe unless grade 1 or 2. Management depends on amount of bleeding, maternal, fetal conditions, placental location, gestation. *Never* perform vaginal examination; EXAMINATION UNDER ANAESTHETIC may be done in operating theatre with facilities to proceed to Caesarean if necessary. *See also* RETAINED PLACENTA.

**placental abruption** premature separation of normally situated placenta after 24 weeks' gestation. May occur in severe pre-eclampsia, membrane rupture due to sudden reduction in uterine size, high parity, smoking, previous Caesarean section, trauma. Bleeding from placental site causes abdominal pain (unlike PLACENTA PRAEVIA), little or no visible bleeding; shock out of proportion with external blood loss. If mild, may resolve spontaneously; if bleeding severe, urgent treatment to combat effects of shock and pain, then to control haemorrhage and plan for birth of baby.

**placental examination** examination of placenta and membranes undertaken by midwife shortly after delivery to assess completeness or identify risk of retained placenta and POSTPARTUM HAEMORRHAGE. Examined for completeness of lobes, membranes, blood clots, extra lobes, cord insertion, general health of placenta, other abnormalities; all findings recorded in mother's notes.

**placental lactogen** hormone affecting breast growth and development, also glucose metabolism in pregnancy; similar to pituitary GROWTH HORMONE but does not actually promote growth.

**placental souffle** *See* SOUFFLE.

**placentophagy** eating placenta, may prevent postnatal depression.

**plagiocephaly** asymmetry of head due to irregular suture closure.

**plantar** pertaining to sole of foot.

**plasma** straw-coloured fluid, constitutes 55% of blood; contains 92% water with plasma proteins, other organic substances, 1% inorganic salts, foods, dissolved gases, waste materials, hormones, secretions, antibodies, enzymes, transported to and from body tissues by plasma; may be transfused to increase plasma proteins or in cases of shock. *P. proteins* albumin, globulin, fibrinogen in serum. Functions: circulatory transport of lipids, hormones, vitamins, metals, enzymes, protease inhibitors, kinin precursors, complement components; regulation of cellular activity, functioning of immune system. Normally 7 g/dL, lower in pregnancy. Albumin decreases colloid osmotic pressure, waters move from plasma to cells or extravascularly, increases

179

blood cell fragility, tendency to oedema.

**plasmapheresis** method of removing portion of plasma from circulation in cases of disease caused by circulating antibodies in plasma; venepuncture is performed, plasma is removed from blood sample and red cells are returned to circulation.

**plasmin** *See* FIBRINOLYSIN; enzyme that dissolves fibrin in thrombus, present in blood as plasminogen before activation.

**Plastibell** plastic device for male circumcision, slipped inside foreskin, string tied around; foreskin becomes gangrenous, drops off.

**platelets** thrombocytes; disc-shaped, non-nucleated blood cells with very fragile membrane, adhere to uneven or damaged surfaces; formed in red bone marrow, average about $250 \times 10^9$ per litre of blood; assist in coagulation, may occlude small breaks in blood vessels and prevent escape of blood.

**platypelloid** flat. *See* PELVIS.

**plethoric** florid colouring due to excess red blood cells; may be seen in baby with large placental transfusion or in one of twins with TWIN-TO-TWIN TRANSFUSION syndrome.

**pleura** serous membrane lining thorax, surrounding each lung, two layers enclosing potential space, pleural cavity.

**pleurisy** inflammation of pleura.

**plexus** network of veins or nerves. *Brachial p.* network of nerves of neck and axilla. *Solar* or *coeliac p.* network of nerves and ganglia at back of stomach, supplying abdominal viscera.

**pneumococcal disease** *Streptococcus pneumonia* disease commonly carried in nose and throat; causes pneumonia, otitis media, sinusitis; meningitis, septicaemia, bacteraemic pneumonia. Most at risk: children under 5 years, elderly, people with chronic disease or non-functioning spleen. 10%–15% mortality rate; 50% of survivors develop chronic hearing loss, learning impairment, cerebral palsy or epilepsy. Bacteria resistant to penicillin, erythromycin; prophylaxis now advocated. *See* IMMUNIZATION.

**pneumonia** inflammation of lung; normally acquired *in utero* or during birth if appearing within 48 hours of birth; later, infection may be iatrogenic. Treatment: antibiotics. *Chlamydial p.* chlamydial infection acquired from mother at birth can cause conjunctivitis, pneumonia, usually occurs between 4 and 12 weeks of age; infants may develop asthma, obstructive lung disease in later life. *Lobar p.* pneumococcal infection of one or more lobes of lung. *Bronchopneumonia* caused by *Staphylococcus aureus*, streptococcus or *Haemophilus influenza*, affecting bronchioles. *Viral p.* RESPIRATORY DISTRESS SYNDROME predisposes neonate to viral pneumonia.

**pneumonitis** inflammation of lungs.

**pneumothorax** accumulation of air in pleural cavity, lung collapses on affected side; may occur spontaneously or after perforation of chest wall, from vigorous resuscitation, ventilation or CONTINUOUS INFLATING PRESSURE, or follow MECONIUM ASPIRATION. Occurs spontaneously, without symptoms, in 1% of neonates; present at birth, due to pressure changes from baby's first breaths, leads to alveolar distension and rupture, allowing air to leak into space between lung pleura. Investigate term babies with respiratory distress, unilaterally reduced breath sounds, displaced heart sounds, distorted chest and diaphragmatic movement. Treatment: immediate medical attention; needle aspiration to drain air leak; insertion of chest drain to prevent further air accumulation; sedation to suppress pain; baby nursed in neonatal unit. *Pl* pneumothoraces.

**P₀₂** partial pressure of oxygen; about 100 mm Hg in an adult and 60–90 mm Hg in baby; if exceeds 100 mm Hg in preterm baby there is danger of RETROLENTAL FIBROPLASIA.

**podalic version** internal correction of transverse lie by grasping foot, converting it to longitudinal lie and breech presentation.

**polarity** gradient of strength of uterine contractions from upper fundal pole, where activity is strongest, to lower segment and cervix, where contractions are weak or absent, which causes cervical dilatation.

**pole** one extremity or end of organ, e.g. uterus.

**policy** general principles or directions; written plan of required action for clinical or managerial situations often set against national recommendations. *See also* PROTOCOL, PROCEDURE.

**poliomyelitis** viral notifiable disease; inflammation of anterior cells of spinal cord, lead to infantile paralysis. Vaccination at 2, 3, 4 months of age and before starting school.

**poly-** prefix meaning 'much' or 'many'.

**polycystic** containing numerous cysts. *P. kidneys* congenitally enlarged kidneys with numerous cysts; may remain undiagnosed,

urinary tract infections and hypertension may occur in pregnancy. In baby, kidneys enlarged at birth, survival unlikely. *P. ovary syndrome* Stein–Leventhal syndrome; affects 6%–10% of women, often asymptomatic; irregular or absent menstrual periods, ovarian cysts, hypertension, acne, infertility, hirsutism, obesity, leading to diabetes. Treatment: weight and diabetes control, ovulation stimulation when pregnancy is desired.

**polycythaemia** excess of red blood cells, as occurs in neonate because of high levels of fetal haemoglobin.

**polydactyly** supernumerary fingers.

**polyhydramnios** HYDRAMNIOS; excess amniotic fluid, above 1500 mL, associated with maternal diabetes, congenital abnormalities, uniovular twins, CHORIOANGIOMA.

**polymerase chain reaction (PCR)** molecular technique to amplify deoxyribonucleic acid (DNA), widely used in medical and biological research; used to identify genetic fingerprints, diagnose infectious diseases, clone genes and for paternity testing. *See also* QUANTITATIVE FLUORESCENCE POLYMERASE CHAIN REACTION (QF-PCR).

**polymorphonuclear** possessing multilobed nuclei as in most white blood cells.

**polyp, polypus** small pedunculated tumour arising from any mucous surface. *Cervical p.* occurs in cervical canal. *Fibroid p.* occurs in uterus, contains fibrous myomatous tissue. *Placental p.* consists of remains of placenta. *Pl* polypi.

**polysaccharide** complex carbohydrate, e.g. starch.

**polyuria** excess secretion of urine, caused by diuretic drugs or diabetes mellitus; normal in first few days of puerperium because of autolysis occurring as part of INVOLUTION.

**pons** 1. part of metencephalon between medulla oblongata and midbrain, ventral to cerebellum. 2. any slip of tissue connecting two parts of organ.

**popliteal** relating to posterior part of knee, *p. fossa* or *p. space*.

**pore** minute circular opening on surface, e.g. of sweat glands.

**porphyria** inherited abnormal red blood cell formation.

**port-wine stain** naevus flammeus; purple-blue capillaries seen on face, occurs in 1 in 3000 births; fully formed at birth, does not regress. Laser treatment, cosmetics may disguise it. If naevus mimics distribution of ophthalmic branch of trigeminal nerve, glaucoma, epilepsy may occur *See* STURGE–WEBER SYNDROME.

**portal vein** large vein carrying nutritive material from digestive tract to liver, formed from gastric, splenic, superior mesenteric veins.

**portfolio** professional midwife is required to maintain portfolio of evidence to demonstrate continuing professional development and updating e.g. reflective practice accounts relating to clinical experiences, certificates of conference attendance, marked course assignments; may be required at annual review.

**position** attitude or posture. *Dorsal p.* lying flat on back. *Genupectoral or knee-chest p.* resting on knees and chest with arms above head or resting on knees and elbows; may relieve pressure on prolapsed cord. *Left lateral p.* lying on left side, right knee drawn up towards chin; avoids

pressure on uterus from RIGHT OBLIQUITY AND ROTUNDITY. *Lithotomy p.* lying on back with thighs raised, knees supported and held widely apart; used for instrumental delivery and operative procedures performed via vagina; both legs must be raised and lowered together to avoid separation of symphysis pubis. *Prone p.* lying face down. *Recumbent p.* lying down. *Sim's p.* similar to *left lateral* but almost on face, semi-prone with right knee, thigh drawn up, resting on bed in front of left one. *Trendelenburg p.* lying on back on tilted plane e.g. operating table, with head lowermost and shoulders supported.

**position of fetus** eight positions relating fetal DENOMINATOR to maternal pelvis. Vertex presentation: denominator is occiput. *Occipitoanterior p.* most favourable position, fetal occiput directed to symphysis pubis, to right or left iliopectineal eminence; *Occipitolateral, occipitotransverse p.* occiput directed to midpoint of left or right iliopectineal line; in *occipitoposterior p.* occiput directed to left or right sacroiliac joint; *Persistent occipitoposterior p.* occiput directed towards sacrum. In breech positions, sacrum is denominator.

**positive predictive value** *See* ODDS OF BEING AFFECTED GIVEN POSITIVE RESULT.

**posseting** regurgitation of small amount of milk after feed.

**post-** prefix meaning 'after', e.g. postnatal clinic.

**postcoital contraceptive** emergency contraceptive measure after unprotected sexual intercourse; may be hormonal oral contraceptive pill, taken within 72 hours, or intrauterine contraceptive device, inserted within

5 days, to prevent embedding of fertilized ovum.

**post-dates pregnancy** prolonged pregnancy beyond 42 weeks' gestation; differentiate from POSTMATURITY. Common indication for labour induction; MEMBRANE SWEEP may be offered at 41 weeks. Predisposing factors: nulliparity, previous post-dates pregnancy, obesity, anencephalic fetus. Perceived risks: increased fetal/neonatal mortality, morbidity from shoulder dystocia, bony and soft tissue trauma, hypoxia from prolonged labour, risk of operative or instrumental birth, postpartum bleeding. Expectant approach: monitor maternofetal condition with NON-STRESS TEST and amniotic fluid volume assessment. Active approach: INDUCTION OF LABOUR. Many women self-administer natural remedies to start labour; inappropriate use can trigger CASCADE OF INTERVENTION as with induction. *See also* NATURAL INDUCTION OF LABOUR.

**post-dural headache** postural headache after 'dural tap' during epidural cannula siting, due to cerebrospinal fluid leakage; may follow spinal anaesthesia, usually less severe. Treatment: epidural injection of maternal blood (blood patch) to seal puncture, relieve pain; mother may need to lie flat for 24 hours.

**posterior** at back.

**posthumous** occurring after death. *P. birth* birth of baby after father's death or by Caesarean section after death of mother.

**postmaturity** in POST-DATES PREGNANCY, refers to neonate affected by prolonged period in uterus; peeling epidermis, long fingernails, alert face,

loose skin suggestive of recent weight loss. Few post-term babies show postmaturity signs but baby presenting as post-mature may indicate late gestation disruption in placental function.

**post mortem** after death. *P.-m. examination* autopsy.

**postnatal** after childbirth, refers to mother. *P. 'blues'* transitory physiological mood changes; occurs in 50%–80% of women commonly days 3–4 after delivery, due to hormone fluctuations after placental expulsion and initiation of lactation; usually resolves spontaneously within 48 hours but may be precursor to postnatal depression. *P. care by midwife* midwife is responsible for psychological support, physiological monitoring, education, care of mother and baby for first few days after birth, in hospital and at home. *P. depression* feelings of sadness, guilt, worthlessness, anxiety; thoughts of suicide, death; difficulty in concentrating, decision making; appetite, sleep disturbances; lack of interest, energy; may occur up to year after delivery; more common if personal or family history of depression or if woman had antenatal depression. May be depression, mania or both (BIPOLAR DISORDER). Treatment: counselling, psychotherapy, medication. May recur in subsequent pregnancy. *P. examination* 1. examination of mother in first 10 days of puerperium to monitor INVOLUTION, lactation, mother's physical, emotional, psychological adjustment. 2. examination at end of puerperium to ensure mother's body has returned to non-pregnant state without complications. *P. exercises* exercises should be done by mother several times daily during puerperium to strengthen pelvic floor, abdominal muscles; deep breathing and leg exercises prevent respiratory infection, deep vein thrombosis.

**postpartum** after labour. *P. haemorrhage* excess genital tract bleeding, any time up to 6 weeks post-delivery. *Primary PPH* occurs in first 24 hours, usually over 500 mL, or any amount detrimental to mother's health; *secondary PPH* occurs after first 24 hours. See APPENDIX 1. *P. shock* collapse from circulatory failure due to ante- or postpartum haemorrhage, uterine inversion or rupture, acid aspiration syndrome, pulmonary or amniotic fluid embolism, hypotension, endotoxic shock from septicaemia. Signs: hypotension, tachycardia, cold, clammy, white skin, air hunger. Treatment: resuscitation to maintain airway, give oxygen, intravenous fluids to raise blood volume, antibiotics if shock is endotoxic.

**post-traumatic stress disorder** reaction to extremely stressful events, can occur after traumatic birth, e.g. urgent Caesarean section, or when mother feels abused by birth experience. Signs and symptoms: acute anxiety, insomnia, nightmares, flashbacks, depression, concentration loss, apathy, guilt, sexual and relationship problems; support and counselling needed.

**potassium** metallic element, symbol K; one of electrolytes of blood and tissue fluids; maintains acid–base and water balance; together with plasma sodium, calcium, potassium, aids cardiac function.

**Potter syndrome** congenital renal agenesis, pulmonary hypoplasia, low-set ears, furrows under eyes; associated with only two umbilical cord vessels; fatal if both kidneys are absent.

**pouch** pocket-like space or cavity. *P. of Douglas* lowest peritoneal fold between uterus and rectum. *Uterovesical p.* peritoneal fold between uterus and bladder.

**Poupart's ligament** inguinal ligament; lower border of external oblique muscle of abdominal wall, passes from anterior superior spine of ilium to pubis bone.

**powers** uterine contractions, which aid progress of labour, enabling fetus (passenger) to negotiate birth canal (passages).

**PPROM** preterm pre-labour rupture of membranes.

**prandial** pertaining to meal, e.g. *postprandial*, after meal.

**pre-** prefix meaning 'before', e.g. prenatal, premature.

**precipitate** 1. settling in solid particles of substance in solution. *P. labour* unduly rapid labour, usually under 2–3 hours from onset to birth, with no real sensation of uterine contractions. Complications: severe vaginal, perineal tears, postpartum haemorrhage, POST-TRAUMATIC STRESS; neonatal intracranial trauma and bleeding due to rapid passage through birth canal.

**preconception** before conception. *P. care* health education and investigation to detect and treat problems before conception; promotes optimum parental health for conception and organogenesis, reduces congenital malformation risk. Includes:

personal, medical, family, reproductive, lifestyle, work history, gynaecological examination, cervical smear; urinalysis; blood tests: rubella antibodies, haemoglobin, haemoglobinopathies, syphilis, HIV antibodies; toxic metal tests; semen analysis; stool tests for infestation. Referral to appropriate physician or genetic counsellor may follow.

**precursor** in medicine, sign or symptom that heralds another.

**pre-diabetes** state preceding diabetes mellitus, before clinically manifested; diabetes may become evident during pregnancy or may present no signs and symptoms but baby's birthweight may be above norm, usually more than 4.5 kg in term baby.

**prednisolone** synthetic glucocorticoid, anti-inflammatory, anti-allergic, act similarly to adrenocortical hormones.

**pre-eclampsia** late pregnancy hypertension; diastolic blood pressure 80 mm Hg or rise of more than 15–20 mm Hg above booking baseline, with oedema, proteinuria; systemic changes affect placenta, kidneys, liver, brain, other organs. *Fulminating p-e.* diastolic pressure ≥160, systolic ≥120, with headache, blurred vision, right-sided abdominal pain, raised urates, low platelet count, abnormal liver enzymes. Untreated or severe cases may develop into ECLAMPSIA. *Superimposed p.-e.* pre-eclampsia developing in women with pre-existing hypertension and/or proteinuria.

**pregnancy** from conception to birth of baby; normal duration 280 days (40 weeks or 9 months, 7 days), counted from first day of last normal menstrual period to birth, or 265 days, from conception to birth. *Ectopic p.* extrauterine pregnancy, commonly in fallopian tube, very rarely in ovary or abdominal cavity. *Adj* pregnant.

**pregnancy-associated plasma protein-A** plasma protein from placental syncytiotrophoblasts, levels rise as pregnancy advances. Average first-trimester levels reduced in DOWN SYNDROME pregnancies. *See also* COMBINED TEST *and* INTEGRATED TEST.

**pregnancy-induced hypertension** gestational hypertension; asymptomatic blood pressure rise, no proteinuria, after 20 weeks' gestation; previous diastolic blood pressure was ≤90 mm Hg; commonly occurs in primigravidae, multiple pregnancy. May progress to superimposed PRE-ECLAMPSIA; must be distinguished from ESSENTIAL HYPERTENSION. Complications: placental abruption, renal, cardiac failure, cerebral haemorrhage, placental insufficiency, intrauterine growth retardation. Resolves in 6–8 weeks postpartum.

**pregnancy tests** urinary biochemical tests measuring HUMAN CHORIONIC GONADOTROPHIN, often purchased for home use.

**pregnanediol** derivative of pregnane, formed by reduction of progesterone, present in urine of pregnant women.

**pre-implantation genetic diagnosis (PGD)** genetic diagnosis performed after in vitro fertilization, before embryo implantation in couples with high risk of baby having inherited condition; avoids selective pregnancy termination. *See also* ANEUPLOIDY diagnosis.

**premature** early, before maturity. *P. labour. See* PRETERM LABOUR.

**prematurity** refers to neonate born before 37 weeks' gestation regardless of birthweight. See PRETERM INFANT.

**premedication** drugs given before general anaesthesia; prior to Caesarean section, mothers are given ranitidine and, for elective surgery, sodium citrate; to inhibit hydrochloric acid secretion from stomach, which may cause MENDELSON SYNDROME.

**premenstrual** preceding menstruation. *P. syndrome* condition occurring 7–10 days before menstruation due to fluctuating hormones; symptoms: irritability, aggression, anxiety, mood changes, headache, breast tenderness, oedema, cravings, poor coordination or concentration; subsides once menstruation commences.

**prenatal** occurring before birth.

**prepuce** foreskin; loose fold of skin covering glans penis.

**pre-registration midwifery education** academic and clinical education to prepare midwives for practice; in UK, 3-year degree programme (18 months for registered nurses). Completion leads to license to practise midwifery and academic degree in midwifery.

**prescription** written or verbal instruction for drug administration; appropriately trained midwives may make diagnosis and prescribe medication, including prescription-only medicines, some controlled drugs relevant to individual's field of expertise and competence. Women in UK receive free prescriptions in pregnancy and for one year after birth. *P.-only medicines* drugs only available with valid prescription specific to patient; pharmacist must legally be present for dispensing. Examples: antibiotics, anti-diabetic medication, strong analgesics, diazepam, corticosteroids.

**presentation** fetal part in lower pole of uterus; normally cephalic; if head flexed, vertex presents; if partially extended, brow presents; if fully extended, face presents; non-cephalic presentations include breech, when sacrum or shoulder presents.

**presenting part** fetal part lying lowest in birth canal, first part felt on examination per vaginam; occiput in vertex presentation. See PRESENTATION.

**pressor** increases blood pressure.

**pressure** stress or strain, exerted by compression, expansion, pull, thrust or shear. See also BLOOD PRESSURE.

**preterm** before term, before 37 completed weeks of pregnancy. *P. infant* baby born before 37 weeks' gestation; low birthweight, may also be SMALL FOR GESTATIONAL AGE. Complications: RESPIRATORY DISTRESS SYNDROME, feeding difficulties due to immature sucking, swallowing, coughing reflexes, hypothermia, jaundice, infection, poor bonding due to prolonged neonatal intensive care unit stay. *P. labour* spontaneous labour before 37 weeks' gestation due to changing hormones, overstretched uterus, weak cervix, infection. Treatment: tocolytics, e.g. ritodrine hydrochloride, to delay birth. If extrauterine environment less hazardous for fetus, labour may be induced before 37 weeks' gestation with controlled forceps delivery to protect delicate fetal head.

**prevalence** total number of cases of specific disease in existence in given population at certain time.

**preventative** prophylactic; means of preventing something. *P. healthcare* strategies to encourage individuals,

## The six presentations

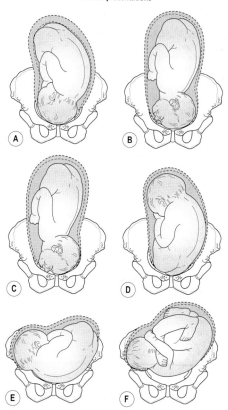

**A,** Vertex presentation; **B,** brow presentation; **C,** face presentation; **D,** breech presentation; **E,** shoulder presentation, dorsoanterior position; **F,** shoulder presentation, dorsoposterior position.

**Features of preterm and small for gestational age babies**

| FEATURE | PRETERM | SMALL FOR GESTATIONAL AGE |
|---------|---------|---------------------------|
| Skin | Reddish pink with lanugo | Grey or yellowish from meconium; dry, sometimes cracked |
| Length | Proportionate to weight | Proportionate to gestation, i.e. long for weight |
| Head | Cranial bones soft | Cranial bones hard, unyielding |
| Face | Eyes closed; peaceful expression | Eyes often open; worried expression |
| Ear pinna | Soft, remains folded | Resistant to folding |
| Breast size | Tissue <1 cm diameter | Palpable tissue ≥1 cm diameter |
| Abdomen | May be prominent | Often scaphoid |
| Behaviour | Weak cry, inactive; no attempt to suck/swallow; flaccid limbs abducted; lies in 'frog' position | Stronger, more mature cry; hungry sucking; swallows; lively, active, good muscle tone |

groups, societies to take steps to prevent disease, or lessen severity, e.g. immunization, health education, screening programmes. In UK, HEALTH VISITORS are responsible for health education and prevention.

**pre-viable** before viability; baby born before 24 weeks' gestation.

**primary** first, in order of time or importance. *P. care* services provided by general practitioners, dentists, community pharmacists, optometrists, community midwives and nurses, health visitors, social workers.

**primigravida** woman pregnant for first time.

**primordial follicle** immature ovarian follicle; oocyte enclosed by single layer of cells.

**primipara** woman who has birthed a viable baby, alive or stillborn.

**primiparous** having borne one viable baby.

**probability** statistical term indicating likelihood of association between variables being due to chance.

**probe** blunt, malleable instrument for exploring sinus tracks, wounds, cavities or passages.

**probenecid** drug that increases uric acid excretion in urine, primarily used for gout, but may be used with antibiotics for GONORRHOEA; inhibits renal excretion of some drugs, thereby increasing their plasma concentration and prolonging effects.

**procaine** hydrochloride salt in solution for local anaesthetic.

**procaine benzylpenicillin** intramuscular antibiotic, commonly used to treat syphilis and gonorrhoea.

**procedure** step-by-step written directions relating to way of performing or effecting outcomes, e.g. actions required in event of fire. *See also* PROTOCOL, POLICY.

**process** 1. prominence or projection, as from bone. 2. series of operations or events leading to achievement of specific result.

**prochlorperazine (Stemetil)** dopamine receptor antagonist, phenothiazine tranquillizer, antipsychotic, antiemetic, may be administered with pethidine for nausea in labour or perioperatively.

**procidentia** complete uterine prolapse; cervix protrudes through vulva.

**procreation** act of producing offspring.

**proctalgia** pain in rectum.

**proctitis** inflammation of anus or rectum.

**proctoscope** instrument for examination of rectum.

**prodromal** preceding. *P. symptom* warning symptom, e.g. visual disturbances occurring before ECLAMPSIA.

**profession** specialized knowledge, skills and attitudes pertinent to practice of a specific role; requires academic preparation in underpinning principles, continuing study to expand body of knowledge, practise autonomously; behaviour in accordance with expected standards.

**professional** pertaining to profession. *Personal p. indemnity insurance* protection from personal financial loss in the event of legal case against practitioner for alleged mistakes, errors, omissions or negligence; employed midwives e.g. in NHS, protected through employer's VICARIOUS LIABILITY. Mandatory for all healthcare professionals in UK.

**profibrinolysin** plasminogen, precursor of fibrinolysin.

**progesterone** female sex hormone essential for maintaining pregnancy, produced from corpus luteum and placenta; promotes formation, maintenance of decidua, glandular breast tissue development; relaxes smooth muscle, aids retention of water and electrolytes in tissues. During menstrual cycle, regulates endometrial secretory changes in preparation for reception of fertilized ovum.

**progestogen** any substance with progestational activity. *P-only pill* See CONTRACEPTION. *P-releasing intrauterine system* plastic device, loaded with progestogen, inserted into uterus so that hormone is steadily released, preventing endometrial proliferation, thickening cervical mucus, possibly suppressing ovulation; developed to overcome problems of conventional intrauterine contraceptive devices which can cause heavy menstrual bleeding.

**prognosis** forecast of course and duration of disease.

**projectile vomiting** *See* VOMITING.

**prolactin** anterior pituitary gland hormone; stimulates lactation.

**prolapse** descent of organ or structure. *Arm p.* serious complication of uncorrected shoulder presentation; fetal arm falls into or through vagina. *Rectal p.* protrusion of rectal mucosa and muscle through anal canal to exterior. *Umbilical cord p.* cord lying below fetal presenting part; occurs after membrane rupture; danger of fetal HYPOXIA or ANOXIA from cord compression; immediate birth of baby required. *Uterine p.* protrusion of uterus into lower vagina due to ligaments and pelvic floor weakening; uterus, vaginal walls, bladder or rectum may be involved.

**proliferation** rapid multiplication of cells, as in malignant growth.

**prolonged labour** labour lasting over 24 hours, due to poor or incoordinate uterine action, cephalopelvic disproportion, malpresentation, malposition. Midwife must ensure mother has adequate pain relief, progress is being made, materno-fetal condition satisfactory. Fetal risks: hypoxia, trauma, excessive skull moulding causing intracranial haemorrhage; maternal risks: exhaustion, dehydration, uterine rupture, physical trauma, long-term uterine, cervical or urinary tract problems. See AUGMENTATION OF LABOUR.

**prolonged pregnancy** pregnancy over 42 weeks (294 days) from first day of last normal menstrual period; induction of labour is only necessary when either maternal or fetal condition is compromised. See INDUCTION OF LABOUR; POST-DATES PREGNANCY.

**promazine hydrochloride (Sparine)** tranquillizer, phenothiazine derivative for schizophrenia treatment.

**promethazine hydrochloride (Phenergan)** antihistamine, phenothiazine for pregnancy sickness, HYPEREMESIS GRAVIDARUM; strong sedative effect, may be used for insomnia. Approved for over-the-counter use in UK, Australia; prescription-only in USA.

**promontory** projection. *Sacral p.* important pelvic landmark formed by projection of upper border of first sacral vertebra.

**pronation** turning downwards. *P. of hand* downwards hand flexion.

**prone** lying face downwards.

**pronucleus** haploid nucleus of sex cell.

**prophylactic** pertaining to prophylaxis, preventative.

**prophylaxis** measures to prevent disease; preventive treatment. *Adj* prophylactic.

**propranolol** beta-adrenergic blocking agent used to treat hypertension and some cardiac conditions.

**propylthiouracil** thyroid inhibitor to treat thyrotoxicosis.

**prostacyclin** potent vasodilator and inhibitor of platelet aggregation; intermediate in metabolic pathway of arachidonic acid, formed from prostaglandin endoperoxides in artery and vein walls.

**prostaglandin** lipid molecules, oxytocic substances in menstrual blood, amniotic fluid, semen, other cells; synthetic prostaglandins, e.g. Prostin, for early termination of pregnancy, and to induce term labour. *P. $E_2$* gel or tablets, administered vaginally act on cervix and myometrium; uterine hyperstimulation may occur with repeated doses; oxytocin should not be given within 3–6 hours of prostaglandin administration. *P. $F_2$* a carboprost to treat postpartum haemorrhage; contracts myometrium; administered intramuscularly or intramyometrically. *P. pessary* dinoprostone, misoprostol, $PGE_2$, vaginal tablets, pessaries, gel and in slow-release form; replicates prostaglandin $E_2$, ripens cervix. See POST-DATES PREGNANCY.

**Insertion of prostaglandin pessary**

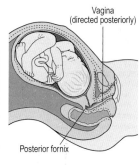

Vagina
(directed posteriorly)

Posterior fornix

**prostate gland** male gland surrounding bladder neck and prostatic urethra, contributes secretions to seminal fluid.

**Prostin E** *See* PROSTAGLANDINS.

**protamine sulphate** antidote to heparin overdosage.

**protease** proteolytic enzyme in digestive juices, causes protein breakdown.

**protein** carbon, hydrogen, nitrogen, oxygen substance; essential constituent of body tissue, found in meat, fish, milk, eggs, peas, beans, lentils; broken down into 20 amino acids, e.g. PHENYLALANINE, TYROSINE, facilitates cell repair, growth; excess amino acids broken down by liver, excreted in urine as urea. Plasma proteins: specific protein carriers aid hormone transport; acute-phase reactants, e.g. alpha-1-antitrypsin, fibrinogen, aid inflammation or clotting; complement components; immunoglobulins. Albumin maintains water distribution by exerting osmotic pressure at capillary membrane, prevents plasma fluid leakage from capillaries into intercellular spaces.

**proteinuria** protein, usually albumin, in urine.

**proteus** gram-negative bacteria in faecal, other putrefying matter.

**prothrombin** plasma protein synthesized in liver, vital for blood clotting: when activated by thromboplastin, which is released when tissues are damaged and platelets broken down; in presence of calcium it forms thrombin, which, with fibrinogen, forms insoluble fibrin. **P. time** seconds required for specimen of blood in contact with thromboplastin to clot.

**prothrombinase** thromboplastin.

**protocol** 1. multidisciplinary written agreement of planned course of action for managing care. 2. action plan for clinical trial.

**proton** positively charged particle forming part of nucleus of atom.

**protoplasm** essential chemical compound of all living cells.

**proximal** in anatomy, central point of system; opposite of distal.

**pruritus** skin irritation; may affect whole body surface or be localized. *P. vulvae* localized vulval irritation, may indicate glycosuria or THRUSH.

**pseudo-** prefix meaning 'false'. *P.-cyesis* false pregnancy; subjective symptoms in absence of conception. *P.-hermaphroditism* apparently having male and female characteristics; INTERSEX. *P.-menstruation* blood-stained vaginal discharge in baby girls; occurs around day 3 of life due to maternal oestrogen withdrawal.

*Pseudomonas* gram-negative, aerobic bacteria, some species of which are pathogenic for plants and vertebrates.

**psoas** muscle forming part of posterior abdominal wall.

**psoriasis** chronic recurrent non-infectious skin disease, unknown cause; reddish marginated patches, profuse silvery scaling on knees or elbows, can be more widespread.

**psyche** conscious and unconscious mind.

**psychiatry** study of mental health disorders and their treatment.

**psychology** science of mind and its functions.

**psychomotor** pertaining to motor effects of cerebral or psychic activity.

**psychoprophylaxis** preparation for birth, aims to modify perception of painful sensations associated with normal birth; Lamaze method.

**psychosexual** relating to mental aspects of sexual activity.

**psychosis** severe mental illness affecting whole personality; organic or emotional origin; personality derangement, loss of contact with reality, delusions, hallucinations, illusions. *Adj* psychotic.

**psychosocial** relating to psychological and social aspects.

**psychosomatic** relating to mind and body. *P. disorders* illnesses in which emotional factors have profound influence.

**psychotherapy** techniques to treat mental illness with psychological methods; relies on establishing communication between therapist and patient as means of understanding and modifying behaviour.

**psychotropics** drugs affecting mind, emotions, behaviour, e.g. lithium.

**ptosis** drooping of upper eyelid from third nerve paralysis; dropping downwards of organ or other structure.

**ptyalin** salivary ENZYME that starts digestion of starches.

**ptyalism** abnormally increased salivation; may occur in pregnancy nausea and vomiting, HYPEREMESIS GRAVIDARUM.

**puberty** age when reproductive organs become functionally active, usually 10–14 years.

**pubes** region over pubic bones.

**pubic** pertaining to pubes, e.g. *p. arch* bony arch formed by junction of *inferior pubic rami*, anterior part of pelvic outlet.

**pubiotomy** cutting through pubic bone to enable birth to take place.

**pubis** anterior portion of hip bone; pubic bone.

**public health** medical field safeguarding and improving physical, mental and social well-being of community; midwives have role in public health and responsibility to provide services and care for socially disadvantaged women, e.g. victims of domestic violence, substance abusers.

**pubococcygeus** one part of levator ani muscle extending from symphysis pubis to coccyx.

**pubovesical** pertaining to pubis and bladder.

**pudenda** external genitalia. *Sing* pudendum.

**pudendal** pertaining to external genital organs. *P. nerve block* local analgesia induced by injecting solution of 0.5% or 1% lidocaine (lignocaine) around pudendal nerve.

**puerperal** pertaining to puerperium. *P. sepsis* infection of genital tract after childbirth.

**puerperium** 6- to 8-week period after birth during which uterus and other organs and structures return to non-pregnant state.

**pulmonary** pertaining to, affecting lungs. *P. circulation.* See CIRCULATION. *P. embolism* See EMBOLISM. *P. infarction* death of tissue due to blood clot in lung. *P. tuberculosis* See TUBERCULOSIS.

**pulsation** beating or throbbing.

**pulse** local rhythmic arterial expansion, felt digitally in artery near body surface, corresponds to each contraction of left ventricle of heart. Normal rate about 72 per minute in adults, 130 in infants, 80 in older children. *P. pressure* difference between diastolic and systolic blood pressures, measured by sphygmomanometer.

**puncture** to pierce. *Lumbar p.* procedure to remove cerebrospinal fluid from between third and fourth or fourth and fifth lumbar vertebrae for diagnostic purposes or to relieve cerebral pressure.

**pupil** opening in centre of iris through which light enters eye.

**purgative** drug that produces evacuation of bowels.

**purple line** See ANAL CLEFT LINE.

**purine** heterocyclic compound, nucleus of purine bases such as adenine and guanine, which occur in DNA and RNA.

**purpura haemorrhagica** extravasation of blood in skin and mucous membranes; causes purple spots and patches; sometimes associated with deficiency of THROMBOCYTES (THROMBOCYTOPENIA).

**purulent** containing or resembling pus.

**pus** thick, semi-liquid substance of dead leucocytes, bacteria, cell debris, tissue fluids, due to inflammation from invading bacteria, which destroy phagocytes and cause local suppuration.

**pustule** small, elevated, circumscribed, pus-containing skin lesion.

**putative** supposed, reputed. *P. father* man believed to be father of illegitimate child.

**pyaemia** condition due to invasion of bloodstream by bacteria; causes blockage of small blood vessels, results in abscess formation, leads to rigors and high fever.

**pyelitis** inflammation of renal pelvis; PYELONEPHRITIS.

**pyelography** radiology of renal pelvis by injection of radio-opaque contrast medium. *Intravenous p.* investigative procedure; water-soluble, iodine-containing contrast medium is injected intravenously; radiographs are taken as contrast medium is excreted by kidneys and passes down ureters into bladder.

**pyelonephritis** kidney and ureter inflammation, usually due to ESCHERICHIA COLI. Symptoms: severe lumbar pain, hyperpyrexia, rigors, tachycardia, vomiting, general malaise, backache, vomiting, anaemia. May occur from 18 and 24 weeks' gestation, due to stasis of urine in dilated ureters and pressure of pregnant uterus, particularly on right side, triggering bacterial growth. In neonates, no obvious signs but condition suspected in pale baby, not feeding well, losing weight, generally not thriving.

**pyelonephrosis** any disease of kidney and its pelvis.

**pyloric stenosis** congenital hypertrophic pyloric stenosis; occurs in 3 in 1000 births. Thickened, strengthened pyloric sphincter, enlarged stomach, palpable pylorus; waves of peristalsis seen abdominally during feeding, persistent projectile vomiting occurs; signs rarely occur before 3–4 weeks of age. Anti-spasmodic drugs e.g. atropine, may be given with feeds; RAMSTEDT OPERATION often necessary for rapid, complete recovery.

**pylorus** opening between stomach and duodenum.

**pyo-** prefix meaning 'pus'.

**pyogenic** producing pus.

**pyometra** pus in uterus.

**pyosalpinx** pus in fallopian tube.

**pyrazinamide** anti-tuberculosis drug.

**pyretic** pertaining to fever.

**pyrexia** fever; rise of body temperature above 37.2°C (99°F).

**pyridoxine** vitamin $B_6$; used to prevent, treat deficiency.

**pyrogen** fever-producing substance, possibly of bacterial origin.

**pyuria** presence of pus in urine, which becomes cloudy; pus cells will be seen if the urine is examined microscopically.

**QRS complex** group of three distinct waves depicted on electrocardiogram, created by passage of cardiac electrical impulses through ventricles; occurs at beginning of each ventricular contraction; R wave normally most prominent.

**quadrant** one quarter of circumference of circle or area, e.g. abdominal surface.

**quadruple test** Down syndrome screening test, TRIPLE TEST with additional serum MARKER, INHIBIN A; also part of INTEGRATED TEST.

**quadruplets** four children born at same labour.

**qualitative research** systematic subjective research approach, used to describe human life experiences and promote understanding of subjective experiences, e.g. pain, caring, powerlessness, comfort.

**quality assurance** pledge to public to work towards optimal achievable degrees of excellence in (health) services, allowing standards of care and norms of professional behaviour to be measured according to predefined criteria so that client care can be improved.

**quantitative fluorescence polymerase chain reaction** diagnostic test to identify TRISOMY and sex chromosome ANEUPLOIDY; results usually available within 48 hours of chorionic villus sampling or amniocentesis. Polymerase chain reaction amplifies small DNA samples labelled with fluorescent dyes; measurements of specific regions on DNA molecules are displayed in graph form, showing number of specific chromosomes in each cell. Heavily blood-stained samples may interfere with analysis.

**quantitative research** formal objective systematic research approach in which numerical data are utilized to obtain information, describe variables, examine relationships among variables, determine cause-and-effect interactions between variables; thought to provide sounder knowledge base for healthcare practice than QUALITATIVE RESEARCH.

**quarantine** period during which known infected persons, contacts and suspects are isolated to prevent infection spread.

**Quetelet index** body mass index calculated by dividing weight in kilograms by height in metres squared. Healthy range: 20–24.9; below 20: underweight; 25–30: overweight; over 30: obesity; over 40: morbid obesity. *See* OBESITY.

**'quickening'** first perceptible fetal movements, felt by mother approximately 18–20 weeks' gestation in primigravidae, 16–18 weeks in multigravidae.

**quinolones** group of synthetic broadspectrum antibiotics.

**quintuplets** five children born at same labour.

**quotient** number obtained by division.

http://dx.doi.org/10.1016/B978-0-7020-6906-2.00017-6

**racemose** grape-like. *R. cells* cells arranged around central duct. *R. glands* compound, lobulated structure e.g. salivary glands, breast cells, cervical glands.

**rachi(o)-** word element meaning 'spine'.

**rachitic pelvis** bony pelvis with flat pelvic brim, similar to platypelloid pelvis, caused by childhood rickets. *See* PELVIS.

**radial** relating to radius. *R. artery* artery at wrist. *R. palsy* wrist drop seen soon after birth, usually resolves spontaneously.

**radical** dealing with root or cause of disease. *R. hysterectomy* complete removal of uterus, cervix, part of vagina, occasionally also ovaries, fallopian tubes, local lymph nodes.

**radioactive** emitting electromagnetic alpha (α), beta (β), gamma (γ) waves naturally, e.g. radium, or artificially e.g. radioactive iodine.

**radiographer** healthcare professional in diagnostic x-ray department or radiotherapy department.

**radiography** diagnostic x-ray examination, rarely performed in pregnancy because of possible adverse fetal effects.

**radioimmunoassay** sensitive assay method to measure minute quantities of specific antibodies or any antigen, e.g. hormone, drug, against which specific antibodies are raised; laboratory test to measure hormones,

therapeutic drug monitoring, drug abuse screening.

**radioisotope** radioactive element; unstable atoms that undergo radioactive decay emitting alpha, beta or gamma radiation, occurring naturally, e.g. radium, uranium, or created artificially.

**radio-opaque** capable of obstructing passage of x-rays, e.g. dyes used for radiographic diagnostic tests.

**radiotelemetry** measurement of data transmitted by radio waves from subject to recording apparatus; radiotelemetry of fetal heart may be used when mother is ambulant in labour.

**radiotherapy** treatment of disease (mainly malignant) with ionizing radiation, either directed from outside patient's body or by isotope implanted or instilled into abnormal tissue or body cavity.

**radium** metallic element, symbol Ra; radioactive metal.

**Ramstedt operation** pyloromyotomy; division of hypertrophied pyloric sphincter to relieve PYLORIC STENOSIS.

**ramus** branch e.g. pubic bone, upper and lower branch. *Pl* rami.

**random blood sugar test** blood glucose test undertaken if unexplained glycosuria in pregnancy; if result is suspicious, glucose load or GLUCOSE TOLERANCE TEST may be performed.

**randomized controlled trial** research trial; study subjects chosen at random from suitable group of potential

http://dx.doi.org/10.1016/B978-0-7020-6906-2.00018-8

participants to increase extent to which sample is representative of target population; usually involves control and experimental groups; difficult to obtain totally random sample because of informed consent requirements.

**ranitidine** H₂ receptor antagonist, given in labour before general anaesthesia to inhibit hydrochloric acid production, reduces risk of MENDELSON SYNDROME.

**rapid diagnostic techniques** *See* FLUORESCENT IN SITU HYBRIDIZATION *and* QUANTITATIVE FLUORESCENCE POLYMERASE CHAIN REACTION.

**raphe** seam or ridge of tissue indicating juncture of two equal parts, e.g. median raphe of perineal body, anococcygeal raphe.

**rash** temporary skin eruption. *Heat r.* miliaria. *Napkin r.* cutaneous localized reaction of baby's buttocks, caused by irritants such as ammonia in decomposed urine, improperly washed nappies, etc.

**raspberry leaf** pharmacological HERBAL MEDICINE thought to tone smooth muscle, prepare uterus for labour from third trimester. Do not use to induce labour. Contraindications: uterine scar, preterm or precipitate labour history, multiple pregnancy, antepartum haemorrhage, hypertension, planned Caesarean section. Midwives must be adequately trained to advise on raspberry leaf.

**raspberry mark** congenital HAEMANGIOMA.

**Rastelli operation** surgery for transposition of great vessels; blood circulation through heart diverted for adequate oxygenation.

**rate** speed or frequency with which event or circumstance occurs per unit of time, population or other standard of comparison. *Glomerular filtration r.* quantity of glomerular filtrate formed each minute in kidney nephrons, calculated by measuring clearance of specific substances, e.g. insulin or creatinine. *See also* BASAL METABOLIC RATE, BIRTH RATE, MORTALITY RATE.

**ratio** expression of quantity of one substance in relation to another; relationship between two quantities expressed as quotient of one divided by other. *Lecithin-sphingomyelin r.* ratio of lecithin to sphingomyelin in amniotic fluid, indicator of fetal lung maturity.

**reabsorption** process of absorbing again, e.g. absorption by kidneys of substances (glucose, proteins, sodium) already secreted into renal tubules.

**reaction** response to application of stimulus; evidence of acidity or alkalinity; pH of solution.

**reagent** substance employed to produce chemical reaction to detect, measure or produce other substances.

**real-time scanner** ultrasound scanner giving moving visual display.

**receptor** 1. molecule on surface of or within cell that recognizes and binds to specific molecules, producing some effect in cell, e.g. cell-surface receptors of immunocompetent cells that recognize antigens, lymphokines or receptors of neurons and target organs that recognize neurotransmitters or hormones. 2. sensory nerve ending that responds to various stimuli.

**recession** receding or drawing back. *Rib r.* or *sternal r.* inwards movement of ribs or sternum, commonly seen in neonatal RESPIRATORY DISTRESS SYNDROME.

**recessive** tending to recede; in genetics opposite of dominant – capable of expression only when carried by both of pairs of homologous chromosomes, i.e. HOMOZYGOUS and not HETEROZYGOUS.

**recipient** one who receives, e.g. blood transfusion, tissue or organ graft. *Universal r.* person able to receive blood of any type without agglutination of donor cells.

**recombinant** 1. new cell or individual resulting from genetic recombination. 2. pertaining or relating to such cells or individuals. *r. DNA technology* process of taking gene from one organism and inserting it into DNA of another; gene splicing.

**record keeping** midwives must keep accurate, comprehensive, contemporaneous records of maternal, fetal/neonatal conditions, all observations, clinical decisions, interactions between mother/baby and midwife/doctor; in UK records must legally be retained for 25 years.

**rectal** relating to rectum. *R. examination* digital examination of rectum or adjacent structures; performed at conclusion of perineal repair to ensure no sutures have penetrated rectal mucosa.

**rectocele** hernia of rectum caused by overstretching of vaginal wall at delivery, treated by posterior colporrhaphy.

**rectovaginal** relating to rectum and vagina. *R. fistula. See* FISTULA.

**rectovesical** pertaining to, communicating with rectum and bladder.

**rectum** lower 15 cm of large intestine from pelvic colon to anal canal.

**rectus abdominis** pair of muscles running vertically on either side of midline from symphysis pubis to xiphisternum, separated by linea alba; in combination with other abdominal muscles raise intra-abdominal pressure, assist in flexing spine and controlling pelvic girdle tilt; poor muscle tone adversely affects lumbar spine flexion, causing difficulty with pelvic tilting, increased lumbar lordosis, postural problems in pregnancy. *Diastasis of r. a.* over-stretching of rectus abdominis by growing uterus may occur in pregnancy, commonly in multiparae; uterus can sometimes be seen bulging through the abdominal wall beneath the skin; treatment: help mother to cope with backache, related discomforts, encourage postnatal exercises.

**recumbent** lying down.

**red blood cells** *See* ERYTHROCYTES.

**referral** directing to sources of help, e.g. to doctor when mother's condition deviates from normal parameters of midwifery practice.

**referred pain** pain at a distance from place of origin, related to distribution of sensory nerve, e.g. right shoulder pain associated with gallbladder disease.

**reflection** process of conscious, systematic thinking about one's actions; review, analysis and synthesis of situations that have occurred, usually after event; active process by which midwives learn from experience, with view to improving future practice.

**reflex** reflected or thrown back. *R. action* involuntary movement relating to stimulus, e.g. knee jerk, withdrawal of limb from pinprick. Reflexes present in term baby include sucking, startle, step, swallowing, MORO REFLEX. *Conditioned r.* action acquired by regular association of physiological event with unrelated outside event, e.g. 'let down' reflex: myoepithelial breast cells contract around acini cells at sight or sound of hungry baby, makes milk supply available.

**reflexology** complementary therapy in which feet represent map of body; pressure to specific points on feet affect distal parts of body. Midwives must be adequately trained to use reflexology.

**regional anaesthesia** EPIDURAL, spinal or caudal analgesia.

**registered midwife** midwife licensed to practise in country in which s/he resides; must comply with mandatory and regulatory requirements of that country.

**registrar of births, marriages and deaths** official recorder of births, marriages, deaths in England, Wales, part of Office for National Statistics; also regulates, records civil marriages, conducts demographic research and analyses material.

**registration** process by which official register can be maintained. *R. of births* all births must be registered within 6 weeks in England, Wales, 3 weeks in Scotland. If parents fail to do this, responsibility falls to any other person present at birth, i.e. midwife. *R. of deaths* family's responsibility; if baby dies shortly after birth, birth and death must be registered. *R. of stillbirths* undertaken by parents before registrar will issue certificate for burial or cremation.

**regulatory body** organization responsible for defining and monitoring preparation and practice of specific professional group, e.g. Nursing and Midwifery Council.

**regurgitation** backward flow, e.g. of food into mouth from stomach; sometimes occurs in newborn babies due to weakness of cardia of stomach. *Aortic r.* backward flow of blood into left ventricle when aortic valve incompetent. *Mitral r. See* MITRAL. *Gastro-oesophageal r. See* HEARTBURN.

**relaxant** causing relaxation. *Muscle r.* agent acting at neuromuscular junction causes muscle paralysis, e.g. anaesthesia, or relieves muscle spasticity, tension, acts directly on muscle or central nervous system.

**relaxation** lessening of tension, e.g. of muscles after contraction. Antenatal classes may teach relaxation techniques to prepare mother for labour.

**relaxin** hormone, in pregnancy causes 'softening' of pelvic tissues and joints, facilitating pelvic capacity; causes lumbar lordosis.

**releasing factor** substance produced in hypothalamus that causes anterior pituitary gland to release hormones.

**reliability** research issue concerned with consistency, dependability, accuracy and comparability of tests or investigations.

**renal** concerning, affecting kidney. *R. agenesis* failure of both kidneys to form in fetus; associated with oligohydramnios. *R. calculus* kidney stone. *R. disease in pregnancy* rare, serious problem; women undergoing dialysis have poor prognosis for successful pregnancy; renal transplant offers better prognosis. May have history of childhood nephritis; proteinuria present from early pregnancy. Risks: miscarriage, pre-eclampsia, placental abruption, intrauterine growth retardation, fetal death, long-term renal impairment. **R. failure** failure of renal function, causes uraemia. **R. threshold** level of substances in blood beyond which they are excreted in urine; normal renal threshold for glucose is 10 mmol/L (180 mg/100 mL): glycosuria results if exceeds this.

**renin** enzyme synthesized, stored, secreted by kidneys; helps blood pressure regulation by catalyzing conversion of angiotensinogen to angiotensin I, then converted to angiotensin II, powerful vasoconstrictor. Also stimulates aldosterone secretion, causes salt and water retention by kidneys. *R-angiotensin-aldosterone system* hormone system, regulates blood pressure, fluid balance; low blood volume causes kidneys to secrete renin, which stimulates angiotensin I production, converted to angiotensin II, causing vasoconstriction, raising blood pressure. Angiotensin II stimulates aldosterone secretion from adrenal cortex, so kidney tubules increase sodium and water reabsorption into blood, increasing fluid volume, blood pressure. If system overactive, blood pressure remains high; drugs can control hypertension, cardiac, renal effects, diabetes.

**rennin** milk-curdling enzyme in gastric juice of babies; catalyzes conversion of casein from soluble to insoluble form.

**Replogle tube** suction tube used for babies with oesophageal atresia to prevent spilling over into trachea, causing aspiration or pneumonia.

**reproduction** process of producing new individual of same kind; creation

of similar object or situation; duplication; replication.

**reproductive organs, female** ovaries, producing ova or eggs, uterine (fallopian) tubes, uterus, vagina, vulva; breasts are secondary sexual organs, enclosing mammary glands.

**reproductive organs, male** penis, testes, scrotum, accessory glands secrete fluids, ducts allow ejaculation of spermatozoa at intercourse.

**research** method of increasing available knowledge through discovery of new information via systematic scientific enquiry. *R.-based practice* clinical practice based on evidence of formal research studies, contributes towards reducing theory–practice gap; mainstay of CLINICAL GOVERNANCE.

**resection** removal of part.

**residential care (for children)** local authority social services department or registered voluntary organization care for children up to age 18; residential nurseries provided for under 5-year-olds, community homes and hostels for children aged 5–18 years; boarding with foster parents is arranged when possible.

**residual** remaining. *R. urine* urine remaining in bladder after micturition.

**resistance** power to overcome; natural power of body to withstand and recover from infection or disease; insensitivity of bacteria to antibiotics, e.g. some staphylococci resistant to penicillin.

**respiration** breathing; exchange of OXYGEN and CARBON DIOXIDE between atmosphere and body cells; inspiration, expiration, diffusion of oxygen from pulmonary alveoli to blood and of carbon dioxide from blood to alveoli, transport of oxygen to and carbon dioxide from body cells. *Inspiration*: contraction of external intercostal muscles, raising ribs and sternum, diaphragm descends. *Expiration*: contraction of internal intercostal muscles, descent of ribs, relaxation of diaphragm. Normal adult respiration rate 16 breaths per minute at rest; in neonates 40–50. **Artificial r.** respiratory movements produced by artificial means.

**respiratory depression** impaired respiration, inhibiting full ventilation and lung perfusion. In neonate, respiratory centre depression may be due to narcotic drugs or cerebral hypoxia in labour, prematurity, intranatal pneumonia after prolonged membrane rupture, severe anaemia from rhesus incompatibility, fetomaternal haemorrhage, congenital abnormalities. *See* CHOANAL ATRESIA.

**respiratory distress syndrome** condition mainly in preterm babies due to lack of SURFACTANT, also in babies of diabetic mothers or if born by Caesarean section. Respiratory difficulty occurs within 4 hours of birth, gradually worsening; also caused by MECONIUM ASPIRATION SYNDROME. **Adult RDS** due to severe hypovolaemic shock, impaired gaseous exchange, reduced oxygen, increased carbon dioxide levels, alveolar collapse, pulmonary oedema, leading ultimately to respiratory failure.

**restitution** restoration, putting right; fetal head rotation after birth, in anteroposterior diameter, realigns position in relation to shoulders.

**resuscitation** restoration from state of collapse. **Neonatal r.** needed if baby fails to breathe after birth;

common in preterm babies due to lung, respiratory centre, respiratory muscle immaturity. Also for medullary depression asphyxia due to maternal intrapartum drugs depressing fetal respiratory centre (reversed by antagonist administration), hypoxia from fetal distress; intracranial intrapartum damage, e.g. excessive, abnormal moulding. *See* APPENDIX 3.

**retained placenta** placenta that fails to be expelled within expected time limits, differing if third-stage labour was actively or passively managed. Commonly due to partial placental separation from poor uterine action, inadequate contraction after baby's birth causing haemorrhage, maternal shock; treatment: manual fundal stimulation *per abdomen*, oxytocic drugs to encourage uterus to contract for placenta separation and delivery. Also caused by PLACENTA ACCRETA, increta, percreta; requires MANUAL REMOVAL under anaesthetic, occasionally hysterectomy. *See also* POSTPARTUM HAEMORRHAGE.

**retained products of conception** tissue retained in utero after baby's birth, or after miscarriage, when evacuation of retained products is required; uterus will feel 'boggy' when palpated abdominally; abnormal vaginal bleeding may occur. *See also* POSTPARTUM HAEMORRHAGE, APPENDIX 1.

**retention** holding back. **R. of urine** inability to pass urine; in obstetrics commonly due to neurological damage from overstretching of urethra and trigone, leading to diminished bladder sensation and perineal discomfort; may also be due to blockage. Catheterization may be necessary but avoid if possible, as chronic urinary tract infection can occur, leading to renal failure in severe cases.

**reticuloendothelial** tissue and cell network throughout body, especially in blood, general connective tissue, spleen, liver, lungs, bone marrow, lymph nodes. Large cells concerned with blood cell formation and destruction, storage of fatty materials, metabolism of iron and pigment, inflammation and immunity; some cells motile, phagocytic; spleen cells aid disposal of disintegrated erythrocytes; Küpffer cells in liver cavities, and cells of general connective tissue and bone marrow transform haemoglobin released by disintegrated erythrocytes into bile pigment.

**retina** inner lining of eyeball; nerve cells and fibres from which optic nerve leaves eyeball, passes to visual area of cerebral cortex; impression of image is focused upon it.

**retinopathy** general pathological conditions of retina occurring in systemic disorders such as hypertension, severe pre-eclampsia, eclampsia, diabetes. *R. of prematurity* neonatal condition; retinal capillary vasoconstriction due to excessive oxygen concentration, producing overgrowth of retinal blood vessels; vascular proliferation and exudation of blood and serum detaches retina, causing scarring, inevitable blindness. Careful monitoring of oxygen tension level is essential in preterm babies.

**retraction** drawing back; permanent progressive shortening of uterine muscle accompanying contractions in labour: dilates cervix, expels fetus, separates placenta, controls bleeding; over-retraction in obstructed labour may cause *r. ring. See* BANDL'S RING.

**retractor** surgical instrument for drawing apart wound edges to make deeper structures more accessible.

**retro-** prefix meaning 'behind' or 'backward'.

**retroflexion** bent backwards, e.g. when uterine body is bent backwards at acute angle with cervix in normal position.

**retrograde** going backwards. *R. pyelography* radiography of kidney and ureter after radio-opaque dye injection into renal pelvis.

**retrolental** behind lens of eye. *R. fibroplasia. See* RETINOPATHY OF PREMATURITY.

**retroplacental** behind placenta. *R. clot* blood clot behind placenta.

**retroversion** turning back, as when uterus is tilted backwards. *cf.* RETROFLEXION.

**retroverted gravid uterus** pregnant uterus tilts backwards; uterus usually spontaneously corrects to anteversion; if persists, INCARCERATION develops with retention of urine, usually around 16–20 weeks' gestation.

**retrovirus** group of RNA viruses, including human T-cell leukaemia viruses, lentiviruses, human immunodeficiency virus (HIV).

**revalidation** three-yearly Nursing and Midwifery Council requirement for registrants to maintain practice; 450 practice hours; 35 hours of professional development; practice-related feedback and reflection, health and character declaration, personal professional indemnity insurance; must be confirmed by suitable colleague.

**rhesus factor** three pairs of antigens (Cc, Dd, Ee) in human blood; if present, blood is rhesus positive, denoted with capitals (C, D, E); if absent, rhesus negative, denoted with c, d, e; D antigen is responsible for rhesus immunity in most cases.

**rhesus incompatibility** occurs in rhesus-negative mother when fetus rhesus-positive; maternal antibodies against fetal cells pass through placenta to fetal circulation, destroys fetal erythrocytes, compensated for by increased bone marrow production and early release of immature red blood cells (erythroblasts). Mother given prophylactic anti-D within 72 hours of delivery to prevent reoccurrence in next pregnancy.

**rheumatic** pertaining to muscular and joint pains; fibrositis. *R. heart disease* acute rheumatic fever associated with streptococcal infection, chorea or acute tonsillitis; can trigger ENDOCARDITIS; myocarditis, pericarditis; MITRAL STENOSIS, aortic incompetence may occur later. Assess pregnant woman with history of childhood rheumatic fever carefully as extra strain exerted on heart. *See also* HEART DISEASE IN PREGNANCY.

**rhinitis** inflammation of nasal mucous membrane, sometimes of staphylococcal origin, occurs in neonate.

**rhomboid/rhombus of Michaelis** diamond- or dome-shaped area at base of spine marked by dimpling of skin, with spinous process of fifth lumbar vertebra beneath superior angle; posterior superior iliac spines palpable under lateral angles; beginning of gluteal cleft inferiorly. May be seen in second-stage labour, represents posterior sacrococcygeal displacement as fetal occiput moves into sacral curve; appears to cause mother to arch back, push buttocks forwards, outstretch her arms. *See also* ANAL CLEFT LINE.

**rhythm** measured movement; recurrence of action or function at regular intervals. *Adj* rhythmic, rhythmical. *R. method of family planning* natural contraceptive method, involves calculation of 'safe' period during which conception least likely, daily temperature monitoring, observation of vaginal discharge, i.e. Billings method.

**ribcage** 12 paired bones from thoracic vertebrae toward median line on ventral aspect of trunk; forms major part of thoracic skeleton; costal bones; acts as protection for heart, lungs. *R. displacement in pregnancy* progesterone and relaxin cause lower ribs to flare outwards, increasing subcostal angle, anteroposterior and transverse diameters increase with corresponding increase in overall chest circumference, diaphragm rises, raising tidal volume.

**riboflavin** vitamin $B_2$, required by certain enzymes that catalyze many oxidation–reduction reactions; present in liver, kidney, heart, brewer's yeast, milk, eggs, greens, enriched cereals.

**ribonucleic acid** nucleic acid of cell, which translates 'code' of DEOXYRIBO-NUCLEIC ACID into action.

**ribosome** minute granule in cell cytoplasm concerned with protein synthesis; can be seen with electron microscope.

**rickets** rachitis; deficient bone calcification due to lack of vitamin D, needed for calcium and phosphorus absorption, causes bony deformities of skull, ribs, legs, pelvis. Prevention: vitamin D administration, exposure to sunlight, ultraviolet light.

**right obliquity and rotundity** change in uterine position in pregnancy; once uterus becomes abdominal organ, it rotates on own axis and tilts to right, avoiding stomach on left. Women encouraged to lie on left side to reduce uterine pressure; for Caesarean section, wedge placed under right side to avoid pressure, SUPINE HYPOTENSIVE SYNDROME.

**rigor** sudden shivering attack with rapidly rising temperature; plateaus then declines after period of sweating; may occur in severe pyelonephritis or puerperal SEPTICAEMIA. *R. mortis* body stiffening soon after death, due to muscle protoplasm coagulation.

**Ringer's lactate** isotonic solution for intravenous administration; not generally used in pregnancy.

**risk management** structured approach to healthcare to reduce identifiable risks, prevent problems arising, reduce incidence of complaints and litigation costs. Standards of care agreed, based on current research to support clinical guidelines; systematic reviews of clinical records undertaken; case discussions, case conferences in event of adverse outcomes to treatment; assessments of health and safety; training programmes for staff.

**ritodrine hydrochloride (Yutopar)** beta-2-adrenergic receptor stimulant; decreases uterine activity, prolongs gestation in preterm labour.

**Ritter disease** exfoliative dermatitis; rare, severe form of PEMPHIGUS NEONATORUM.

**Robert pelvis** abnormal pelvis with bilateral absence of sacral alae, fusion of sacrum to ilium on each side; prevents engagement of fetal head. *See also* PELVIS.

**rockerbottom feet** prominent heels in babies with chromosomal disorders e.g. EDWARD SYNDROME, PATAU SYNDROME.

**rogitine** phentolamine; adrenolytic test for phaeochromocytoma.

**Röntgen rays** *See* X-RAYS.

**rooting reflex** neonatal reflex elicited by stroking cheek or side of mouth: baby turns to stimulated side, opens his mouth to suckle.

**rotation** turning of body on its long axis, e.g. presenting part for proper orientation to pelvic axis; usually occurs naturally, occasionally achieved through manual or instrumental manipulation.

**rotator** muscle that causes rotation of any part.

**rotavirus** virus, looks like wheel under microscope; common cause of acute infantile diarrhoea, often preceded by respiratory signs.

**Rothera test** test for presence of acetone in urine.

**roughage** indigestible vegetable fibre; cellulose; gives bulk to diet, stimulates peristalsis; found in bran, cereals, fruit, vegetable fibres.

**round ligaments** ligaments from uterine cornua to labia majora.

**Royal College of Midwives (RCM)** midwives' professional body and trade union founded 1881, concerned with education, professional practice standards, negotiation of conditions of service and salaries.

**Royal College of Nursing – Midwifery Society** division of Royal College of Nursing for members who are midwives.

**RU86** *See* MIFEPRISTONE.

**rubella** German measles; mild infective disease causing faint macular body rash, enlargement of posterior cervical lymph nodes; spread by droplets from infected person 7 days before rash appears but of low infectivity. Uncommon in pregnancy, but virus crosses placenta to fetus, may cause abortion, stillbirth, congenital rubella, malformations, e.g. cardiac, ear, eye defects, especially if infection acquired in first 4 weeks of pregnancy. Infection later in pregnancy may cause fetal growth retardation, congenital thrombocytopenic purpura, learning difficulties, physical disabilities, deafness; baby may be source of infection for up to 2 years. First-trimester exposure to rubella requires blood to be taken to test for immunity; termination may be considered if there is evidence of infection. Vaccination is given (with mumps and measles) at 1 year, repeated for girls between 12–13 years.

**Rubin test**    test for patency of uterine tubes, made by transuterine inflation with carbon dioxide gas; also called *tubal insufflation*.

**Rubin manoeuvre**    rotational manoeuvre to relieve shoulder dystocia; pressure applied over fetal back to adduct and rotate shoulders. *See* APPENDIX 4.

**rugae**    ridges or creases, e.g. stomach mucosa, vaginal squamous epithelium.

**Rules    and    Standards    for Midwives**    Nursing and Midwifery Council document stating rules by which all UK midwives must abide; failure to do so may result in allegations of professional misconduct.

**rupture**    tearing or bursting, e.g. of aneurysm, of membranes in labour, of tubal pregnancy. *Uterine r.* bursting apart of uterus after obstructed labour; BANDL'S RING, ridge running obliquely across abdomen, marks junction between grossly thickened upper uterine segment and dangerously thinned, overstretched lower segment. Also, tearing of uterine scar from previous Caesarean section – DEHISCENCE – may occur insidiously towards term or rapidly in labour due to powerful contractions. Treat shock and blood loss before suturing rupture; hysterectomy may be required.

**Ryles tube**    thin rubber tube with weighted end, introduced via nose into stomach to withdraw gastric contents or administer fluids.

**Sabin vaccine** oral poliomyelitis vaccine developed by Albert Salk, in 1961; on World Health Organization List of Essential Medicines.

**sac** pouch-like cavity.

**saccharide** carbohydrate: monosaccharides, disaccharides, trisaccharides, polysaccharides.

**sacculation of uterus** rare complication of incarcerated RETROVERTED GRAVID UTERUS; fundus remains under sacral promontory, anterior uterine wall grows to accommodate fetus.

**sacral** relating to sacrum. *S. promontory* upper anterior border of body of prominent first sacral vertebra.

**sacro-** concerning sacrum. *Sacroanterior* and *sacroposterior* positions in breech presentation, sacrum is DENOMINATOR.

**sacrococcygeal** concerning sacrum and coccyx. *S. joint* slightly mobile pelvic joint between sacrum and coccyx.

**sacrocotyloid** relates to sacrum and acetabulum. *S. diameter* sacral promontory to nearest point of iliopectineal eminence; 9.5 cm.

**sacroiliac** concerning sacrum and ilium. *S. joint* or *s. synchondrosis* slightly movable joint between sacrum and ilium.

**sacrum** wedge-shaped bone; five united vertebrae between lowest lumbar vertebra and coccyx; forms posterior pelvic wall.

**safeguarding** child protection agencies working with children, young people, families must ensure risks of harm to children are minimized or take appropriate actions if concern about a child's welfare.

**Safe Motherhood Initiative** World Health Organization campaign to reduce worldwide maternal mortality and morbidity.

**sagittal** arrow-shaped. *S. section* anteroposterior midline section. *S. suture* junction of parietal bones; sagittal or third fontanelle may be noted in sagittal suture, may be linked to DOWN SYNDROME.

**salbutamol** beta-sympathomimetic drug; suppresses preterm labour, avoid in pre-eclampsia, antepartum haemorrhage.

**salicylate** salt or salicylic acid ester, e.g. aspirin; analgesic, antipyretic, anti-inflammatory drug; inhibits prostaglandin synthesis, blocks pyretic and inflammatory processes mediated by prostaglandins.

**saline** containing salt or salts. *Isotonic s. normal s.* 0.9% sodium chloride solution, isotonic with blood, given intravenously to replace fluid in shock and haemorrhage; rapidly excreted.

**saliva** secretion of salivary glands, poured into mouth when food is eaten; moistens, dissolves certain substances, begins carbohydrate digestion with action of enzyme, ptyalin, salivary amylase.

**salivation** normal flow of saliva. *Excessive s.* hypersalivation or PTYALISM,

http://dx.doi.org/10.1016/B978-0-7020-6906-2.00019-X

physiological disorder occurs in some pregnant women, particularly those of West African origin; cause unknown.

**Salk vaccine** intramuscular poliomyelitis vaccine developed by Albert Salk, in 1955; rarely used now *See* SABIN VACCINE.

**Salmonella** genus of bacteria responsible for GASTROENTERITIS.

**salpingectomy** excision of one or both fallopian tubes.

**salpingitis** fallopian tube inflammation.

**salpingogram** radiological outline of fallopian tube interior, used to detect patency and other disorders.

**salpingography** fallopian tube radiography after intrauterine injection of radio-opaque medium.

**salpingo-oophorectomy** removal of fallopian tube and ovary.

**salpingotomy** surgical incision of uterine tube.

**salpinx** fallopian tube.

**salt** 1. sodium chloride, common salt, used in solution as cleansing agent or as intravenous infusion to replace fluid. 2. any compound of acid with alkali or base. **S. depletion** loss of salt from body due to sweating, persistent vomiting or diarrhoea.

**salutogenesis** sociological term; approach focusing on factors that support health and well-being, rather than factors causing disease.

**salutogenic model** relationship between health, stress and coping.

**sample** selected group of population.

**sandal gap** exaggerated gap between first and second toes.

**sanguinous** pertaining to or containing blood.

**saphenous** two superficial veins carrying blood up leg from foot.

**sarcoma** highly malignant tumour of connective or other non-epithelial tissue cells. **Kaposi s.** malignant skin tumour, occurs in those with poor immune system e.g. in ACQUIRED IMMUNE DEFICIENCY SYNDROME.

**saturated solution** liquid containing largest amount of solid that can be dissolved in it without forming precipitate.

**Saving Lives: Improving Mothers' Care** confidential enquiry into maternal and child health, explores causes and contributing factors to maternal and perinatal deaths, offering suggestions on how situations could be avoided or management improved.

**Saving Newborn Lives** global initiative led by Save the Children to raise awareness, conduct research, support global efforts to improve newborn health.

**scalp** layer of tissue over cranial bones. **S. electrode** transducer applied *per vaginam* to fetal scalp to monitor fetal heart in labour.

**scan** image of internal structures and tissues. *See also* COMPUTED TOMOGRAPHY, MAGNETIC RESONANCE IMAGING, ULTRASONOGRAPHY.

**scapula** large, flat, triangular bone forming shoulder blade.

**scar dehiscence** rupture of existing scar from previous surgery, as in uterus; cause of ruptured uterus.

**Schilling test** test to confirm diagnosis of pernicious anaemia by estimating absorption of ingested radioactive vitamin $B_{12}$.

**schizophrenia** psychosis of unknown cause but showing hereditary links; sufferers feel influenced by external forces, experiencing delusions and hallucinations; pregnancy aggravates condition.

**Schultze expulsion** normal placental expulsion; inverted fetal surface presents at vulva; more common and less bleeding than with MATTHEWS DUNCAN EXPULSION.

**sciatic nerve** large nerve fibre; begins in lower back, runs through buttock, down leg; supplies leg skin, muscles, foot, back of thigh; derived from spinal nerves lumbar 4 to sacral 3.

**sciatica** severe pain down back of leg along course of sciatic nerve, due to pressure of heavy uterus on nerves, ligaments. Treatment: ergonomic advice, physiotherapy; acupuncture; usually resolves spontaneously after delivery.

**sclera** white outer coat of eyeball, continuous anteriorly with cornea and posteriorly with external sheath of optic nerve. *Adj* scleral.

**sclerema** uncommon neonatal condition, occurs in HYPOTHERMIA; involves hardening of skin and subcutaneous fat.

**sclerosis** hardening of fibrous and connective tissue, often due to chronic inflammation.

**scoliosis** lateral spine curve deviation. See LORDOSIS, KYPHOSIS.

**scopolamine** prescription anticholinergic drug sometimes used for hyperemesis gravidarum, usually in the form of skin patches.

**screening test** means to identify individuals in a defined population at higher risk than normal from certain conditions; some tests incorrectly identify proportion of unaffected individuals (false positives) or fail to detect affected individuals (false negatives).

**Scriver test** biological test used to diagnose inborn errors of metabolism, e.g. PHENYLKETONURIA. See also GUTHRIE TEST.

**scrotum** in men, pouch of skin and soft tissues, contains testicles.

**scurvy** vitamin C deficiency disease; anaemia, mucous membrane bleeding, joint swelling, mouth ulcers; treatment: dietary vitamin C.

**sebaceous** fatty or pertaining to sebum. *S. glands* sebum-secreting glands in skin communicating with hair follicles.

**sebum** fatty secretion of sebaceous glands.

**second-degree perineal lacerations** See PERINEAL LACERATIONS.

**second stage of labour** from full dilatation of uterine cervix to complete birth of baby.

**secondary** second in order of time or importance. *S. care* medical or surgical care, either elective or emergency, usually after referral from PRIMARY CARE professional. *S. postpartum haemorrhage* excessive genital tract bleeding occurring any time from 24 hours up to 6 weeks after delivery; usually due to retained products of conception and/or infection. Treatment: dependent on cause: evacuation of retained products, intravenous or oral oxytocics, antibiotics. See also POSTPARTUM HAEMORRHAGE.

**secretin** hormone secreted by duodenal and jejunal mucosa when acid chyme enters intestine, carried by blood, stimulates secretion of pancreatic juice, bile and intestinal secretion.

**secretion** substance produced by gland.

**sedative** calming substance, e.g. drug, often facilitating sleep.

**sedimentation** formation of sediment. *S. rate* See ERYTHROCYTE SEDIMENTATION RATE.

**segment** section, part. *Upper uterine s.* upper three-quarters of uterus, contracts and retracts in labour. *Lower uterine s.* lower quarter of uterus and cervix; stretches and dilates in first stage labour.

**segmentation** division of fertilized ovum into 2 cells, then 4, 8, 16, etc., as it traverses fallopian tube.

**seizure** convulsion, attack of epilepsy.

**selective feticide** medical destruction of seriously abnormal fetus in multiple pregnancy; enables healthy fetus to develop normally. *See also* MULTI-FETAL PREGNANCY REDUCTION.

**selective serotonin reuptake inhibitors** antidepressant drugs; adverse effects in pregnancy: fetal anomalies, miscarriage; needs supervised discontinuation to avoid withdrawal effects.

**Sellick manoeuvre** cricoid cartilage pressure during anaesthesia initiation to occlude oesophagus, preventing regurgitation of stomach contents into pharynx with risk of aspiration into lungs; pressure maintained until endotracheal tube inserted and respiratory tract sealed off.

**semen** male secretion of seminal fluid from prostate gland and spermatozoa from testis, produced at ejaculation.

**seminiferous tubules** testicular tubes where spermatozoa produced.

**semipermeable** property of membrane, permitting passage of some molecules, hindering others.

**semi-prone** lying face down with knees turned to one side.

**senna** (Senokot) cassia plant laxative; safe in pregnancy but advise small doses, as can be too purgative.

**sense** faculty of perception, e.g. hunger, thirst, pain, well-being. Five major senses: vision, hearing, smell, taste, touch.

**sensitive** reacting to stimulus.

**sensitivity of tests** measure of accuracy of screening test in identifying individuals with condition; proportion of people with condition found to be positive (high risk) on screening test; DETECTION RATE.

**sensitization** 1. initial exposure of individual to specific antigen, resulting in immune response. 2. antibody cell coating, preparatory step in eliciting immune reaction. 3. action of hormone on tissue or organ so it responds functionally to another hormone. *Adj* sensitized i.e. rendered sensitive.

**sensory** pertaining to sensation. *S. nerve* peripheral afferent nerve, conducts impulses from sense organ to spinal cord or brain.

**sepsis** infection by pathogenic bacteria. *Puerperal s.* genital tract infection in puerperium. *Adj* septic. *S. shock See* TOXIC SHOCK.

**septicaemia** multiplication of pathogenic bacteria in blood; rapid temperature rise, later fluctuating, rigors, sweating, signs of acute fever. *See also* ENDOTOXIC SHOCK, PUERPERAL SEPSIS.

**septum** division, partition e.g. between right and left heart ventricles.

**septuplets** seven offspring produced at one birth.

**sequela** morbid long-term consequences of disease. *Pl* sequelae.

**serology** study of antigen–antibody reactions *in vitro*. *Adj* serological.

**serotonin** vasoconstrictive amine in platelets, intestines, central nervous system, derived from amino acid tryptophan; inactivated by monoamine oxidase.

**serrated** with saw-like edge, e.g. fetal skull bones.

**sertraline** SELECTIVE SEROTONIN REUPTAKE INHIBITOR antidepressant drug, considered safe in pregnancy in UK when benefits outweigh risks. *See also* PAROXETINE, FLUOXETINE.

**serum** clear, straw-coloured fluid in blood; residue with corpuscles and fibrin are removed. Serum from infected person may be used to protect another with same disease, e.g. diphtheria, tetanus.

**serum bilirubin** bile pigment from breakdown of haem, reduced biliverdin; circulates in plasma; taken up by liver, conjugated to form BILIRUBIN. High concentrations may cause jaundice. All neonates have transient bilirubin rise. *See also* KERNICTERUS.

**Maximum Serum Bilirubin Levels**

| Under 27 weeks | 250 µmol/L |
|---|---|
| 28–30 weeks | 280 µmol/L |
| 31–34 weeks | 310 µmol/L |
| 35–38 weeks | 350 µmol/L |
| 39+ weeks | 380 µmol/L |

**sex** fundamental distinction based on type of gametes produced by individual. *S. chromosomes* chromosome pair, X or Y; determine sex and sex-linked characteristics; XX in female; XY in male.

**sextuplets** six offspring produced at same birth.

**sexual** pertaining to sexual act. *S. abuse* sexual contact or rape; may cause prolonged psychological trauma and difficulty making and maintaining relationships. *S. behaviour, risky* sexual activity increasing risk of sexually transmitted disease e.g. numerous sexual partners, unprotected sex, anal sex.

**sexual intercourse** coitus. *S. i. to initiate labour* may trigger contractions due to prostaglandin in semen, local cervical prostaglandin release, increased oxytocin from breast stimulation, orgasm, not supported by research but acceptable unless medical reasons to avoid intercourse in late pregnancy, e.g. grade 4 PLACENTA PRAEVIA.

**sexually transmitted infection** infection transmitted through sexual intercourse or intimate genitals, mouth, rectal contact; treat early in pregnancy to avoid preterm labour, stillbirth due to vertical transmission from mother to baby. Routine screening performed at booking to detect SYPHILIS, HEPATITIS B, HUMAN IMMUNODEFICIENCY VIRUS, CHLAMYDIA.

**shaken baby syndrome** *See* NON-ACCIDENTAL HEAD INJURY.

**shared care** antenatal care shared between midwife and obstetrician or general practitioner.

**sheath** tubular case. *See* CONDOM.

**Sheehan syndrome** hypopituitarism; uncommon complication of severe prolonged shock after PLACENTAL ABRUPTION or POSTPARTUM HAEMORRHAGE; anterior pituitary gland necrosis leads to AMENORRHOEA, genital atrophy, senility.

**shigellosis** intestinal disease due to *Shigella* bacteria, passed through direct contact with stool e.g. due to poor hand washing. Causes diarrhoea, often bloody, commonly occurs in children aged 2–4 years. May resolve spontaneously or require antibiotics.

**shingles** *See* HERPES ZOSTER.

**shock** collapse from acute peripheral circulatory failure after ante- or postpartum haemorrhage, uterine rupture or inversion, acid aspiration syndrome, pulmonary or amniotic fluid embolism, severe hypotension, septicaemia. Signs: hypotension, tachycardia, fluctuating central venous pressure; cold, clammy skin, pallor, air hunger. Treatment: urgent resuscitation: maintain airway; oxygen, intravenous fluids to combat dehydration; plasma substitutes. Foot of bed raised if baby is born; position mother on left side to prevent inferior vena cava pressure. Sedatives; avoid overheating. *Endotoxic s.* occurs in gram-negative infection, e.g. *Escherichia coli*, *Clostridium welchii*; widespread arteriole dilatation, reduced venous return; signs similar to hypovolaemic shock but rigors may also occur; treat infection urgently with appropriate antibiotics.

**shoulder dystocia** rare complication after birth of fetal head; shoulders fail to rotate, descend and deliver, usually due to large baby or contracted pelvic outlet. Mother adopts left lateral position or squatting to enlarge outlet, deliver baby. *See also* MCRO-BERTS MANOEUVRE, WOOD'S MANOEUVRE, SYMPHYSIOTOMY, ZAVANELLI MANOEUVRE, APPENDIX 4.

**shoulder presentation** may develop if fetus in oblique lie: one fetal shoulder driven into maternal pelvis, labour obstructed; may occur in second stage of twin labour, after birth of first baby. Examination: uterus appears broad, fundal height less than expected; vaginally, fetal ribs may be felt, arm may prolapse into vagina. Treatment: Caesarean section or internal podalic version with breech extraction if baby alive; possibly

destructive operation if baby dead, but risk of uterine rupture very high.

**'show'** blood-streaked vaginal discharge from shedding of part of cervical OPERCULUM, prior to labour onset.

**shunt** diversion, bypass; anastomosis between two natural channels, especially blood vessels; may occur naturally occurring or as surgical intervention.

**Siamese twins** colloquial term for CONJOINED TWINS.

**sibling** one of two or more children having same parents.

**sickle cell disease, anaemia** recessively inherited HAEMOGLOBINOPATHY; commonly occurs in Afro-Caribbean, sub-Saharan African people. Red blood cells become deoxygenated, form rigid, sickle-shaped structures unable to pass through small capillaries; causes chronic anaemia, increased infection risk; vaso-occlusive crisis with pain, ischaemic damage. *S. c. trait* individual carries one sickle haemoglobin (HbS) gene, one normal adult haemoglobin (HbA) gene (healthy carrier); if both genes abnormal disease is present. If both parents are carriers 25% chance of affected baby; neonates screened via NEWBORN BLOOD-SPOT SCREENING PROGRAMME.

**sign** objective evidence or manifestation of changes in physiology or pathology; signs of pregnancy include abdominal growth, palpation of fetal parts; subjective experience of nausea is a SYMPTOM.

**SILC cup** *See* VACUUM EXTRACTOR.

**silent (missed) miscarriage** loss of pregnancy with no pain or bleeding, may be due to blighted ovum, detected on ultrasound scan.

**Silverman–Anderson score** breathing performance scoring system for preterm babies; assesses five categories, graded 0, 1 or 2: chest retraction compared with abdominal retraction at inspiration; lower intercostal muscle retraction; xiphoid retraction; flaring of nares with inspiration; expiratory grunt. Score of 0 indicates adequate ventilation; 10 indicates severe respiratory distress.

**Simmond disease** complete PITUITARY GLAND, HYPOPITUITARISM; affects total endocrine system. *See also* SHEEHAN SYNDROME.

**Simpson forceps** obstetric forceps for low- or mid-cavity delivery if sagittal suture in anteroposterior diameter of pelvic outlet or cavity.

**Sims position** semi-prone with right knee and thigh drawn up, resting on bed in front of left leg.

**sinciput** brow of skull between coronal suture and orbital ridges.

**Singer's test** blood test to distinguish fetal from maternal blood.

**single-blind trial** clinical trial in which researchers, but not subjects, know who receives treatment being studied; eliminates subjective bias (placebo effect). *See also* DOUBLE-BLIND.

**sinoatrial node** specialized muscle fibres in wall of right atrium where cardiac contraction rhythm usually established; heart's pacemaker.

**sinus** cavity in cranial bones or dilated channels for venous blood, also found in cranium. *See* INTRACRANIAL MEMBRANES.

**skeleton** bony body structure, supports and protects organs, soft tissues.

**Skene duct** largest female urethral gland, opening within urethral orifice; homologous with prostate.

**skills drills** annual midwifery and medical updating; mock-up practical sessions enable practice of emergency procedures, manipulations, other techniques, e.g. breech delivery, shoulder dystocia.

**skin-to-skin contact** placing of baby on mother's chest or abdomen at birth; aids heat retention, prevents complications from heat loss.

**skin tags** benign excess pieces of normal skin; in neonates, usually tissue remaining from embryological development; easily removed; if located in front of ears, may indicate potential hearing problems.

**skull** bony structure of head, encloses, protects brain. Base and face bones united, incompressible. Vault: two frontal bones, two parietal bones, two temporal bones, one occiput; not fully ossified at birth. Membranous sutures between bones; three or more sutures together form FONTANELLE. *See also* FETAL SKULL, MOULDING.

**slapped cheek syndrome** *See* PARVOVIRUS B19.

**sleeping position, neonate** current research baby should be placed in cot supine (on back) to reduce sudden infant death risk.

**slough** dead tissue mass in, or separating from, adjacent tissue.

**small for gestational age baby** baby below 10th centile for population norms, or $\geq$ two standard deviations below mean, i.e. 50th centile for gestational age. Baby is proportionately small, weight, length, head circumference. *See* PRETERM for comparison, LOW-BIRTHWEIGHT BABY, INTRAUTERINE GROWTH RESTRICTION.

**smear** superficial vaginal or cervical cell specimen; microscopic examination to detect hormone levels or early malignant disease.

**smegma** secretion of sebaceous glands of clitoris and prepuce.

**smoking in pregnancy** carbon monoxide reduces oxygen transport, nicotine causes arteriole vasoconstriction, diminishes oxygen supply to fetus, causes poor fetal growth, development; predisposes baby to asthma, other allergenic and respiratory conditions.

**snuffles** noisy breathing, nasal catarrh in babies with congenital SYPHILIS.

**social services** local authority community services to meet certain individual needs; responsible for children, young persons, elderly, physically disabled, those with learning disabilities, socially inadequate, unsupported parents; some provision may be delegated to voluntary organizations; may also act as adoption agency.

**social worker** professional who assesses social need, provides necessary resources.

**sociology** scientific study of relationships and phenomena.

**sodium** positively charged ion element, determines osmolality of extracellular fluid. Normal serum level 140 mEq/L; low level reduces posterior pituitary antidiuretic hormone, decreases water absorption in renal collecting ducts. Increased sodium and osmolality stimulates hypothalamic thirst centre, prompting fluid intake. Fluid volume deficit, e.g. diarrhoea, vomiting, renal failure reduces serum sodium. Excess level (HYPERNATRAEMIA) occurs when insensible water loss is not replaced by drinking; also when artificial infant feeds made with excess milk powder concentration. Symbol Na. *S. bicarbonate* used to reverse metabolic ACIDAEMIA after tissue hypoxia. *S. citrate* added to donor blood to prevent clotting.

**sodium valproate** anticonvulsant, anti-epileptic drug, also to control manic episodes in bipolar disorder. In pregnancy, poses highest risk of birth defects of any commonly used anti-epilepsy drugs.

**soft chancre** non-syphilitic venereal ulcer caused by *Haemophilus ducreyi* (Ducrey bacillus).

**soft palate** fleshy structure at back of mouth; with hard palate, forms roof of mouth; in swallowing, soft palate drawn up against back of pharynx to prevent food, fluids entering nasal passage.

**solar plexus** See COELIAC PLEXUS.

**solute** substance dissolved in solution.

**solvent** liquid that dissolves, or has power to dissolve.

**somatic** relating to body as opposed to mind.

**somatosensory system** diverse sensory system of receptors and processing centres to produce sensory modalities e.g. touch, temperature, proprioception (body position), nociception (pain).

**somatotrophin** growth hormone. *Adj* somatotrophic.

**somite** one of paired segments along neural tube of vertebrate embryo, formed by transverse subdivision of thickened mesoderm next to midplane; develops into vertebral column and muscles.

**sore buttocks** perianal excoriation in neonate due to frequent loose stools, infrequent nappy changing, poor hygiene, incorrect laundering of napkins, diet (extra sugar), infection, e.g. candidiasis.

**souffle**  sounds heard on auscultation in antenatal ABDOMINAL EXAMINATION. *Placental s.* muffled, ocean-like sound of blood coursing through placenta, synchronous with fetal heart, usually in vicinity of placenta. *Uterine s.* soft blowing sound due to blood passing through uterine arteries, heard most distinctly in lower part of uterus synchronous with maternal pulse.

**soya-based infant formulae**  milk substitute for babies unable to tolerate breast or cows' milk constituents such as lactose; contains only vegetable fats.

**Spalding sign**  gross fetal cranial bone overlapping, seen on x-ray; indicates intrauterine death several days previously.

**spasm**  sudden involuntary muscle contraction.

**specific gravity**  weight of substance compared with that of equal volume of another substance, e.g. SG of water is 1000, urine 1010–1020, blood 1055.

**specificity**  measure of accuracy of screening test identifying people who do not have condition; proportion of people not affected by disorder who will be found to be negative (low risk) on screening test for that disorder; linked to true-positive rate.

**spectinomycin**  aminocyclitol antibiotic, given intramuscularly for gonorrhoea, especially to those allergic to penicillin.

**specular reflection**  reflecting from surface; in ULTRASOUND, interface giving a strong reflection or echo, e.g. fetal skull.

**speculum**  instrument to open up cavity, normally not visible, to enable inspection. *Pl* specula.

**Spencer Wells forceps**  type of artery forceps.

**sperm, spermatozoa**  male reproductive cells, essential part of semen, normally 50 million cells per mL; *Sing* spermatozoon. *S. count* determination of spermatozoa concentration in semen sample. *S. donation* seminal fluid provided by donor to enable woman with sterile partner, or in single-sex relationship, to conceive.

**spermatic**  pertaining to spermatozoa, semen. *S. cord* structure from abdominal inguinal ring to testis; comprises pampiniform plexus, nerves, ductus deferens, testicular artery, other vessels.

**spermatogenesis**  development of mature spermatozoa.

**spermicide**  agent that destroys spermatozoa; cream, foam or paste applied to vaginal or cervical caps for contraceptive purposes.

**sphenoid**  wedge-shaped. *S. bone* bone forming part of skull base.

**spherocyte**  small, globular, completely haemoglobinated erythrocyte without usual central pallor; characteristically found in hereditary spherocytosis but also in acquired haemolytic anaemia.

**spherocytosis**  presence of spherocytes in blood.

**sphincter**  ring-shaped muscle; contracts to close a natural orifice.

**sphingomyelin**  complex molecule of protein and fatty acid used to measure ratio of LECITHIN in amniotic fluid.

**sphygmomanometer**  instrument to measure blood pressure.

**spigot** small peg or bung to close opening of tube.

**spina bifida** congenital condition; arches at back of spine are incomplete; may be a bony gap (spina bifida occulta) or spinal cord may be exposed; presence of sac over spinal cord is MENINGOCELE; if nerves exposed, involved in sac, MENINGOMYELOCELE.

**spinal** relating to spine. *S. cord* See CORD. *S. anaesthesia* single-dose, fast-acting, short-lived, reliable, local anaesthetic for labour, injected directly into cerebrospinal fluid using lower doses of anaesthetic than epidural analgesia. Risks: dramatic hypotension, nausea, vomiting, post-spinal headache, infection.

**spine** 1. vertebral column. 2. sharp process of bone.

**spinnbarkeit** thread of mucus secreted by cervix uteri; used to determine ovulation, which usually coincides with time when the mucus can be drawn out on glass slide to its maximum length.

**spirochaetae** micro-organisms with flexible, spiral filament, e.g. *Treponema pallidum*, cause of SYPHILIS.

**spirograph** apparatus to measure and record respiratory movements.

**spirometer** instrument to measure air intake and expulsion.

**splanchnic** pertaining to viscera. *S. nerves* three nerves from thoracic sympathetic ganglia distributed to viscera.

**spleen** vascular lymphoid organ in left hypochondrium under border of stomach; assists in formation of erythrocytes in fetal life only; production of lymphocytes throughout life; control of red cell breakdown, excretion of resulting products; ANTIBODY formation.

**splenomegaly** enlargement of spleen.

**splint** wood or metal piece to support and immobilize injured limb.

**spondylolisthesis** forward displacement of fifth lumbar vertebra on first sacral segment; narrows true conjugate by formation of false promontory; rare cause of DYSTOCIA in labour. See PELVIS.

**spondylosis** vertebral joint ankylosis; degenerative spinal changes.

**spontaneous** occurring naturally with no external aid. *S. onset of labour* start of labour naturally, without intervention or induction. *S. version* change of fetal lie without obstetric interference.

**spore** reproductive element of certain plants, fungi, bacteria. Tetanus bacilli are spore-bearing; spores resistant to high temperatures, strong antiseptics, can remain dormant for years.

**Sprengel deformity** congenital high scapula. Rare skeletal abnormality; one scapula higher than the other; may be associated with other congenital abnormalities or syndromes.

**spurious labour** false labour. See LABOUR.

**squamous** scaly or plate-like. *S. bone* thin part of temporal skull bone articulating with parietal bone. *S. epithelium* thin-celled skin, e.g. lining of vagina.

**squatting position** with hips, knees flexed, buttocks resting on heels; may facilitate birth by enlarging pelvic outlet, gravity.

**standard deviation (σ)** measure of dispersion of random variable: square root of average squared deviation from mean. For data with normal distribution, about 68% fall within one standard deviation from mean and about 95% fall within two standard deviations.

**Staphylococcus** pyogenic bacteria genus; cause skin infections e.g. PEMPHIGUS NEONATORUM, MASTITIS, PUERPERAL SEPSIS. *S. aureus* or *S. pyogenes* cause severe infections, may be resistant to antibiotics. *S. albus* skin COMMENSAL, may cause urinary tract infection.

**stasis** stagnation, stoppage. *Intestinal s.* sluggish intestinal muscle movement, causes constipation. *S. of urine* physiological in pregnancy due to kinking of ureters by action of progesterone, may lead to urinary tract infection. *See* PYELONEPHRITIS.

**stat** *statim* (immediately).

**station** location of presenting fetal part in birth canal, according to number of centimetres above or below an imaginary plane at the level of ischial spines; calculated from $-5$ to $-1$ if above; 0 when at level of ischial spines and from $+1$ to $+5$ if below ischial spines.

**statistical** pertaining to statistics. *S. significance* research conclusion that results have little probability of occurring by chance; if below 1 in 20 or 0.05 probability level, something other than chance produced result.

**statistics** 1. numerical facts pertaining to particular subject or body of objects. 2. science dealing with collection, tabulation, analysis of numerical facts.

**status** condition, state. *S. epilepticus* rapid succession of epileptic spasms, no intervals of consciousness; brain damage may result.

**statutory body** organization controlling practice by law, e.g. NURSING AND MIDWIFERY COUNCIL controls midwifery practice.

**Statutory Maternity Pay** payment made by employer to enable working pregnant women to take time off work before and after the birth.

**Stein–Leventhal syndrome** female condition of AMENORRHOEA or OLIGOMENORRHOEA, hirsutism, infertility, enlarged cystic ovaries from which excessive male hormones may be produced.

**stem cells** cells in all multicellular organisms; divide through mitosis, differentiate into diverse specialized cell types; can self-renew. Embryonic stem cells are isolated from inner cell mass; adult stem cells found in various tissues.

**Stemetil** *See* PROCHLORPERAZINE.

**stenosis** narrowing or contraction of channel or opening. *Aortic s.* aortic heart valve narrowing due to scar tissue from inflammation. *Mitral s.* of mitral orifice from same cause. *Pyloric s.* generally due to congenital hypertrophy.

**stercobilin** bile pigment derivative formed by oxidation of stercobilinogen; brown/orange/red pigmentation colouring faeces, urine.

**sterile** 1. barren; incapable of producing young. 2. free from micro-organisms.

**sterilization** 1. process of making sterile by operation, e.g. ligation of fallopian tubes. 2. rendering sterile dressings, instruments, etc.

**sterilizer** apparatus in which objects can be sterilized.

**sternum** bone plate in middle anterior thoracic wall, articulates with clavicles and cartilages of first seven ribs; by 36 weeks' gestation uterine fundus normally reaches xiphoid process (xiphisternum) at lower end of sternum.

**steroids** carbon and hydrogen substances with particular chemical structure; include adrenocortical and sex hormones, cholesterol, bile acids.

**stethoscope** instrument to auscultate sounds in body, e.g. heart, lungs. *Binaural s.* branches into two flexible tubes, one for each ear of examiner. *Fetal or monaural s.* metal trumpet-shaped instrument placed on abdomen over area pertaining to fetal shoulders to hear fetal heart sounds; Pinard's stethoscope.

**stiletto** fine wire probe to keep lumen of hollow structures clear.

**stillbirth** baby born after 24 weeks' gestation who has not, at any time after being completely expelled from mother, breathed or shown any sign of life. *Adj* stillborn. Midwife must by law ensure notification, certification, registration of stillbirth.

**stillbirth certificate** certificate issued by registered medical practitioner (or midwife if no medical practitioner involved in care) who was present at birth of dead baby or who examined body; must legally be given to qualified informant (usually father or mother) so birth can be registered and certificate of burial or cremation issued; if there is inquest, coroner issues order for burial.

**stomach** dilated portion of alimentary canal between oesophagus and duodenum, just below diaphragm; wall consists of serous, muscular, submucous and mucous coats; gastric juice contains HYDROCHLORIC ACID and enzymes PEPSIN and RENNIN.

**stomatitis** inflammation of lining of mouth.

**stool** bowel motion or discharge; in newborn baby, first meconium, gradually changing to brown, then to soft bright yellow stool.

**strabismus** squint; deviation of eye.

**straight sinus** venous sinus in fetal skull at junction of falx cerebri and tentorium cerebelli; may rupture, causing intracranial haemorrhage if excessive or abnormal fetal head moulding during birth.

**'strawberry mark'** congenital capillary haemangioma.

***Streptococcus*** genus of haemolytic or non-haemolytic, aerobic or anaerobic bacteria. *Group beta-haemolytic s.* bacteria present in vagina in many women. Usually asymptomatic, but may have adverse neonatal effects at birth, may cause severe infection in first week of life, particularly if mother pyrexial, starts labour before term or has early membrane rupture. Mother is given preventative antibiotics in labour, or at membrane rupture, if earlier.

**streptokinase** enzyme produced by streptococci; catalyzes conversion of plasminogen to plasmin; when administered as thrombolytic careful use needed to avoid haemorrhage; may also trigger severe antigenic reactions on re-administration.

**streptomycin** aminoglycoside antibiotic administered intramuscularly, may cause otitis, including in fetus if used in pregnancy.

**stress** undue strain of mind or body, may impair mental or physical function. In acute stress adrenaline increases heart rate, blood pressure, blood glucose, dilates blood vessels in muscles for immediate energy ('fight or flight'); in chronic stress, continued hormone output, apparently increasing body's resistance. Prolonged stress causes coronary artery disease, high blood pressure, cancer. **S. incontinence** involuntary leakage of urine; due to hormonal laxity of pelvic floor muscles, internal urethral sphincter relaxation, reduced bladder capacity, overstretched pelvic floor muscles. Treatment: pelvic floor exercises; specialist medical treatment, physiotherapy.

**striae gravidarum** stretch marks, skin marks due to stretching, often on abdomen, breasts, thighs in pregnancy, first as reddish marks, later fading to silvery white colour (permanent).

**stridor** harsh vibrating respiratory noise due to laryngeal obstruction.

**stroke volume** blood volume pumped with each beat from one heart ventricle; increases 10% in first half of pregnancy, peaks at 20 weeks' gestation, maintained until term; facilitates second-trimester increase in cardiac output in conjunction with plasma volume expansion.

**Sturge–Weber syndrome** encephalotrigeminal angiomatosis, rare congenital, not hereditary, neurological and skin disorder; associated with PORT-WINE STAIN, glaucoma, epilepsy, mental retardation; proliferation of cerebral arteries causing multiple angiomas. Treatment is symptomatic according to individual presentation.

**sub-** prefix meaning 'under' or 'below'; denotes factors below normal limit. **S.-acute** moderately acute; disease progresses moderately rapidly but does not become acute. **S.-cutaneous** beneath skin, e.g. subcutaneous injection.

**subaponeurotic haemorrhage** rare neonatal haemorrhage under scalp, due to excess traction on local veins, associated with vacuum-assisted birth, primigravida, severe dystocia, malposition, preterm or precipitate birth, macrosomia, coagulopathy, male infant.

**subarachnoid** below arachnoid. **S. space** space between arachnoid and pia mater in which cerebrospinal fluid circulates.

**subclavian** beneath clavicle. **S. artery** main artery to arm.

**subdermal implants** contraceptive implants containing progestogen capsules, inserted under local anaesthetic in inner upper arm; hormone released into circulation changes cervical mucus to prevent spermatozoa penetration, disturbs endometrial maturation, suppresses ovulation.

**subdural** under dura mater. **S. haemorrhage** intracranial bleeding under dura mater; seen in neonate after traumatic birth; subdural tap may be used to withdraw blood to relieve pressure.

**subfertility** less-than-normal fertility.

**subinvolution** incomplete, delayed return of uterus to non-pregnant size in puerperium, due to retained conception products, infection.

**subluxation** partial dislocation.

**submentobregmatic diameter** on fetal skull, measured from point where chin joins neck to highest point on vertex, 9.5 cm.

**suboccipital region** area of fetal skull below occipital protuberance.

**subtotal hysterectomy** See HYSTERECTOMY.

**substance misuse** abnormal dependence on alcohol, nicotine, recreational addictive drugs, other substances, e.g. glue.

**succenturiate** additional or accessory. **S. lobe** See PLACENTA.

**sucking reflex** natural reaction of term baby to suck when teat or finger is inserted in mouth, often immature in preterm babies.

**sudden infant death syndrome (SIDS)** sudden unexpected death of apparently healthy asymptomatic infant or one with only a slight cold, typically between 3 weeks and 5 months of age, unexplained by post-mortem examination; more common in preterm babies, less common in breastfed babies. Predisposing factors: prone position, tobacco smoke, overheating.

**sugar** carbohydrates: monosaccharides, e.g. glucose, fructose, galactose; disaccharides, e.g. sucrose, lactose.

**sulcus** groove, furrow, as between cotyledons of placenta. *Pl* sulcii.

**sulfonylureas** antidiabetic drugs; increase insulin release from pancreas; potentially teratogenic; avoid in pregnancy.

**sulphonamides** group of chemotherapeutic drugs used orally to treat bacterial infections, e.g. streptococci, gonococci, *Escherichia coli* and other bacteria.

**super-** prefix, 'over' or 'above'. *S.-fecundation* fertilization of two ova from same ovulation by spermatozoa from two different individuals. *S.-fetation* fertilization of an ovum occurring in pregnancy.

**superior** 1. higher than, above. 2. better than. 3. one in charge of others. *S. longitudinal sinus* upper venous sinus between layers of falx cerebri; separates two hemispheres of brain.

**supervisor of midwives** experienced midwife, appointed by LOCAL SUPERVISING AUTHORITY (LSA) for supervision of midwives in local area. Receives and records notifications of intention to practise from all midwives working in area; monitors standards of midwifery practice, provides professional, clinical, educational support and guidance; issues supply orders for and witnesses destruction of controlled drugs, ensures midwives competent to administer medicines; investigates allegations of malpractice, negligence or misconduct; where appropriate, refers midwives to Nursing and Midwifery Council, notifies LSA of midwives liable to be source of infection.

**supination** turning upwards. *S. of hand* palm upward cf. PRONATION.

**supine** lying on back. *S. hypotensive syndrome* pressure of gravid uterus on inferior vena cava reduces venous return, cardiac output, blood pressure, causes faintness, adversely affects fetal oxygenation; may occur in late pregnancy if woman lies supine, aggravated by EPIDURAL ANALGESIA. Treatment: sit woman upright.

**supplementary** pertaining to supplement, addition to compensate deficiency. *S. feed* feed given to baby instead of or in addition to breastfeed. cf. COMPLEMENTARY. *S. prescribers* when doctor has made initial assessment, midwives may review and change medication if appropriate to mother's clinical care plan.

**supply order** procedure method by which community midwives obtain drugs for home births. If mother is transferred to hospital, drugs obtained under supply order procedure may not be used. Women anticipating home birth may be advised to request doctor's prescription for analgesics, in which case, drugs belong to mother.

**suppository** solid cone-shaped medicated compound introduced into rectum, either to cause bowel action (e.g. glycerine, bisacodyl) or to administer drugs, particularly analgesics.

**suppression** complete cessation of secretion. Mother unable or unwilling to breastfeed, lactation is suppressed naturally, i.e. by not removing milk, or with drugs e.g. bromocriptine.

**suppuration** formation or discharge of pus.

**supra-** prefix meaning 'above'. **S.-pubic** above pubic bones.

**suprarenal** above kidney. **S. glands** adrenal glands, two small triangular endocrine glands, one above each kidney, which secrete ADRENALINE and NORADRENALINE from medulla, hormones from cortex.

**surfactant** LECITHIN in lungs; helps alveoli to remain open; deficient in RESPIRATORY DISTRESS SYNDROME, which may be predicted by estimating LECITHIN–SPHINGOMYELIN RATIO before birth.

**surrogate** substitute. **S. mother** woman who bears baby for another with intention that child be handed over after birth.

**survey** systematic collection of information, not normally forming part of scientific epidemiological study.

**suture** 1. stitch or series of stitches to close wound. 2. fibrous joint in which opposed bony surfaces closely united by thin connective tissue, permitting movement; only in neonate. See FETAL SKULL.

**Swan Ganz catheter** soft, flow-directed catheter with balloon at tip for measuring pulmonary arterial pressures.

**symmetrical cortical necrosis** rare complication of severe concealed PLACENTAL ABRUPTION; destruction of renal cortex due to internal spasm of renal cortical arteries. Impaired renal function, renal failure, death may follow. See also TUBULAR NECROSIS.

**symmetrical growth restriction** fetal growth restriction, less common (25%–30%) than ASYMMETRICAL GROWTH RESTRICTION, indicates slow growth from early stage due to chromosomal abnormalities, maternal smoking or alcohol abuse, severe anaemia or intrauterine infection e.g. cytomegalovirus, rubella; head in proportion to body; risk of neurological compromise.

**sympathetic** exhibiting sympathy.

**sympathetic nervous system** part of autonomic system; when stimulated, prepares body for emergency or flight; pulse rate increases, blood pressure rises, pupils dilate, peristalsis slows.

**symphysiotomy** symphysis pubis division to facilitate birth in cases of disproportion; used when Caesarean section not possible, to avoid repeated Caesarean section and in regions where midwifery services are inadequate, to avoid leaving woman with uterine scar.

**symphysis pubis** pelvic joint; bone surfaces joined by fibrocartilage, movement very slight. **S. fundal height** measurement (in centimetres) taken between upper symphysis pubis border and uterine fundus; sequential measurements, plotted on growth chart, show changes in uterine or fetal growth rates. **S. pubis discomfort** See PELVIC GIRDLE PAIN.

**symptom** evidence of disease or condition observed by woman herself, e.g. AMENORRHOEA, certain breast changes are symptoms of pregnancy. *See also* SIGN.

**symptothermal** contraceptive method involving temperature charting, observing cervical mucus changes, calendar calculation and optional cervical palpation to identify time when woman is most fertile.

**syn-** prefix meaning 'together'.

**synapse** junction between processes of two neurons or between neuron and effector organ; neural impulses transmitted by chemical means, causing release of neurotransmitter, e.g. acetylcholine, noradrenaline from presynaptic membrane of axon terminal.

**synclitism** state when fetal head enters pelvic brim with both parietal eminences at same level. *See* ASYNCLITISM.

**syncope** fainting; loss of consciousness due to reduced cerebral blood flow.

**syncytium, syncytiotrophoblast** outer TROPHOBLAST layer; persists through pregnancy, covers CHORIONIC VILLI, unlike CYTOTROPHOBLAST cells.

**syndactyly** webbed fingers or toes.

**syndrome** group of symptoms and signs typical of distinctive disease.

**synthesis** joining together of substances, naturally or artificially.

**Syntocinon** *See* OXYTOCIN.

**Syntometrine** oxytocic drug; 0.5 mg ergometrine and 5 units Syntocinon in 1 mL, administered intramuscularly to manage third-stage labour actively; causes rapid sustained uterine contraction and separation of placenta from uterine wall.

**syphilis** SEXUALLY TRANSMITTED INFECTION due to spirochaete *Treponema pallidum*. Primary syphilis: small painless ulcer (chancre), usually on vulva, easily missed. Secondary syphilis: occurs 3–12 weeks later: pyrexia, malaise, rash, lymphadenopathy. Tertiary syphilis: can last several years; gummatous tumours develop; neurological and cardiac involvement. Vertically transmitted from mother to fetus from 9 weeks' gestation; causes miscarriage, stillbirth, neonatal death, long-term morbidity. All pregnant women offered Venereal Disease Research Laboratory and rapid plasma reagin tests; if results positive, diagnosis confirmed by syphilis-specific FLUORESCENT TREPONEMAL ANTIBODY-ABSORBED TEST (FTA-ABS). Treatment: penicillin.

**syringocele** cavity containing herniation of spinal cord through bony defect in spina bifida.

**syringomyelocele** hernial protrusion of spinal cord through bony defect in spina bifida, mass containing cavity connected with central canal of spinal cord.

**Système International d'Unités** international measurement system; weight in grams; length in metres; fluid in litres; all drugs must be prescribed and dispensed in SI units. *See also* INDEX NOTATION.

**systemic** pertaining to, affecting whole body. *S. lupus erythematosus* autoimmune connective tissue disease, commonly presents as arthritis, affects skin, kidneys, nervous system. Diagnosis made on clinical features, presence of autoantibodies, which increase pregnancy complications, fetal loss, e.g. ANTIPHOSPHOLIPID ANTIBODIES may cause abnormal clotting, thrombolysis.

**systematic review** in-depth literature review, collating and analysing critically a range of research papers on a given subject.

**systole** contraction of heart. *cf.* DIAS-
TOLE. *Ventricular s.* contraction of
ventricles, so blood pumped into
aorta, pulmonary arteries.

**systolic** pertaining to systole. *S. murmur* abnormal sound produced dur-
ing systole in heart affections. *S.
pressure See* BLOOD PRESSURE. *S. sound*
dull sound of heart in ventricular systole, caused by its movement against
chest wall.

**Mass**

| | |
|---|---|
| 1 kilogram (kg) | =1000 grams (g) |
| 1 gram (g) | =1000 milligrams (mg) |
| 1 milligram (mg) | =1000 micrograms (µg) |
| 1 microgram (µg) | =1000 nanograms (ng) |
| 1 nanogram (ng) | =1000 picograms |

**Measurements Smaller than a Unit**

| PREFIX | SYMBOL | MEANING | EXAMPLE |
|---|---|---|---|
| Deci- | d | One-tenth | dL = one-tenth of a litre |
| Centi- | c | One-hundredth | cm = one-hundredth of a metre |
| Milli- | m | One-thousandth | mL = one-thousandth of a litre |
| Micro- | µ | One-millionth | µg = one-millionth of a gram |

**Multiples of Units**

| PREFIX | SYMBOL | MEANING | EXAMPLE |
|---|---|---|---|
| Deca- | da | 10 | daL = 10 litres |
| Hector- | h | 100 | hg = 100 grams |
| Kilo- | k | 1000 | kg = 1000 grams |
| Mega- | M | 1 million | MJ = 1 million joules |

**T cell** lymphocyte derived from thymus, responsible for cell-mediated immunity.

**TAB** vaccine against typhoid, paratyphoid A and B. *TABT* also protects against tetanus.

**tachycardia** abnormally rapid heart and pulse rate.

**tachypnoea** abnormally rapid respiration.

**tactile** pertaining to touch.

**taking up of cervix** effacement of cervical canal early in labour.

**talipes** clubfoot; congenital deformity, usually found on first examination; foot develops at abnormal angle to leg. Oligohydramnios may cause fetus to become cramped *in utero*, leading to positional talipes, either equinovarus or calcaneovalgus combination. Treatment: immediate physiotherapy if mild; stretching, massage, splinting or surgery if severe.

**talipomanus** clubhand.

**talus** ankle bone; highest tarsal bone.

**tamoxifen** non-steroidal oral anti-oestrogen palliative drug for post-menopausal women with breast cancer; also used to stimulate ovulation in subfertility.

**tarsus** 1. bone articulation between foot and leg: talus, calcaneus, navicular, medial, intermediate and lateral cuneiform, cuboid; ankle or instep. 2. cartilaginous plate forming framework of either (upper or lower) eyelid.

**taurine** crystallized acid from bile; also in lung and muscle tissue; present in high quantities in breast milk; needed for bile acid conjugation in first week function, and for nervous system development.

**Taussig–Bing syndrome** transposition of great vessels of heart with ventricular septal defect straddled by large pulmonary artery.

**taxonomy** orderly classification of organisms into appropriate categories (taxa) with application of suitable and correct names.

**Tay–Sachs disease** inherited autosomal-recessive condition; primarily affects Ashkenazi Jews; progressive brain and macular degeneration, dementia, blindness, death. At 14 weeks' gestation tests reveal absence of enzyme hexosaminidase A; indicates conclusive diagnosis. Carriers have lower level of enzyme in blood.

**tea tree oil** highly anti-infective, antibacterial, antifungal, antiviral, antimicrobial aromatherapy essential oil; midwives must be adequately trained to use or advise on aromatherapy.

**team midwifery** management system in which midwives are divided into teams to care for identified groups of women; aims to improve communication and continuity of care. *See also* CASELOAD MIDWIFERY.

**tears** 1. liquid product from lacrimal ducts, which cleanse eyes 2. *See* PERINEAL LACERATION, TENTORIAL TEARS.

http://dx.doi.org/10.1016/B978-0-7020-6906-2.00020-6

**teat** 1. breast nipple. 2. manufactured nipple on infant feeding bottles.

**teething** eruption of teeth through gums; first tooth usually erupts between 6 and 9 months. *See also* DENTITION.

**telemetry** remote fetal heart and uterine contraction recording, enabling ambulation in labour.

**temazepam** hypnotic drug; avoid in first trimester.

**temperature** degree of heat measured by thermometer, taken via mouth, rectum, axilla, groin or via mechanical apparatus. *Normal body t.* 36–37°C (97–98.4°F); higher during luteal phase of menstrual cycle. *See* PYREXIA *and* FEVER.

**temporal** pertaining to side of head. *T. bone* irregular skull bone with squamous part forming part of vault.

**tendon** cord, band of strong white fibrous tissue connecting muscle to bone; muscle contracts it pulls tendon, which moves bone.

**TENS** *See* TRANSCUTANEOUS ELECTRICAL NERVE STIMULATION.

**tension** 1. act of stretching. 2. pressure or concentration of gas; see $PO_2$. *Premenstrual t.* symptoms due to hormonal changes in 5–7 days before menstruation, e.g. abdominal distension, headaches, emotional lability, poor coordination, fluid retention.

**tentorial tear** laceration of TENTORIUM CEREBELLI from excess moulding in labour or PRECIPITATE LABOUR, causes bleeding from GREAT VEIN OF GALEN.

**tentorium cerebelli** septum of dura mater, separating cerebral hemispheres from cerebellum. *See* INTRACRANIAL MEMBRANES.

**teras** malformed fetus or infant. *Adj* teratic.

**teratogen** agent causing physical defects in developing embryo. *Adj* teratogenic.

**teratogenicity** ability to cause defects in developing embryo/fetus; including drugs: anticonvulsants, anticoagulants, heroin, alcohol, nicotine; environmental factors: radiation, chemicals: pesticides; infective agents: rubella, cytomegalovirus; maternal disease: diabetes; distinct from mutagenicity, which causes genetic mutations.

**teratoma** congenital tumour containing teeth, hair and cells of other tissues not normally found in place where situated.

**terbutaline** bronchodilatory drug used to treat asthma.

**term** end of pregnancy, any time after 37th week of pregnancy.

**termination of pregnancy (TOP)** abortion induced, legally or illegally.

**tertiary** third. *T. syphilis See* SYPHILIS.

**testicles, testes** two glands in scrotum; produce spermatozoa and male sex hormones. *Undescended t.* testicle remains in pelvis or inguinal canal.

**testosterone** hormone produced by testes; stimulates development of male characteristics.

**tetanus** notifiable disease due to *Clostridium tetani*, anaerobe found in cultivated soil, manure; tetanus antitoxin confers passive immunity if exposed to infection. *Adj* tetanic.

**tetany** condition of calcium deficiency, alkalaemia or impaired parathyroid gland function; tonic contraction of hand and feet muscles, hypersensitivity of other muscles; artificially fed neonates with low serum calcium may develop tetany. *See also* HYPOCALCAEMIA.

**tetracycline** antibiotic effective against many micro-organisms; if prescribed in second or third trimester, may cause yellow discoloration and subsequent premature degeneration of baby's bones and first teeth.

**tetradactyly** four digits on hand or foot.

**tetralogy** series of four. *Fallot t.* four congenital heart defects: pulmonary stenosis; ventricular septal defect; right ventricular hypertrophy; dextroposition of aorta; surgery required.

**thalamus** part of brain at base of cerebrum; most sensory impulses pass from body to thalamus, transmitted to cortex and forebrain.

**thalassaemia** recessive inherited HAEMOGLOBINOPATHY prevents normal haemoglobin production. Trait: individual with one thalassaemia gene, one normal adult haemoglobin gene (healthy carrier, no symptoms). If both genes are abnormal, disease is present. *Alpha t.* common in Chinese, Southeast Asian, Mediterranean people; incompatible with life, causes BARTS HYDROPS. *Beta t.* occurs in Mediterranean and some Asian groups; carrier status suspected if erythrocytes small, anaemia present; *beta t. major* not apparent at birth but as fetal haemoglobin declines baby becomes anaemic. Treatment: blood transfusions 4–6 weekly for life, with risk of transfusion reactions, infection, iron overload; iron chelation therapy from age 2 to prevent toxic iron accumulation. Pregnant women, and partners, if appropriate, screened for carrier status; if both are carriers, 25% chance of having affected baby.

**thalidomide** sedative, hypnotic, immunomodulatory drug for multiple myeloma and leprosy; causes serious fetal deformities if taken in pregnancy, e.g. absence or foreshortening of one or more limbs.

**theca externa, interna** two layers of ovarian follicle.

**theophylline** respiratory stimulant, no known long-term side effects; reduces incidence of apnoeic attacks in small preterm babies.

**therapeutic abortion** legally induced termination of pregnancy before 24 weeks' gestation if fetus grossly malformed or if mother's physical or mental health is jeopardized if pregnancy continues. *See* ABORTION.

**thermogenesis** production of body heat.

**thermometer** instrument for measuring temperature.

**thermoneutral environment** range of environmental temperature over which heat production, oxygen consumption, nutritional requirements for growth are minimal, provided body temperature is normal.

**thermoregulation** balance between heat production and heat loss.

**thiamine** vitamin $B_1$; found in food, plasma, cerebrospinal fluid; deficiency causes neurological symptoms, cardiovascular dysfunction, oedema, reduced intestinal motility.

**thiazole** benzothiadiazine sulphonamide derivatives, e.g. chlorothiazide; diuretic; inhibits reabsorption of sodium in proximal renal tubule and stimulates chloride excretion.

**thiopental** sodium pentothal, intravenous barbiturate to induce general anaesthesia; not recommended in pregnancy.

**third-degree perineal laceration** complete tear of whole perineal body

225

extending through anal sphincter into rectum.

**third stage of labour** from birth of baby to separation and complete expulsion of placenta and membranes, may be managed physiologically (duration 5 minutes to 2 hours, average 20–30 minutes) or actively, with oxytocic drug to expedite placental separation and control haemorrhage (duration 5–10 minutes). Placenta and membranes may be delivered actively with CONTROLLED CORD TRACTION.

**thoracic** relating to thorax. *T. duct* large lymphatic vessel situated in thorax along spine, opening into left subclavian vein.

**thorax** chest; cavity containing heart, lungs, bronchi, oesophagus, bounded by diaphragm below, sternum in front and dorsal vertebrae behind; enclosed by ribs as protective framework.

**threatened            miscarriage** *See* MISCARRIAGE.

**thrill** tremor or vibration elicited by tapping wall of cavity containing fluid, e.g. pregnant uterus with POLYHYDRAMNIOS.

**thrombo-** pertaining to blood clot.

**thrombectomy** surgical removal of clot from blood vessel.

**thrombin** substance formed in blood by action of thromboplastin on PROTHROMBIN in presence of calcium; thrombin then converts plasma protein fibrinogen into fibrin, forming clot.

**thrombocyte** blood platelet.

**thrombocythaemia** increase in circulating blood platelets.

**thrombocytopenia** uncommon deficiency of PLATELETS, with purpuric haemorrhages; usually resolves

spontaneously; occurs in neonates of mothers with purpura and congenital RUBELLA.

**thromboembolism** obstruction of blood vessel with thrombotic material carried in blood from site of origin to plug another vessel; major cause of maternal death. *Adj* thromboembolic.

**thromboembolitic D stockings** compression stockings that reduce risk of thromboembolic disorders; used prior to, during, after Caesarean section to reduce deep vein thrombosis.

**thrombokinase** activated clotting factor X.

**thrombolysis** dissolution of thrombus.

**thrombophilia screen** tests to identify familial or acquired disorders that increase thrombosis risk, e.g. antithrombin, protein C, protein S, activated protein C resistance, factor V Leiden, factor II variant lupus type inhibitor. Women with personal or family history of venous thromboembolism tested to identify those at increased risk of INTRA UTERINE GROWTH RESTRICTION, PRE-ECLAMPSIA, fetal loss.

**thrombophlebitis** inflammation of vein with clot formation, usually adherent to vein wall; rarely separates; minimal danger of EMBOLISM. *Femoral t.* may occur postnatally after pelvic infection. *cf.* PHLEBOTHROMBOSIS.

**thromboplastin** substance liberated by injured tissue and platelets. *See* THROMBIN *and* PROTHROMBIN.

**thrombosis** formation of THROMBUS. *Coronary t.* clot in coronary vessel; heart muscle deprived of blood according to size of blockage; if thrombus detaches from wall and carried along in bloodstream, may lead to EMBOLISM.

**thrombus**  stationary blood clot produced by coagulation of blood, usually in vein, often due to PHLEBITIS.

**thrush**  *Candida albicans* infection; may occur in vagina in pregnancy due to altered pH suppressing normal vaginal flora; babies may acquire it orally when passing through vulva, or develop napkin rash with small, white-headed pustules; spreads quickly in bottle-fed babies. Treatment: antibiotics, fungicidal drugs.

**thymine**  principal component of DNA, paired with adenine.

**thymus**  gland between lungs, above heart; grows until puberty, then involutes; cortex contains small T lymphocytes, contributing to immunological reactions.

**thyroid-binding globulin**  blood protein, combines with thyroxine. *TBG test* diagnostic test to determine cause of abnormal thyroid hormones.

**thyroid function test**  screening test for thyroid disorder; measures thyroid-stimulating hormone; if high, indicates hypothyroidism; if low, hyperthyroidism, although levels may be low in first trimester.

**thyroid gland**  endocrine gland in neck in front of trachea; secretes thyroxine and triiodothyronine, which control metabolism; overactivity causes thyrotoxicosis, underactivity causes myxoedema; babies with inadequate thyroid function suffer from cretinism.

**thyroiditis**  inflammation of thyroid gland, may occur postpartum involving hyperthyroidism and/or hypothyroidism.

**thyroid-stimulating hormone**  thyrotropin; secreted from anterior pituitary; stimulates thyroid gland to produce and release thyroid hormones; HUMAN CHORIONIC GONADOTROPHIN may trigger thyroid activity, although serum TSH is reduced; transient HYPOTHYROIDISM may develop; may affect severity of MORNING SICKNESS, leading to HYPEREMESIS GRAVIDARUM.

**thyroid storm**  rare, serious emergency due to uncontrolled or poorly managed HYPERTHYROIDISM; spontaneous or due to infection, surgery or stress of labour; hyperthermia, dehydration, tachycardia, acute respiratory distress, cardiovascular collapse. Treatment: oxygen administration, antipyretics, cooling blanket, hydration, antibiotics, medication to reduce thyroid hormone effects. High risk of maternal heart failure, neonatal hyperthyroidism, stillbirth.

**thyrotoxicosis**  hyperthyroidism; excessive activity of thyroid.

**thyrotrophin**  anterior pituitary gland hormone that stimulates thyroid gland; thyroid-stimulating hormone.

**thyroxine**  thyroid gland hormone; contains iodine, amino acid TYROSINE derivative; affects growth and development; metabolism of carbohydrates, fats, proteins, electrolytes, water; vitamin requirements; reproduction; resistance to infection; prescribed for HYPOTHYROIDISM and GOITRE.

**tidal volume**  amount of gas passing into and out of lungs in each respiratory cycle.

**tinidazole**  anti-parasitic drug used to treat protozoan, amoebic, parasitic infections.

**tissue**  cells or fibres uniting to perform particular function in body. *Connective t.* tissue that connects, e.g. adipose (fatty), areolar (elastic supporting), bone, blood, cartilage. *Brown adipose t., brown fat t.* thermogenic adipose tissue with dark pigment, arises in embryonic life between shoulder blades, behind sternum, in neck, around kidneys and suprarenal glands; utilized by neonate to produce heat. *Epithelial t.* covers all inner and outer body surfaces, e.g. ciliated, some columnar, some squamous. *Erectile t.* spongy tissue, expands, becomes hard when filled with blood. *Granulation t.* formed in repair of wounds and soft tissue, consists of connective tissue cells and ingrowing young capillaries; ultimately forms fibrous tissue; scar. *Muscular t.* skeletal, voluntary striated, plain, involuntary unstriated and striated, involuntary cardiac tissue. *Nervous t.* nerve cells and their processes. *Subcutaneous t.* loose connective layer under skin.

**tissue fluid** fluid in tissue spaces between cells; extracellular fluid; excess constitutes OEDEMA.

**titre** amount of substance, e.g. antibody, in blood, estimated by finding amount needed to correspond with known amount of another substance.

**toco-, toko-** childbirth, labour.

**tocograph** instrument to measure pattern and pressure of uterine contraction, usually in conjunction with fetal heart monitoring.

**tocolytics** drugs to arrest threatened preterm labour, including beta sympathomimetics: ritodrine hydrochloride salbutamol; non-steroidal anti-inflammatories: indomethacin; calcium channel blockers: nifedipine; magnesium sulphate; OXYTOCIN ANTAGONISTS.

**tocopherol** vitamin E, present in wheat germ, green leaves, milk.

**tocophobia** extreme fear of childbirth, may be relieved by providing information, antenatal education, relaxation strategies, e.g. HYPNOTHERAPY.

**tomography** method of producing images of single tissue planes. *Computed t.* radiological imaging modality using computer processing of x-ray photons detected after passing through patient; image represents tissue densities within 'slice', 1–10 mm thick, through patient's body; computed axial tomography. *Ultrasonic t.* ultrasonographic visualization of cross-section of predetermined plane of body.

**tone** normal degree of tension, e.g. muscle tone.

**tongue tie** shortening of frenulum anchoring tongue to floor of mouth; does not usually interfere with feeding. Treatment: FRENULOTOMY.

**tonic uterine contraction** sustained abnormal uterine contraction; generalized may lead to fetal anoxia; or localized CONSTRICTION RING, most commonly around fetal neck, adversely affecting labour progress; deep anaesthesia may be required to relax muscles.

**tonic seizures** sudden attack, spasm, convulsion.

**tonus** muscle tone.

**topical** in medicine, direct application to body or skin e.g. topical drugs.

**topiramate** anticonvulsant (anti-epileptic) drug; not recommended in pregnancy as may cause cleft lip and/or palate in fetus.

**'topping up' epidural anaesthesia** repeat administration of bupivacaine for epidural anaesthesia after cannula insertion and administration of first dose by anaesthetist; midwives permitted by Nursing and Midwifery Council to perform this subject to training, assessment, cross-checking with colleague, written instructions from anaesthetist. Maternal blood pressure must be recorded frequently to identify hypotension.

**TORCH** acronym for intrauterine or neonatal infection due to TOXOPLASMOSIS, RUBELLA, CYTOMEGALOVIRUS, HERPES SIMPLEX or other agents.

**torsion** twisting; ovarian cyst complication: pedicle produces venous congestion and gangrene.

**torticollis** contraction of cervical muscles, causes neck torsion; may be congenital, psychosomatic or due to accessory nerve pressure, inflammation or muscle spasm.

**total parenteral nutrition** nutrition for neonate unable to feed, to ensure all nutritional requirements are met; normally administered through central line, either long line or umbilical catheter; prolonged use may be needed for very immature babies, infants with gastroschisis or NECROTIZING ENTEROCOLITIS, but long-term use may cause conjugated hyperbilirubinaemia or cholestasis.

**tourniquet** instrument applied to limb to arrest bleeding or to make vein more prominent for venepuncture.

**toxic** poisonous, relating to toxin. *T. shock* acute infection, hyperpyrexia, sunburn-like rash, vomiting, diarrhoea, shock; caused by toxin-producing strain of *Staphylococcus aureus* bacterium, may occur if vaginal tampon retained in vagina for prolonged period.

**toxin** poison, usually bacterial; does not produce symptoms until after incubation period, when microbes multiply and overwhelm leucocytes and other antibodies; cause antitoxins to form, establishing immunity to certain diseases.

**toxoid** toxin rendered non-toxic but retains its protective qualities, e.g. APT for diphtheria immunization.

**toxoplasmosis** infection with *Toxoplasma gondii*, parasitic protozoa; causes glandular fever-like symptoms in mother; if fetus infected, risk of hydrocephalus, intracranial calcification, splenomegaly, anaemia, jaundice, retinal damage.

**trachea** windpipe; cartilaginous tube lined with ciliated epithelium, extending from lower part of larynx to bronchi.

**trace elements** chemical elements required in minute quantities to maintain proper functioning.

**tracheo-oesophageal fistula** congenital defect, opening between trachea and lower oesophagus. *See also* OESOPHAGEAL ATRESIA.

**tracheostomy** emergency creation of opening into trachea through neck; insertion of indwelling tube to restore airway in acute obstruction or improve airway and aspirate secretions.

**traction response** neonatal neurological test; when pulled upright by wrists to sitting position, baby's head will initially lag, then correct itself momentarily before falling forward onto chest.

**traditional birth attendant** unqualified birth supporter, usually women in developing countries where midwifery/obstetric help may be unavailable; also, indigenous midwife, *hilot, dunken, dai*.

**trait** characteristic behaviour pattern. *Sickle cell t.* tendency for red blood cells to sickle, without accompanying anaemia, in someone who is HETEROZY-GOUS for the condition.

**tranexamic acid**  synthetic drug that inhibits fibrin breakdown in blood clots, used to treat haemorrhage.

**tranquillizers**  anti-anxiety drugs e.g. chlorpromazine, promethazine.

**transcervical ligaments**  *See* CARDINAL LIGAMENTS.

**transcription**  process by which information in a strand of deoxyribonucleic acid is copied into a new molecule of messenger ribonucleic acid.

**transcutaneous blood gas monitor**  measures neonatal $PO_2$, $PCO_2$ via skin probe; accuracy depends on peripheral circulation; usually used in conjunction with intermittent arterial sampling.

**transcutaneous electrical nerve stimulation**  self-administered analgesia suitable for labour; mild electrical stimulation applied via skin transducers over lumbo-sacral area; intercepts nerve pathways for vagina, cervix, uterus; aids release of endorphins in cerebrospinal fluid, reduces pain perception as in GATE CONTROL THEORY. Risks: affects cardiotocograph monitoring, skin allergy from electrodes; preterm labour if used before term; contraindicated in women with pacemaker. Appropriately-trained midwives may use it in labour.

**transducer**  device that transforms one form of energy into another, e.g. ULTRASOUND; TENS.

**transferase**  enzyme; catalyzes transfer of chemical group, not existing in free state during transfer, from one molecule to another.

**transferrin**  serum globulin that binds and transports iron.

**Position of electrodes for transcutaneous electrical nerve stimulation**

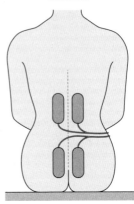

**transfusion**  direct administration into bloodstream of blood or other solutions to increase blood volume, stabilize body chemistry, give drugs. *Exchange t.* repeated small withdrawals and replacement of blood to alter constituents but not blood volume, e.g. in haemolytic disease of newborn to decrease bilirubin. *Transplacental t.* flow of blood from fetus to mother via placenta.

**transient tachypnoea of newborn**  common neonatal condition after Caesarean birth; respirations up to 120 per minute for up to 5 days; cyanosis, with mostly normal blood gases; little rib recession or expiratory grunt. Treatment: oxygen therapy; eliminate other causes of respiratory distress.

**transillumination** passage of strong light through body structure to permit inspection by observer on opposite side.

**transition** phase at end of first-stage labour, from about 8 cm to full cervical dilatation, or until expulsive contractions of second stage felt by mother; there is often a brief lull in intensity of uterine activity.

**translocation** in genetics, transfer of material from one chromosome to one of different kind. If occurs during meiosis, balanced or reciprocal translocation occurs: total chromosomal complement is normal, no clinical manifestation, discovered only during karyotyping. If occurs during mitosis, unbalanced translocation results in either excess or deficient chromosomal material in gamete.

**transmigration** wandering. *External t.* passage of ovum from ovary to fallopian tube on opposite side.

**transplacental** through placenta.

**transport** movement of materials in biological systems, particularly into and out of cells and across epithelial layers. *Active t.* movement of materials across cell membranes and epithelial layers resulting directly from expenditure of metabolic energy.

**transposition of great vessels** group of congenital heart defects; pulmonary artery arises from left ventricle instead of right; poorly oxygenated blood leaves right ventricle by aorta; patent ductus or creation of atrioseptal shunt are required to maintain life.

**transudate** fluid passing through membrane, has high fluid content, low protein and cellular content, e.g. vaginal fluid. *Opp* exudate.

**transvaginal scan** ultrasound scan using probe inserted into vagina, commonly performed in first trimester of pregnancy as intrauterine detail often much clearer than via abdominal route. Also used to visualize fetal parts in pelvic cavity in late pregnancy.

**transverse arrest** deflexed fetal head caught above level of ischial spines, sagittal suture in transverse diameter of pelvis; causes cephalopelvic disproportion, OBSTRUCTED LABOUR. *See* DEEP TRANSVERSE ARREST.

**transverse lie** longitudinal fetal axis lies across maternal uterus; due to lax abdominal, uterine muscles, as in grande multiparae, multiple pregnancy, placenta praevia, contracted pelvic outlet; may cause SHOULDER PRESENTATION, obstructed labour. Abdominal examination: uterus appears broad, asymmetrical with low fundus, fetal head felt in flank or iliac fossa. Persistent transverse lie may need external version near term, controlled labour induction or elective Caesarean section.

**transverse sinuses** venous sinuses in tentorium cerebelli by which blood is drained from head.

**traumatic haemorrhage** vaginal bleeding, commences immediately after birth of baby; continues despite good uterine contractions, due to cervical, vaginal or perineal body lacerations. Treatment: direct pressure to bleeding point with artery or sponge-holding forceps or digitally until lacerations can be sutured.

**travail** labour, childbirth.

**travellers** generic term describing nomadic families; some health authorities provide designated maternity services to offer some element of continuity of care.

**treatment** mode of dealing with patient or disease. *Active t.* specific medical or surgical intervention. *Conservative t.* natural means, e.g. rest, fluid replacement, rather than active or radical treatment. *Palliative t.* relieves distressing symptoms but not disease.

**Trendelenburg position** *See* POSITION.

**Treponema pallidum** SPIROCHAETAE causing syphilis.

**trial labour** conducted in obstetric unit when fetal head not engaged due to slight cephalopelvic disproportion to see if vaginal birth possible; if good contractions occur, head may flex and descend through pelvic brim, facilitating normal birth; lack of progress in descent of head and dilatation of cervix despite good contractions, or signs of fetal or maternal distress, requires Caesarean section.

**trial of scar** controlled, often induced labour to observe mother's condition and progress when she has uterine scar from previous Caesarean or other uterine surgery; increased risk of scar dehiscence, particularly in multigravidae, labour must be carefully monitored in obstetric unit with facilities for emergency measures.

**Trichomonas vaginalis** sexually transmitted flagellate protozoon; causes trichomoniasis: frothy, thin, watery or yellow-green vaginal discharge, vulval pruritus, inflammation. Treatment: metronidazole for both partners.

**tricuspid atresia** congenital heart disease; complete absence of tricuspid valve, absence of right atrio-ventricular connection, leads to hypoplastic or absent right ventricle; heart unable to oxygenate blood; atrial-septal, ventricular-septal defects present; treatment: creation of patent ductus arteriosus to increase pulmonary flow.

**tricyclic antidepressants** antidepressant drugs, largely replaced by SELECTIVE SEROTONIN REUPTAKE INHIBITORS (SSRIs) with fewer side effects.

**trifluoperazine** antipsychotic, sedative drug related to phenothiazine.

**triglyceride** compound; three molecules of fatty acid bound with one molecule of glycerol; neutral fat, usual storage form of lipids.

**trigone** triangular area. *T. of bladder* triangular non-elastic base of bladder between ureteric openings and urethral orifice; embedded in anterior vaginal wall, which, if distended in labour, may adversely affect bladder function.

**tri-iodothyronine** thyroid hormone similar to thyroxine.

**trimester** period of 3 months.

**trimethoprim** oral or intravenous antibiotic for urinary and respiratory tract infections; contraindicated in pregnancy and neonates.

**tripartite placenta** placenta divided into three lobes, each with cord leaving it that join to form one cord a short distance from the lobes.

**triple test** biochemical Down syndrome blood screening test performed between 15 and 20 weeks' gestation. ALPHA-FETOPROTEIN (AFP), HUMAN CHORIONIC GONADOTROPHIN, UNCONJUGATED OESTRIOL measured and compared with median value for gestational age; higher-than-average hCG, lower-than-average AFP and $UE_3$ levels may mean increased Down syndrome risk. Maternal age, gestation, biochemical marker levels calculated to give combined Down syndrome risk; if more than 1 in 250 at term, mother offered AMNIOCENTESIS, CHORIONIC VILLUS SAMPLING.

**triple vaccine** combined diphtheria, tetanus, pertussis vaccines.

**triplets** three children born at one labour.

**triploidy (69XXX, 69XXY)** syndrome with three HAPLOID sets of chromosomes present; may occur when two sperm fertilize one egg. Normal human karyotype contains 46 chromosomes. Spontaneous miscarriage common; liveborn babies may have craniofacial abnormalities, eye defects, developmental delay.

**trisomy** additional chromosome on one particular pair. **Trisomy 21** extra chromosome with 21st pair; DOWN SYNDROME. **Trisomy 18** EDWARD SYNDROME; **trisomy 13** PATAU SYNDROME.

**trizygotic** formed from three separate zygotes.

**trocar** sharply pointed surgical instrument in metal cannula for aspiration or removal of fluids from cavities.

**trochanter** two prominences below neck of femur; **greater t.** on outer side; **lesser t.** on inner side.

**trophoblast** outer covering of blastocyst from which placenta and chorion develop.

**trophoblastic tissue** SYNCYTIOTROPHOBLAST, CYTOTROPHOBLAST.

**true conjugate** See CONJUGATE.

**true pelvis** bony canal through which fetus must pass during birth, brim, cavity and outlet. See PELVIS.

**trypsin** pancreatic enzyme; aids digestion of proteins to amino acids.

**tubal** pertaining to fallopian tubes. **T. insufflation** test assessing fallopian tube patency by transuterine inflation with carbon dioxide gas. **T. ligation** sterilization method; fallopian tubes tied by laparoscopy and diathermy or with clips on tubes. **T. mole** blood clot mass retained in fallopian tube after tubal pregnancy. **T. pregnancy** pregnancy in fallopian tube lining. See ECTOPIC PREGNANCY.

**tube feeding** administration of liquid (or semi-solid foods in adults) through nasogastric, gastrostomy or enterostomy tube; method of feeding preterm babies who tire easily when suckling and have immature swallowing and gag reflexes.

**tuberculosis** notifiable infection due to *Mycobacterium tuberculosis*, commonly in lung but any part of body may be affected. Treatment: streptomycin, isoniazid, para-aminosalicylic acid or ethambutol; rifampicin contraindicated in first trimester. Antenatal: shared care from obstetrician, chest physician; if mother has positive sputum, hospital admission, isolation; care provided by staff immune to TB. Labour: epidural anaesthesia, forceps delivery, intravenous ergometrine to limit blood loss. Postnatal: if maternal sputum positive, lactation suppressed, baby segregated until mother is Mantoux test positive. Baby given bacille Calmette–Guérin vaccination soon after birth.

**tuberosity** expanded portion of bone or protuberance; transverse diameter of pelvic outlet measured between ISCHIAL TUBEROSITIES.

**tubular necrosis (acute)** 1. protein deposited in collecting and distal convoluted renal tubules, as with incompatible blood transfusion or septic abortion; epithelium damaged and urine dammed back, preventing further activity of GLOMERULUS; usually clears in 7–14 days. 2. proximal, convoluted tubule becomes ischaemic or bacterial toxins released; epithelium may necrose with tubular death; kidney function may recover in 10–30 days if only partial necrosis.

**tubule** microscopic tube forming one part of nephron.

**tumescence** swelling or enlargement; penile erection.

**tumour** growth or swelling.

**tunica** coat. *T. albuginea* dense layer of connective tissue below germinal epithelium of ovary. *T. vasculosa* vascular layer. *T. vaginalis* serous covering of testis.

**Tuohy needle** cannula and needle to site catheter in epidural space.

**Turner syndrome (XO, monosomy X, 45X)** chromosome disorder due to absence of one X chromosome; occurs in approximately 1 in 2500 female births. Characteristics: short stature, neck webbing, normal vagina, uterus, fallopian tubes, nonfunctional ovaries, no pubertal development, infertility; aortic narrowing; learning difficulties. Suspected in pregnancy from abnormal ultrasound findings, e.g. CYSTIC HYGROMA, heart defects, ascites, renal abnormalities; diagnosis confirmed with karyotyping.

**twin reversed arterial perfusion** in twin pregnancy, one fetus presents without well-defined cardiac structure, is kept alive through placental anastomoses to circulatory system of viable fetus; occurs in 1 in 30,000 births; also known as *acardiac twin*.

**twin-to-twin transfusion syndrome** monochorionic placental multiple pregnancy condition, high mortality.

Chronic TTTS: placenta transfuses blood from donor fetus, causes anaemia, growth restriction in donor, polycythaemia with circulatory overload (hydrops) in recipient. Suspect condition if mother reports second trimester rapid abdominal girth increase and continuously hard painful uterus with polyhydramnios. Treatment: early diagnosis, repeated amnio-reduction, laser ablation therapy of communicating placental vessels or septostomy. Acute TTTS occurs in labour; both fetuses die of cardiac failure if not treated urgently.

**twins** two babies developing in uterus together. Genetically identical (monozygous) twins arise from division of single fertilized egg; if this occurs in MORULA within 4 days of fertilization, twins will be dichorionic, diamniotic (DC-DA) with separate placentae, possibly fused; if BLASTOCYST divides 4–8 days after fertilization, monochorionic (one placenta) diamniotic twins (MC-DA) result. Vascular connections in common placenta may cause TWIN-TO-TWIN TRANSFUSION SYNDROME. Occasionally blastocyst divides 8–13 days after fertilization with monochorionic monoamniotic twins (MC-MA); shared amniotic cavity causes high fetal mortality, morbidity. Dizygotic nonidentical twins occur when two separate eggs are fertilized: two placentae, two amniotic sacs (DC-DA). *See also* MULTIPLE PREGNANCY.

**typing** method to measure degree of organ, solid tissue or blood compatibility between two individuals; specific histocompatibility antigens, e.g. those present on leucocytes or erythrocytes, are detected by means of suitable isoimmune antisera.

**tyramine** enzyme in cheese, game, yeast extracts, wine, beer, broad bean pods; has adrenaline-like effects; should be avoided by those taking monoamine oxidase inhibitor drugs.

**tyrosine** naturally occurring amino acid found in most proteins; product of phenylalanine metabolism, precursor of melanin, catecholamines, thyroid hormones.

**ulcer** skin or mucous membrane lesion resulting from trauma, infection, pressure or nerve injury.

**ultrasonic** beyond audible range; relates to sound waves with frequency above 20,000 cycles per second.

**ultrasound scan, ultrasonography** technique enabling deep body structures to be visualized by recording reflections (echoes) of ultrasonic waves directed into tissues; used in pregnancy to confirm gestation, placental location, estimate fetal size, weight, maturity, liquor volume, identify fetal abnormalities, examine uterine contents, measure fetal and uteroplacental blood flow, observe fetal movements and functions; also used during amniocentesis, chorionic villus biopsy to avoid fetal or placental damage.

**umbilical** relating to umbilicus. *U. catheterization* insertion of catheter into baby's umbilical vein or artery to administer drugs or fluids, continuously monitor blood gases, exchange transfusion, obtain blood samples. *U. hernia* protrusion of intestine through umbilicus. *See* EXOMPHALOS.

**umbilical cord** cord connecting fetus and placenta, about 50–60 cm long; two arteries carry deoxygenated blood, one vein carries oxygenated blood; surrounded by Wharton's jelly covered by amnion. Cord clamped and cut after birth, leaving stump, which separates naturally through dry, aseptic necrosis within 5–7 days. *U. c. presentation, U. c. prolapse* See CORD.

**umbilicus** navel; abdominal point at which umbilical cord attached.

**unassisted birth** 'freebirthing', planned birth at which mother gives birth without professional assistance; a legal choice in UK.

**unconjugated oestriol (UE₃)** biochemical marker produced by placenta and fetal adrenals; used in second-trimester serum Down syndrome screening; reduced in affected pregnancies. *See also* QUADRUPLE TEST *and* TRIPLE TEST.

**unconscious** 1. insensible; incapable of responding to sensory stimuli. 2. part of mental activity concealed from consciousness.

**uni-** prefix meaning 'one'. *U.-lateral* on one side only. *U.-ovular* from one ovum. *See* MONOZYGOTIC.

**universal donor** *See* ABO BLOOD GROUPS.

**universal recipient** *See* ABO BLOOD GROUPS.

**unstable lie** continual alteration of fetal lie after 36 weeks' gestation; predisposes mother and baby to life-threatening complications. Treatment options: external version, controlled membrane rupture, induction of labour, Caesarean section.

**urachal** pertaining to urachus. *U. cyst* congenital abnormality of small cysts developing along urachus. *U. fistula* fistula forming when urachus fails

http://dx.doi.org/10.1016/B978-0-7020-6906-2.00021-8

to close, causing urine leakage from umbilicus.

**urachus** fibrous band uniting apex of bladder to umbilicus; vestigial remnant of fetal canal.

**uraemia** renal failure; high blood urea, headache, vertigo, vomiting, convulsions, coma; complication of nephritis, concealed PLACENTAL ABRUPTION, ECLAMPSIA.

**urea** protein metabolism end product, excreted in urine. *Blood u.* normally 2.5–58 mmol/L (15–35 mg/100 mL); in pregnancy, usually 2.3–5.0 mmol/L (14–30 mg/100 mL).

**ureters** two fibromuscular tubes conveying urine from kidneys to bladder; dilatation occurs in pregnancy due to smooth muscle relaxation by PROGESTERONE, leading to urinary stasis and multiplication of micro-organisms. *See* PYELONEPHRITIS. *Adj* ureteric.

**ureterovesical** pertaining to ureter and vagina. *U. fistula* abnormal passage between ureter and vagina; complication of prolonged or obstructed labour due to prolonged pressure by fetal head.

**urethra** canal through which urine is discharged from bladder; 20–22.5 cm long in men, 3.7 cm in women. *Adj* urethral.

**urethritis** inflammation of urethra. *Non-specific u.* male sexually transmitted disease, unknown origin.

**urethrocele** female urethral wall prolapse, from pelvic floor damage.

**uric** pertaining to urine. *U. acid* end product of purine metabolism or oxidation, present in blood, excreted in urine.

**urinalysis** physical and/or chemical examination urinary to detect disorders, investigate symptoms. Dark urine indicates dehydration; cloudy urine indicates infection. Reagent dipsticks used to detect protein, glucose, ketones, pH. Regular urine tests in pregnancy aid diagnose of urinary tract infection, PRE-ECLAMPSIA, dehydration, diabetes mellitus. Microbiological examination identifies bacteria, blood cells and other microorganisms.

**urination** micturition.

**urine** fluid secreted by kidneys, excreted by bladder in micturition; normal pH 6; 96% water containing dissolved waste products, e.g. UREA, CREATININE, sodium chloride, phosphates. *Adj* urinary.

**urinometer** instrument to measure urinary specific gravity.

**urobilinogen** by-product of bilirubin reduction formed in intestines by bacterial action on bilirubin; approximately half is reabsorbed, taken up via portal vein to liver, enters circulation, excreted by kidney.

**urodynamics** dynamics of propulsion and flow of urine in urinary tract.

**urolithiasis** bladder or urinary tract stones.

**urticaria** vascular skin reaction; transient slightly elevated patches, redder or paler than surrounding skin, often accompanied by severe itching; caused by food intolerance, infection or stress.

**uterine** pertaining to uterus. *U. souffle See* SOUFFLE. *U. ligaments* two ligaments; passing backwards from cervix to sacrum, encircling rectum; maintain uterus in anteverted position. *U. tubes See* FALLOPIAN TUBES.

**utero-** pertaining to uterus. *U.-placental* pertaining to uterus and placenta. *U.-sacral* pertaining to uterus and sacrum. *U.-salpingography* radiography of uterus and uterine tubes; hysterosalpingography. *U.-tonics* drugs that stimulate uterine muscle e.g. Syntocinon.

**uterovesical** referring to uterus and bladder. *U. pouch* fold of peritoneum between uterus and bladder.

**uterus** hollow, muscular organ in pelvic cavity between bladder and rectum. Inner ENDOMETRIUM, termed DECIDUA in pregnancy; muscle layer, MYOMETRIUM; outer PERIMETRIUM hangs loosely over FUNDUS to form UTEROVESICAL POUCH anteriorly, POUCH OF DOUGLAS posteriorly. *Bicornuate u.* congenital malformation; uterus has two horns. *U. didelphys* double uterus caused by failure of the two sides to unite during development. *U. unicornus* uterus with only one horn. *Adj* uterine.

**vaccination** injection of bacterial vaccine. See BACILLE CALMETTE–GUÉRIN, HUMAN PAPILLOMAVIRUS, TRIPLE VACCINE.

**vaccine** suspension of killed organisms in normal saline. *Attenuated v.* prepared from living organisms that have lost their virulence. *Bacille Calmette-Guérin v.* attenuated bovine bacillus to protect against tuberculosis. *Salk v.* prepared from poliomyelitis virus strain.

**vacuum aspiration** method of first-trimester termination of pregnancy; also used to remove hydatidiform mole.

**vacuum extractor** alternative to forceps delivery; suction cup attached to fetal scalp; traction synchronized with uterine contractions is exerted. Types of extractor: Malmström, modified Bird extractor, SILC.

**vagal** pertaining to vagus nerve.

**vagina** squamous epithelium–lined canal between vulva and cervix; part of birth canal. Anterior wall 6.5–7.5 cm long, with urethra and bladder base embedded in it; posterior wall 9–10 cm, in contact with perineal body, rectum, pouch of Douglas; lateral walls are in contact with levator ani muscles.

**vaginal** pertaining to vagina. *V. bleeding* See ANTEPARTUM HAEMORRHAGE; POST-PARTUM HAEMORRHAGE. *V. discharge* See DISCHARGE. *V. examination/examination per vaginam* digital assessment of obstetric/gynaecological condition. *V. orifice* introitus, vaginal opening.

*V. seeding* practice of covering baby born by Caesarean section with vaginal fluid in belief that exposure to vaginal bacteria will boost baby's immune system; no proven benefits to date.

**vaginismus** painful vaginal muscle spasm.

**vaginitis** vaginal inflammation, often due to infection, e.g. *Candida albicans*, *Trichomonas vaginalis*.

**vagus** tenth cranial nerve; parasympathetic nerve widely distributed throughout body, supplies heart, lungs, liver, alimentary tract.

**validation** approval process, e.g. academic courses such as midwifery: UK pre-registration programmes are approved by NURSING AND MIDWIFERY COUNCIL to ensure consistent standards.

**validity** research term used to determine extent to which a process actually reflects construct being examined when used for specific group or purpose.

**Valsalva manoeuvre** increase of intrathoracic pressure by forcible exhalation against closed glottis. Baby with respiratory distress adopts partial Valsalva manoeuvre by grunting, maintaining positive pressure in chest even during exhalation, i.e. CONTINUOUS POSITIVE AIRWAY PRESSURE.

**value** quantitative measurement of activity, concentration, etc., of specific substances.

**valve** membranous fold in canal or passage that prevents backward flow of material passing through it.

http://dx.doi.org/10.1016/B978-0-7020-6906-2.00022-X

## Identification of fetal position on vaginal examination

### Occipitoanterior positions viewed from the pelvic outlet

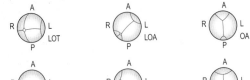

### Occipitoposterior positions viewed from the pelvic outlet

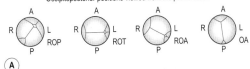

(A)

Identifying the position of the fetus on vaginal examination by identifying the position of the sutures and fontanelles in relation to the pelvis

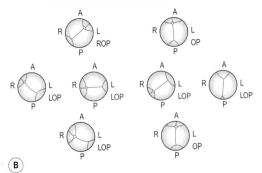

(B)

**vancomycin** antibiotic drug used to treat neonatal sepsis.

**vanillylmandelic acid** excretory catecholamine product, tests for adrenaline metabolism; raised with adrenal tumours, e.g. PHAEOCHROMOCYTOMA.

**vanishing twin syndrome** reabsorption of one twin fetus, usually before 12 weeks' gestation.

**variable** in epidemiology, any measurement that can have different values. *Dependent v.* affected by other variables in epidemiological studies. *Independent v.* not influenced by other variables but may cause alterations in these variables.

**variance** measure of variation seen in set of data.

**varicella-zoster virus (chickenpox)** viral infection commonly acquired in childhood, spread by respiratory droplets; non-specific malaise, abdominal, facial vesicular rash. Infective from 2 days before rash appears until last vesicle crusts over. Virus remains latent, reactivation leads to shingles; previous infection usually confers lifelong immunity to chickenpox. Pregnant women with no previous infection should avoid contact with infected people; delay birth as long as possible if primary infection after 36 weeks' gestation, so fetus develops passive immunity from maternal antibodies. Maternal complications: encephalitis, hepatitis, pneumonia; congenital varicella syndrome before 20 weeks' gestation can affect fetal skin, eyes, limbs, brain; infection after 36 weeks causes severe neonatal varicella; immunoglobulin administration reduces severity.

**varicose** swollen or dilated. *V. veins* abnormally distended, tortuous veins, usually in leg, due to inefficient valves allow back- or cross-flow of blood, particularly in superficial and deep veins; progesterone in pregnancy relaxes vein walls, causing stasis and inefficient venous return; also occur in vulva or rectum.

**variola** smallpox.

**varices** enlarged tortuous veins, arteries or lymphatic vessels. *Sing* varix.

**vas** vessel. *Pl* vasa. *V. deferens* tube through which spermatozoa pass from testis to seminal vesicle.

**vasa praevia** presentation in front of fetal head in labour of umbilical cord vessels, which enter placenta in velamentous cord insertion; when membranes rupture, bleeding may lead to fetal distress.

**vascular** relating to vessels.

**vasectomy** removal of part of VAS DEFERENS through small scrotal incision, usually for sterilization.

**vasoconstriction** contraction of blood vessels.

**vasodepressor** lowers blood pressure through reduced peripheral resistance.

**vasodilation** dilatation of blood vessels.

**vasomotor** controlling muscles of blood vessels, dilator and constrictor.

**vasopressin** pressor agent produced in pituitary gland; antidiuretic hormone.

**vasopressor** stimulates capillary and arterial muscular tissue contraction.

**vault** part of fetal skull containing cerebral hemispheres; two frontal, two parietal, two temporal, one occipital bone separated by membranous sutures; facilitates skull moulding in labour and brain growth. *V. cap* contraceptive bowl-shaped device attached to vaginal vault by suction to prevent spermatozoa entering cervix; best used with spermicidal agent. *Vaginal v.* upper part of vagina into which cervix protrudes.

**vegan** vegetarian who excludes all foods of animal origin from diet.

**vegetarian diet** diet in which no meat is eaten. *Lacto-vegetarian diet* prohibits intake of meat, poultry, fish and eggs.

**vein** vessel carrying blood from capillaries back to heart; thin walls and lining endothelium from which venous valves are formed.

**velamentous insertion** umbilical cord vessels divide before reaching placenta, increasing risk of tearing of vessels and bleeding in third-stage labour. *See also* VASA PRAEVIA.

**vena cava** one of two trunk veins returning venous blood to right atrium of heart.

**venepuncture** vein puncture to obtain blood or administer drugs.

**venereal** concerning or resulting from sexual intercourse. *V. diseases* syphilis, gonorrhoea, soft chancre. *V. Disease Research Laboratory test* booking blood test for SYPHILIS. False-negative results can occur in early stages of disease. Positive results also arise from infectious mononucleosis, antiphospholipid antibody syndrome, lupus, hepatitis A, leprosy, malaria. Syphilis-specific test, e.g. FLUORESCENT TREPONEMAL ANTIBODY-ABSORBED TEST confirms diagnosis of syphilis.

**venesection** opening vein to withdraw blood to relieve congestion.

**ventilation** neonatal process of air exchange between lungs and ambient air for preterm babies, those with RESPIRATORY DISTRESS SYNDROME, severe APNOEA, PO$_2$ below 5 kPa despite high oxygen in inspired air, PCO$_2$ above 12 kPa if acidosis fails to respond to treatment. If very low birthweight, routine for 24 hours to prevent respiratory distress syndrome. Complications: pneumothorax, infection, bronchopulmonary dysplasia, retinopathy due to high oxygen and carbon dioxide levels. *Pulmonary v.* total exchange of air. *Alveolar v.* ventilation of alveoli where gas exchange with blood takes place. *See also* CONVENTIONAL MECHANICAL VENTILATION, CONTINUOUS POSITIVE AIRWAY PRESSURE, HIGH-FREQUENCY OSCILLATION VENTILATION, EXTRACORPOREAL MEMBRANE OXYGENATION, CONTINUOUS NASAL END EXPIRATORY PRESSURE.

**ventilator** respirator; apparatus which qualifies air breathed through it or which controls pulmonary ventilation.

**ventouse** *See* VACUUM EXTRACTOR.

**ventricle** small pouch or cavity, especially lower chambers of heart and four cavities of brain.

**ventricular septal defect** congenital heart defect; persistent patency of ventricular septum allows direct blood flow from one ventricle to the other, bypassing pulmonary circulation, causing cyanosis due to OXYGEN deficiency.

**ventrosuspension** operation to shorten round ligaments to correct a RETROVERTED GRAVID UTERUS.

**venule** minute vein.

**vernix caseosa** greasy substance covering fetus from 30–32 weeks' gestation; sebaceous gland secretion with desquamated cells; some present on skin at birth, more if baby is preterm.

**version** turning fetus *in utero* to alter lie or presentation to a more favourable one. *Cephalic v.* turning fetus to head presentation. *External v.* turning fetus by manipulation via abdominal wall. *External cephalic v.* performed from 34 weeks' gestation to turn breech presentation. *Internal v.*

turning fetus with one hand in uterus, other on abdomen. *Podalic v.* turning fetus to breech presentation; may be performed when labouring multipara has oblique fetal lie or if second twin in oblique lie.

**vertebrae** irregular bones of spinal column: 7 cervical, 12 thoracic, 5 lumbar, 5 sacral, 4 coccygeal (coccyx) bones. Sing vertebra.

**vertex** area of head bounded by anterior and posterior fontanelles, laterally by parietal eminences. *V. presentation* vertex lies over internal os, fetal head well flexed; optimal presentation for birth.

**vesica** bladder, usually urinary bladder; See ECTOPIA VESICAE.

**vesical** relating to bladder.

**vesicle** blister or small sac usually containing fluid.

**vesico-ureteric reflux** loss of efficiency at junction of ureter and bladder due to ureteric shortening and perpendicular angle from displacement by enlarging uterus; occurs in approximately 3% of women towards term due to ascending urinary tract infection.

**vesicovaginal** pertaining to bladder and vagina. *V. fistula* abnormal opening between bladder and vagina; rare complication of prolonged or obstructed labour when bladder tissues are devitalized by prolonged pressure of fetal head.

**vesicular** relating to, or containing, vesicles. *V. mole* HYDATIDIFORM MOLE.

**vestibule** entrance; part of vulva lying between labia minora.

**vestige** remnant of structure that functioned in previous stage of species or individual development. *Adj* vestigial.

**viable, viability** capable of life; in pregnancy, fetal heart pulsations seen on ultrasound; gestation at which baby is capable of independent life, legally 24 weeks' gestation.

**Viagra (sildenafil citrate)** oral drug to treat erectile dysfunction.

**vicarious** substituted for another. *V. liability* employer is liable for torts of employees during employment.

**villi** fine hair-like processes projecting from surface. *Chorionic v.* branched processes on trophoblast, dip into maternal blood of placental site. See PLACENTA and CHORIONIC VILLI. *Intestinal v.* minute projections on intestinal mucosa, with blood capillaries and lacteals; sites of absorption of fluids, nutrients. Sing villus.

**vimule** rubber occlusive cap placed over cervix for contraception.

**viraemia** presence of viruses in blood.

**viral** caused by or having nature of a virus.

**virilization** abnormal development of male characteristics in female.

**virus** small complex infective agent; causes smallpox, poliomyelitis, influenza, rabies, measles, rubella, etc.; cross placenta, may cause fetal abnormalities, especially in first trimester.

**viscera** internal organs in body cavities, e.g. heart, uterus.

**viscid** sticky, glutinous.

**visual analogue scale** method to quantify subjective feelings, e.g. pain; a line graded numerically from 'no sensation' to 'maximum sensation'.

**visualization** technique using imagination and relaxation to create desired changes in person's life.

**vital** relating to or necessary to life. *V. capacity* maximum amount of air forcibly expelled from respiratory tract after maximum inspiration. *V. statistics* births and death records among populations: causes and factors influencing rise and fall.

**vitamins** food nutrients essential to health; vitamins A, D, E, K are fat soluble; B and C are water soluble. Deficiencies lead to numerous conditions, e.g. ANAEMIA (B$_{12}$), pregnancy sickness (B$_6$), HYPOCALCAEMIA (D), HAEMORRHAGIC disease (K), etc.

**vitelline duct** VESTIGIAL remains of yolk sac in umbilical cord base.

**volvulus** intestinal loop torsion, causes obstruction, strangulation.

**vomiting** expulsion of stomach contents via mouth. *V. of blood* HAEMATEMESIS. *V. in newborn* blood-stained vomit: due to swallowing maternal blood at birth or from cracked nipples, or to baby's own blood in HAEMORRHAGIC disease. Milk: due to feeding problems, infection, GASTROENTERITIS, MENINGITIS, relaxed cardia, raised intracranial pressure. In intestinal obstruction: bile-stained vomit, no meconium. *V. in pregnancy* severe vomiting in pregnancy may leads to weight loss and dehydration, HYPEREMESIS GRAVIDARUM. Differential diagnosis may be PYELONEPHRITIS, other gastrointestinal conditions or severe illness. Vomiting with hypertension, oedema and proteinuria in late pregnancy may indicate impending ECLAMPSIA caused by liver oedema and/or haemorrhage. *Projectile v.* profuse, sudden, forceful vomiting, as occurs in hypertrophic PYLORIC STENOSIS.

**vomitus** material vomited.

**voriconazole** antifungal drug.

**vulsellum** *See* FORCEPS.

**vulva** external female genital organs. *Adj* vulval.

**vulvectomy** excision of vulva.

**vulvitis** inflammation of vulva.

**'waiter's tip'** characteristic position of forearm and hand in ERB'S PARALYSIS.

**walking reflex** primitive neonatal reflex, in which baby simulates walking if supported upright with feet touching flat surface.

**warfarin** anticoagulant drug to control prothrombin time to 2.5–3.5 times above normal. Crosses placenta, is teratogenic, particularly at 6–9 weeks' gestation. Risk of FETAL WARFARIN SYNDROME, central nervous system abnormalities. Women should convert to heparin as soon as they become pregnant, except those with metal prosthetic heart valves and high risk of thromboembolic complications if risks of changing treatment outweigh fetal risks of remaining on warfarin. Women on anticoagulants should be advised not to take herbal remedies, which may potentiate anticoagulation.

**wart** epidermal tumour of viral origin. *See* GENITAL WARTS.

**water birth** practice in which mother chooses to labour and/or give birth in water for relaxation and pain relief; midwives should be adequately trained before taking responsibility for water births.

**water embolism** in water birth, theoretical risk of water entering maternal circulation when placental bed sinuses are torn during third-stage labour. Third stage should be managed without oxytocin or controlled cord traction, preferably avoiding cutting cord until placenta delivered.

**weaning** detaching from accustomed habit, e.g. changing infant feeding from breast to bottle or cup feeding, or from milk feeds to solid food.

**webbed** connected by membrane or tissue strand. *W. hands* or *feet* congenital abnormality in which digits are not separated from each other; syndactyly. *W. neck* folds of neck skin giving webbed appearance; may be congenital e.g. Turner syndrome.

**weight gain** normal weight gain in pregnancy is 10–12 kg, approximately 2.5 kg in first 20 weeks, 0.5 kg per week thereafter; due to term fetus, placenta, amniotic fluid, uterus, blood, breasts, plus tissue fluid, fat, protein deposition. Excess weight gain may be due to OEDEMA, PRE-ECLAMPSIA, multiple pregnancy, large baby; poor weight gain may indicate INTRAUTERINE GROWTH RESTRICTION. *W. g. in babies* neonate loses up to 10% of birthweight in first few days of life due to passage of meconium; should regain birthweight by 10–14 days; thereafter approximately 200 g per week.

**Weil's disease** spirochaetal jaundice caused by *Leptospira icterohaemorrhagiae*, transmitted in rat urine; acquired through skin or from infected food or water.

**well woman clinic** clinic to screen women early for breast and cervical cancer, anaemia, diabetes, hypertension, etc.

http://dx.doi.org/10.1016/B978-0-7020-6906-2.00023-1

**Wernicke encephalopathy** acute haemorrhagic encephalitis, occurring occasionally in severe HYPEREMESIS GRAVIDARUM due to vitamin B₁ deficiency.

**Wertheim operation** *See* HYSTERECTOMY.

**Wharton's jelly** connective tissue of umbilical cord.

**whey** fluid part of milk, separated from curd after addition of rennet; easily digested as casein and fat are removed. *W.-dominant infant formula* small amount of skimmed milk combined with demineralized whey, with 60:40 ratio of proteins. More easily digested than CASEIN-DOMINANT INFANT FORMULA.

**white blood cell** *See* LEUCOCYTE.

**white coat hypertension** syndrome in which anxiety in a medical environment results in abnormally high reading when blood pressure is measured.

**white leg** *See* PHLEGMASIA ALBA DOLENS.

**white matter, white substance** white nervous tissue, myelinated nerve fibres; constitutes conducting portion of brain and spinal cord.

**WHO International Code of Marketing of Breast Milk Substitutes** World Health Organization and UNICEF code to promote breastfeeding and control marketing of products for artificial feeding, especially in developing countries. *See* BABY FRIENDLY HOSPITAL INITIATIVE.

**whooping cough** *See* PERTUSSIS.

**Wilson–Mikity syndrome** pulmonary dysmaturity occurring in babies ventilated for long periods or who need prolonged OXYGEN therapy, characterized by early development of cystic interstitial emphysema.

**withdrawal bleed** vaginal bleeding due to hormone withdrawal.

**withdrawal method** contraceptive method in which penis is withdrawn from vagina before ejaculation; not 100% reliable because semen can be deposited within vagina before full ejaculation.

**wolffian bodies** two small organs in embryo, primitive kidneys.

**Wood's manoeuvre** method of facilitating delivery of baby in SHOULDER DYSTOCIA by inserting hand into vagina to identify fetal chest, then exerting pressure on posterior fetal shoulder to rotate it, enabling delivery to be completed. *See* APPENDIX 4.

**World Health Organization** specialized United Nations agency concerned with international health.

**wound** physically induced bodily injury causing disruption of normal function of local structures. *W. healing by first intention* restoration of tissue function occurring directly without granulation. *W. healing by second intention* repair by closure of wound with granulation tissue. *W. healing by third intention* closure of contaminated wound is delayed until 4–5 days after injury.

**Wrigley's forceps** obstetric forceps for very low forceps deliveries, assisting delivery of aftercoming head of breech or at Caesarean section.

**X chromosome** sex chromosome. Female cells carry two X chromosomes (XX), male cells one X, one Y chromosome (XY). During maturation of ovum and spermatozoon, one of two chromosomes is cast off; at fertilization two remaining chromosomes determine baby's sex: two X chromosomes produce girl, X and Y chromosomes produce boy. *See also* TURNER SYNDROME, KLINEFELTER SYNDROME.

**X-linked** transmitted by genes on X chromosome; sex-linked.

**xiphisternum** XIPHOID PROCESS; base of sternum.

**xiphoid process** small cartilaginous process at lower end of sternum; xiphisternum; ensiform cartilage.

Landmark to which uterine fundal height is related during abdominal examination to assess gestation.

**XO** *See* TURNER SYNDROME.

**x-ray** photographic or digital image of internal composition of parts of the body, produced by x-rays being passed through it and being absorbed to different degrees by different materials.

**XYY syndrome (47XYY)** genetic condition, occurring in approximately 1 in 1000 men, in which an additional Y chromosome is inherited; physical development is normal, although men may be taller than normal; mental maturity and speech development may be delayed; excessive violent criminal tendencies may also occur.

http://dx.doi.org/10.1016/B978-0-7020-6906-2.00024-3

**Y chromosome** sex chromosome; male cells carry one Y and one X chromosome.

**yaws** non-venereal, tropical, treponemal infection; local lesions similar to those of SYPHILIS; serological tests for syphilis are positive.

**yeast** fungus producing fermentation; e.g. yeast-like fungus *Candida albicans* causes THRUSH infection.

**yolk sac** one of two spaces in inner cell mass of trophoblast, surrounded by entodermal cells; other space is amniotic cavity; between two is intervening layer of mesoderm. Embryo is formed from area where ectoderm, mesoderm and entoderm lie in apposition.

**Yutopar** *See* RITODRINE HYDROCHLORIDE.

http://dx.doi.org/10.1016/B978-0-7020-6906-2.00025-5

**Zavanelli manoeuvre** final choice of manoeuvre in management of SHOULDER DYSTOCIA which has not responded to other manoeuvres; fetal head is returned to pre-restitution position, then flexed back into vagina; delivery by Caesarean section is required.

**zidovudine** antiviral drug used to slow progress of AIDS; azidothymidine, AZT.

**Zika virus** disease caused by virus transmitted by *Aedes* mosquitoes, found particularly in Africa, Americas, Asia and Pacific. Symptoms: mild fever, skin rashes, conjunctivitis, muscle and joint pain, malaise or headache, lasting 2–7 days, can lead to Guillain Barré syndrome. May also be sexually transmitted. Pregnant women exposed to virus at risk of having babies with MICROCEPHALY.

**zinc** trace element, component of several enzymes, found in red meat, shellfish, liver, peas, lentils, beans, rice; severe deficiency causes low sperm count in men, miscarriage, growth retardation, slow wound healing.

**zona pellucida** transparent, noncellular, secreted layer surrounding OVUM. SPERM release enzymes allowing penetration of zona pellucida; only one sperm enters ovum at fertilization.

**zygosity** describing genetic make-up of children in multiple births.

**zygote** ovum before segmentation, formed by gametes combining at fertilization. *Z. intrafallopian transfer* infertility treatment involving artificial stimulation of ovulation, harvesting of oocytes with ultrasound-directed follicle aspiration, transvaginally or at laparoscopy; once fertilization has occurred, zygote is transferred at laparoscopy into mid-ampullary section of fallopian tube.

**The Zavanelli manoeuvre**

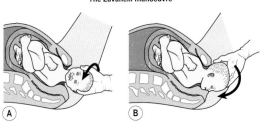

**A,** Head being returned to direct anteroposterior position. **B,** Head being returned to the vagina.

http://dx.doi.org/10.1016/B978-0-7020-6906-2.00026-7

# **Appendices**

# Appendix 1

## Management of primary postpartum haemorrhage

Basic principles of management – be aware that several aspects can occur concurrently:

1. Call for medical aid
2. Stop bleeding
   A. Rub up contraction
      - massage fundus until uterus is firm and contracted
      - ensure bladder is empty, leave Foley catheter in situ
      - baby may be put to breast to encourage natural oxytocin production
      - bimanual compression if necessary, until intravenous infusion set up
   B. Administer uterotonic drug
      - syntocinon 5 or 10 units by slow intravenous infusion
      - or combined ergometrine/oxytocin 1 mL
      - or ergometrine 0.5 mg by slow intravenous infusion; contraindicated if hypertensive
      - syntocinon infusion (40 units in 500 mL Hartmann's at 125 mL/hour) unless fluid restriction necessary
      - carboprost 0.25 mg intramuscularly, repeated at 15-minute intervals; maximum 8 doses; contraindicated in women with asthma; obstetrician may give intramyometrially
      - misoprostol 1000 micrograms rectally
   C. Empty uterus
      - deliver placenta if possible, using controlled cord traction (CCT)
      - expel any clots by applying firm gentle pressure on fundus
      - if placenta undelivered and in vagina or cervix, grasp and remove
      - catheterize to empty bladder, facilitating uterine contraction
      - if placenta undelivered and partially separated and bleeding continues, use CCT
      - if placenta undelivered and completely adherent, usually there is no bleeding, but MANUAL REMOVAL OF PLACENTA required
3. Resuscitate mother
   - assess airway, breathing, circulation
   - administer oxygen by mask at 10–15 L/min

- position mother flat and keep warm
- commence intravenous infusion using 14-gauge cannula
- if $\leq$1000 mL, 1–2 L crystalloid infusion
- if $\geq$1000 mL, 3.5 L warmed crystalloid Hartmann's solution, then 1–2 L of colloid infusion until blood available
- take blood for cross-matching; transfuse blood as soon as possible; use group 0 rhesus negative if necessary
- fresh frozen plasma: 4 units for every 6 units of red cells or prothrombin time/ activated
- partial thromboplastin time (PLT) >1.5 $\times$ normal (12–15 mL/kg or total 1 litre)
- platelets concentrate if PLT count <50 $\times$ $10^9$
- cryoprecipitate if fibrinogen <1 g/L

Reference: RCOG 2009 Green Top Guideline 52.

# Appendix 2

## Basic life support (mother)

1. Shake and shout to establish mother's level of consciousness and whether she can hear.
2. Summon medical aid as soon as possible.
3. Position mother on back without pillows; if pregnant, use padding for left lateral tilt to prevent autoclaval compression.
4. Tilt mother's head backwards, with chin upwards to open airway.
5. Clear mucus or vomit; listen for breath sounds; look for chest movement.
6. Chest (sternal) compressions 100 times per minute.
7. After 30 chest compressions, give 2 breaths by bag and mask or mouth-to-mouth, pinching mother's nose to make seal, 1 second per breath.
8. Maintain 2 breaths to 30 compressions until help arrives.

**Endotracheal intubation**

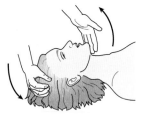

Tilt head backwards and lift chin upwards to open airway

# **3** Appendix

## Neonatal resuscitation

**Resuscitation action plan**

1. Establish and maintain clear airway.
2. Ensure effective circulation.
3. Correct acidosis.
4. Prevent hypothermia, hypoglycaemia and haemorrhage.
   - Airway – clear with oro- and nasopharyngeal suction if no respiratory effort; under direct vision if meconium present.
   - Dry baby and transfer to resuscitation table with overhead heater if available.
   - Position baby on back, neck slightly, but not fully, extended.
   - If no response, use face mask with airway inserted: commence with 5 sustained inflations of oxygen or air, pressure 30 cm $H_2O$ for 2–3 seconds, then ventilate at 40 respirations per minute (IPPV).

**Endotracheal intubation**

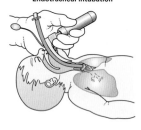

   - If equipment not available, use mouth-to-face resuscitation, using air in cheeks at rate of 20–30 breaths per minute.
   - If no response or bradycardia is present, intubate with endotracheal tube.
   - If heart rate $\leq$60 bpm or 60–100 but falling, start chest compressions at 100–120 per minute at depth of 2–3 cm.
   - If slow or no response, drugs may be required to correct acidosis.

# Appendix 4

## Management of shoulder dystocia

| HELPERR MNEMONIC | ACTION |
|---|---|
| HELP | Call for urgent help; note time |
| EVALUATE NEED FOR EPISIOTOMY | Assess need for episiotomy to access fetus without undue trauma to perineum and vaginal walls |
| LEGS IN McROBERTS POSITION | Lie mother flat, with knees to chest to rotate angle of symphysis pubis superiorly |

**Effects:**
- Straightens the lumbosacral lordosis
- Increases the AP diameter of the pelvis
- Flexes the fetal spine
- Reduces more than 40% of shoulder dystocias

**McRoberts manoeuvre position**

Alternatively, mother can adopt all-fours position (Gaskin manoeuvre), if posterior shoulder is impacted behind sacral promontory, to optimize space in sacral curve

| | |
|---|---|
| PRESSURE SUPRAPUBICALLY | Apply suprapubic pressure on side of fetal back, towards fetal chest — to adduct shoulders and push anterior shoulder away from symphysis pubis into oblique or transverse diameter – continuously for up to 30 seconds, then intermittent or rocking for up to 30 seconds |
| ENTER VAGINA – INTERNAL ROTATION | On *examination per vaginam,* identify *anterior* shoulder from behind. Exert pressure on scapula to adduct shoulder and rotate to oblique position (RUBIN MANOEUVRE) |
| | Continue McRoberts manoeuvre |
| | Alternatively, on vaginal examination, identify fetal chest, exert pressure on anterior aspect of *posterior* shoulder, gently rotate shoulder towards symphysis (WOOD'S MANOEUVRE) |
| | Combine Rubin manoeuvre: midwife will have one hand on each shoulder, rotating together |
| | Approach *posterior* shoulder from *behind.* Gently rotate fetus in opposite direction to previous attempts (reverse Wood's screw manoeuvre) |
| | May be successful when all previous manoeuvres have failed |
| REMOVE POSTERIOR ARM | Insert hand into vagina, using space in sacral hollow; two fingers splint humerus, flex elbow, sweep forearm over chest to deliver hand |
| ROLL MOTHER OVER AND TRY AGAIN | If all previous manoeuvres have been unsuccessful, roll woman over into all fours and try again (Gaskin manoeuvre)<br>• increases pelvic diameters<br>• movement and gravity may dislodge the impaction<br>• deliver the *posterior* shoulder with gentle traction |

# Appendix 5

## Management of cord prolapse

**Diagnosis** – cord felt in front of or alongside presenting part on vaginal examination, or within vagina or cervical os, or seen externally.

### Management

1. Note time.
2. Summon medical aid urgently.
3. Stop oxytocin infusion if in progress.
4. Replace cord in vagina to prevent spasm, if necessary, keeping hand in vagina to hold presenting part off cord.
5. Administer oxygen to mother.
6. Assist mother into position which relieves pressure on cord; raise foot of bed, knee–chest or exaggerated Sim's position.
7. Insert urinary catheter and instil sterile saline; full bladder elevates presenting part above ischial spines, further relieving cord pressure.
8. Expedite delivery of baby; Caesarean section is method of choice if fetus is still alive and vaginal birth not imminent.
9. If cord prolapse occurs in second stage in multipara, perform episiotomy to expedite birth, possibly with forceps or vacuum extraction.
10. In community, transfer to hospital for emergency Caesarean section is essential.

## Cord prolapse

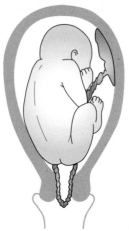

## Knee-chest position

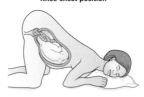

# Appendix 6

## Abbreviations

| | |
|---|---|
| AABR | automated auditory brainstem response |
| AADC | aromatic amino acid decarboxylase deficiency |
| ABO | blood group classifications |
| ACA | anticardiolipin antibody |
| ACE | angiotensin-converting enzyme |
| ACH | aftercoming head (of breech) |
| ACTH | adrenocorticotrophic hormone |
| ADH | antidiuretic hormone |
| AF | artificial feeding |
| AFI | amniotic fluid index |
| AFLP | acute fatty liver of pregnancy |
| AFP | alpha-fetoprotein |
| AHF | anti-haemophilic factor |
| AID | artificial insemination by donor |
| AIDS | acquired immune deficiency syndrome |
| AIH | artificial insemination by husband |
| ALP | alkaline phosphatase |
| ALSO | Advanced Life Support in Obstetrics |
| ALT | alanine aminotransferase |
| AMU | alongside midwifery unit |
| AN(C) | antenatal (clinic) |
| AP | anteroposterior |
| AP(E)L | accreditation of prior (experiential) learning |
| APH | antepartum haemorrhage |
| APT | alum-precipitated toxoid |
| ARM | artificial rupture of membranes |
| ART | 1. antiretroviral therapy. 2. assisted reproduction techniques |
| ARDS | adult respiratory distress syndrome |
| AST | aspartate aminotransferase |
| ASD | atrial septal defect |
| | |
| BBA | born before arrival (of the midwife) |
| BCG | bacille Calmette–Guérin (vaccine) |

| | |
|---|---|
| b.d. | twice daily |
| BF | breastfeeding |
| BFI | Baby-Friendly Initiative |
| BMI | body mass index |
| BMR | basal metabolic rate |
| BNF | British National Formulary |
| BP | 1.blood pressure. 2. British Pharmacopoeia |
| BPD | biparietal diameter |
| BSD | bisacromial diameter |
| BV | bacterial vaginosis |
| | |
| C | Celsius |
| Ca | calcium |
| CAH | congenital adrenal hyperplasia |
| CAM | complementary and alternative medicine |
| CAT | computed axial tomography |
| CCT | 1. controlled cord traction. 2. controlled clinical trial |
| CDH | congenital dislocation of the hip |
| CEMACH | Centre for Maternal and Child Health Enquiries |
| CEMD | Confidential Enquiry into Maternal Deaths |
| CESDI | Confidential Enquiry into Stillbirth and Deaths in Infancy |
| CF | cystic fibrosis |
| CHD | congenital heart disease |
| CHRE | Council for Healthcare Regulatory Excellence |
| CHT | congenital hypothyroidism |
| CIN | cervical intraepithelial neoplasia |
| CIP | continuous inflating pressure |
| CMV | 1. controlled mechanical ventilation. 2. cytomegalovirus |
| CNEEP | continuous nasal end expiratory pressure |
| CNP | continuous negative pressure |
| CNS | central nervous system |
| CNST | Clinical Negligence Scheme for Trusts |
| COC | combined oral contraceptive |
| CONI | Care of Next Infant scheme |
| COSHH | Control of Substances Hazardous to Health |
| CPAP | continuous positive airway pressure |
| CPD | 1. cephalopelvic disproportion. 2. continuing professional development |
| CPR | cardiopulmonary resuscitation |
| CQC | Care Quality Commission |
| CRL | crown–rump length |
| CRP | C-reactive protein |
| CSF | cerebrospinal fluid |

| CSU | catheter specimen of urine |
| CT | 1. computed tomography. 2. complementary therapy(ies) |
| CTG | cardiotocograph |
| CVP | central venous pressure |
| CVS | 1. chorionic villus sampling. 2. cardiovascular system |
| Cx | cervix |
| | |
| D&C | dilatation and curettage |
| D&V | diarrhoea and vomiting |
| DAT | direct antiglobulin test |
| DBS | Disclosure and Barring Service |
| DH/DoH | Department of Health |
| DHA | docosahexaenoic acid |
| DIC | disseminated intravascular coagulation |
| DMPA | depot, medroxyprogesterone acetate |
| DNA | 1. did not attend. 2. deoxyribonucleic acid |
| DOMINO | domiciliary in and out (scheme) |
| DTA | deep transverse arrest |
| DVT | deep venous thrombosis |
| | |
| $E_1$ | estrone (oestrone) |
| $E_2$ | estradiol-17β (oestradiol) |
| $E_3$ | estriol (oestriol) |
| EBM | expressed breast milk |
| ECG | electrocardiogram |
| ECMO | extracorporeal membrane oxygenation |
| ECV | external cephalic version |
| EDD | estimated date of delivery/estimated due date |
| EEG | electroencephalogram |
| EFM | electronic fetal heart monitoring |
| EPA | examination *per abdomen* |
| EPAU | early pregnancy assessment unit |
| EPV | examination *per vaginam* |
| ERPC | evacuation of retained products of conception |
| ESR | erythrocyte sedimentation rate |
| EUA | examination under anaesthetic |
| | |
| F | Fahrenheit |
| FBS | fetal blood sampling |
| FDPs | fibrin degradation products |
| Fe | iron |
| FGM | female genital mutilation |
| FH (HR) | fetal heart (heard and regular) |

| | |
|---|---|
| FIGO | International Federation of Gynaecologists and Obstetricians |
| FISH | fluorescent in situ hybridization |
| FSH (RF) | follicle-stimulating hormone (releasing factor) |
| FTA-ABS | fluorescent treponemal antibody-absorbed test |
| | |
| g | gram |
| G | gravida |
| GBS | group B streptococcus |
| GFR | glomerular filtration rate |
| GIFT | gamete intrafallopian transfer |
| GIT | gastrointestinal tract |
| GP | general practitioner |
| G6PD | glucose-6-phosphate dehydrogenase |
| GROW | gestation-related optimal weight |
| GTT | glucose tolerance test |
| | |
| H | hydrogen |
| HAART | highly active antiretroviral therapy |
| HAI | hospital-acquired infection |
| Hb | haemoglobin |
| hCG | human chorionic gonadotrophin |
| HCl | hydrochloric acid |
| HDN | haemolytic disease of the newborn |
| HEI | higher education institution |
| HELLP | haemolysis, elevated liver proteins and low platelets |
| HELPERR | Help; Episiotomy; Legs; Pressure; Enter; Remove; Roll |
| HFEA | Human Fertilisation and Embryology Authority |
| HFOV | high frequency oscillation ventilation |
| Hg | mercury |
| HG | hyperemesis gravidarum |
| Hib | Haemophilus influenza B |
| HIV | human immunodeficiency virus |
| hPL | human placental lactogen |
| HPLC | high-performance liquid chromatography |
| HPV | human papillomavirus |
| HSV | herpes simplex virus |
| HV | Health Visitor |
| HVS | high vaginal swab |
| | |
| IAT | indirect antiglobulin test |
| ICP | 1. intracranial pressure. 2. intrahepatic cholestasis of pregnancy |

| ICSH | interstitial cell-stimulating hormone |
| ICSI | intracytoplasmic sperm injection |
| ICU/ITU | intensive care unit/intensive therapy unit |
| IEM | inborn errors of metabolism |
| IFG | impaired fasting glucose |
| Ig | immunoglobulin |
| IGT | impaired glucose tolerance |
| IHD | ischaemic heart disease |
| IM | intramuscular |
| IMV | intermittent mandatory ventilation |
| IOL | induction of labour |
| IPPV | intermittent positive pressure ventilation |
| IRT | immune-reactive trypsin |
| ITP | Intention to Practise (form) |
| IUCD | intrauterine contraceptive device |
| IUD | intrauterine death |
| IUGR | intrauterine growth restriction |
| IU(C)S | intrauterine (contraceptive) system |
| IUT | intrauterine fetal transfer |
| IV (I) | intravenous (infusion) |
| IVF | in vitro fertilization |
| IVH | intraventricular haemorrhage |
| IVP/IVU | intravenous pyelogram/urogram |
| | |
| J | joule |
| | |
| K | potassium |
| k | kilo |
| kcal | kilocalorie |
| kJ | kilojoule |
| | |
| LARC | long-acting reversible contraception |
| LBW | low birthweight |
| LSCS | lower segment Caesarean section |
| LFD | light for dates |
| LFT | liver function tests |
| LGA | large for gestational age (baby) |
| LH | luteinizing hormone |
| LMA | left mentoanterior |
| LML | left mentolateral |
| LMP | 1. left mentoposterior. 2. last menstrual period |
| LOA | left occipitoanterior |
| LOL | left occipitolateral |

| | |
|---|---|
| LOP | left occipitoposterior |
| LOT | left occipitotransverse |
| LP | lumbar puncture |
| LSA | left sacroanterior |
| LSCS | lower segment Caesarean section |
| LSL | left sacrolateral |
| LSP | left sacroposterior |
| L/S | lecithin–sphingomyelin ratio |
| | |
| m | milli, meta |
| M | mega |
| MAOI | monoamine oxidase inhibitor |
| MBRRACE-UK | Mothers and Babies: Reducing Risk through Audits and Confidential Enquiries in the UK |
| MCA | middle cerebral artery |
| MCADD | medium-chain acyl-coenzyme A dehydrogenase deficiency |
| MCH | mean corpuscular haemoglobin |
| MCHC | mean corpuscular haemoglobin concentration |
| MCV | mean corpuscular volume |
| MDMA | methylenedioxymethamphetamine (ecstasy) |
| MFPR | multi-fetal pregnancy reduction |
| mg | milligram |
| Mg | magnesium |
| MgSO$_4$ | magnesium sulphate |
| MHRA | Medical and Healthcare products Regulatory Agency |
| mL | millilitre |
| mm | millimetre |
| mmol | millimole |
| MMR | mumps, measles, rubella (vaccination) |
| MOET | Managing Obstetric Emergencies and Trauma |
| MOM | multiple of the median |
| MRI | magnetic resonance imaging |
| MRSA | methicillin-resistant *Staphylococcus aureus* |
| MSLC | Maternity Services Liaison Committee |
| MSH | melanocyte-stimulating hormone |
| MSU | midstream specimen of urine |
| MSUD | maple syrup urine disease |
| MSW | maternity support worker |
| MV | mentovertical |
| | |
| Na | sodium |
| NAD | nothing abnormal detected |
| NAI | non-accidental injury |

| NAHI | non-accidental head injury |
|------|---------------------------|
| NBFD | Neville Barnes forceps delivery |
| ND | normal delivery |
| NCT | National Childbirth Trust |
| NEC | necrotizing enterocolitis |
| NHS | National Health Service |
| NICE | National Institute for Healthcare and Clinical Excellence |
| NICU | neonatal intensive care unit |
| NIPE | newborn and infant physical examination |
| NIPT | Non-invasive Prenatal Testing |
| NMC | Nursing and Midwifery Council |
| NMR | nuclear magnetic resonance |
| NN4B | NHS Number for Babies |
| NND | neonatal death |
| NNU | neonatal unit |
| $N_2O$ | nitrous oxide |
| NSAIDs | non-steroidal anti-inflammatory drugs |
| NSC | National Screening Committee |
| NSF | National Service Framework |
| NST | non-stress test |
| NSU | non-specific urethritis |
| NT | nuchal translucency |
| NTD | neural tube defect |
| | |
| O | oxygen |
| OA | occipitoanterior |
| OAE | otoacoustic emissions (test) |
| OAPR | odds of being affected given a positive result |
| OCD | obsessive compulsive disorder |
| ODA | operating department assistant |
| OL | occipitolateral |
| OP | occipitoposterior |
| OPD | outpatient department |
| OT | occipitotransverse |
| OTC | over-the-counter (drugs) |
| | |
| P | 1. phosphorus. 2. para, parity |
| *P* | probability |
| Pa | pascal |
| PA | *per abdomen* |
| $P_aO_2$ | partial pressure of oxygen in arterial blood |
| PAP | Papanicolaou (smear) |
| PAPP-A | pregnancy-associated plasma protein-A |

| | |
|---|---|
| PCA | patient-controlled analgesia |
| PCC | post-coital contraception |
| PCEAS | patient-controlled epidural analgesic system |
| PCO$_2$ | partial pressure of carbon dioxide |
| PCOS | polycystic ovarian syndrome |
| PCR | polymerase chain reaction |
| PCV | 1. packed cell volume. 2. pneumococcal conjugate vaccine |
| PDA | patent ductus arteriosus |
| PG | prostaglandin |
| Pg | picogram |
| PGD | 1. pre-implantation genetic diagnosis. 2. patient group directions. 3.pelvic girdle dysfunction |
| pH | acid–alkali balance |
| PID | pelvic inflammatory disease |
| PIH | pregnancy-induced hypertension |
| PIN | personal identification number |
| PKU | phenylketonuria |
| PM | post-mortem |
| PMR | perinatal mortality rate |
| PND | postnatal depression |
| PO$_2$ | partial pressure of oxygen |
| POMs | prescription-only medicines |
| POP | 1. persistent occipitoposterior. 2. progestogen-only pill |
| PPH | postpartum haemorrhage |
| PPHN | persistent pulmonary hypertension of newborn |
| PPR | Price precipitation reaction |
| PPROM | preterm per-labour rupture of membranes |
| PR | *per rectum* |
| PREP | post-registration education and practice |
| prn | as required, when necessary |
| PROMPT | PRactical Obstetric Multi-Professional Training |
| PTSD | post-traumatic stress disorder |
| PUBS | percutaneous umbilical cord blood sampling |
| PUO | pyrexia of unknown origin |
| PV | *per vaginam* |
| PVH | periventricular haemorrhage |
| PVI | periventricular haemorrhage infarction |
| | |
| Q | quadrant |
| q.d. | every day |
| q.d.s. | four times a day |
| QF-PCR | quantitative fluorescence polymerase chain reaction |
| q.h. | every hour |

| | |
|---|---|
| q.i.d. | four times daily |
| q.q.h. | every 4 hours |
| | |
| RBC | 1. red blood cells. 2. red blood count |
| RCM | Royal College of Midwives |
| RCN | Royal College of Nursing |
| RCT | randomized controlled trial |
| RDS | respiratory distress syndrome |
| R(G)N | Registered (General) Nurse |
| Rh | rhesus (factor) |
| RIA | radioimmunoassay |
| RM | Registered Midwife |
| RMA | right mentoanterior |
| RML | right mentolateral |
| RMP | right mentoposterior |
| RNA | ribonucleic acid |
| ROA | right occipitoanterior |
| ROL | right occipitolateral |
| ROP | right occipitoposterior |
| RPCF | Reiter's protein complement fixation |
| RPR | rapid plasma reagin |
| RSA | right sacroanterior |
| RSL | right sacrolateral |
| RSP | right sacroposterior |
| Rx | treatment |
| | |
| S | sulphur |
| SB | stillbirth |
| SBR | serum bilirubin |
| SC | subcutaneous |
| SCBU | special care baby unit |
| SCD | sickle cell disease |
| SFD | small for dates |
| SGA | small for gestational age |
| SGOT | serum glutamate oxaloacetate transaminase |
| SGPT | serum glutamate pyruvate transaminase |
| SI | Système International d'Unités |
| SIDS | sudden infant death syndrome |
| SLE | systemic lupus erythematosus |
| SMP | Statutory Maternity Pay |
| SPD | symphysis pubis diastasis/discomfort |
| SRM | spontaneous rupture of membranes |
| SSRI | selective serotonin reuptake inhibitor |

| | |
|---|---|
| STI/STD | sexually transmitted infection/disease |
| SVD | spontaneous vaginal delivery |
| | |
| TB | tuberculosis |
| TBA | 1. traditional birth attendant. 2. to be advised |
| TBG | thyroid-binding globulin |
| t.d.s. | three times daily |
| TED | thromboembolitic D (stockings) |
| TENS | transcutaneous electrical nerve stimulation |
| TFT | thyroid function test |
| TOP | termination of pregnancy |
| TORCH | toxoplasmosis, rubella, cytomegalovirus, herpes |
| TPHA | *Treponema pallidum* haemagglutination |
| TPN | total parenteral nutrition |
| TPT | transplacental transfusion |
| TRAP | twin reversed arterial perfusion |
| TSH | thyroid-stimulating hormone |
| TTA/TTO | to take away/to take out |
| TTN | transient tachypnoea of the newborn |
| TTTS | twin-to-twin transfusion syndrome |
| TV | 1. transvaginal. 2. *Trichomonas vaginalis* |
| | |
| U&E | urea and electrolyte (estimations) |
| UDFA | ultrasound-directed follicle aspiration |
| UDP-GT | uridine diphosphoglucuronyl transferase |
| UE$_3$ | unconjugated oestriol |
| UNICEF | United Nations Children's Emergency Fund |
| URTI | upper respiratory tract infection |
| US (S) | ultrasound (scan) |
| UTI | urinary tract infection |
| | |
| VBAC | vaginal birth after Caesarean |
| VDRL | Venereal Disease Research Laboratory (syphilis test) |
| VE | vaginal examination |
| VLBW | very-low-birthweight |
| VMA | vanillylmandelic acid |
| VZ | varicella zoster |
| | |
| WBC | white blood cell/count |
| WHO | World Health Organization |
| WR | Wassermann reaction |
| | |
| ZIFT | zygote intrafallopian transfer |